Hùnyuán Xīnfǎ

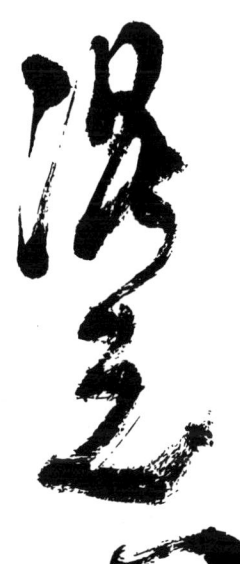

The Lost Heart of Medicine

Special Edition

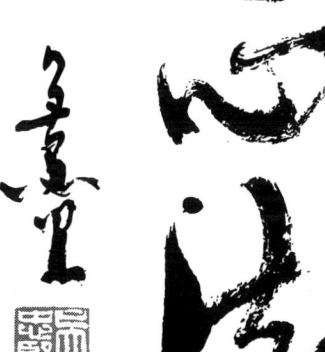

Yaron Seidman
&
Teja A. Jaensch

Hùnyuán Research Institute for Chinese Classics

"There is nothing outside of Tàijí. More so when making a picture of Tàijí, we simply draw an empty circle. This is the image of complete pureness...Only after this realization can there be harmony, as without this Center there is never, and will never be true peace."

Liú Yuán

Copyright © 2013 by Yaron Seidman.

All rights reserved. No portion of this book may be reproduced, stored in a retrieval system, or transmitted in any form or by any means – electronic, mechanical, photocopy, recording, scanning or any other – except for brief quotations in printed reviews, without the prior written permission of the publisher.

NOTE: Every effort has been made to ensure that the information contained in this book is complete and accurate. However, neither the publisher, nor the authors are engaged in rendering professional advice or services to the individual reader and no portion of this book is intended to diagnose, treat, or cure the individual reader. Neither the publisher nor the authors shall be liable or responsible for loss, injury, or for the damage allegedly arising from any information or suggestion in this book.

Hùnyuán Xīnfǎ: The Lost Heart of Medicine
Y. Seidman & T. A. Jaensch
Published by: Hunyuan Group Inc.
Greenwich, Connecticut, USA
Email: info@hunyuan.org
Website: www.hunyuan.org and www.chineseclassics.org
Teja A. Jaensch: www.pointspecifics.com

Library of Congress catalog number: 2013905610
ISBN: 978-0-9891679-1-8
Special Edition (April 2013)
Printed in the United States of America

Cover calligraphy by Master Wú Zhōngxián (吴忠賢).
The cover calligraphy reads *Hùnyuán Xīnfǎ* (混元心法).

Cover and book layout and illustrations by Michael Andre Musa-Tapia.
(Miguel Andres – Design & Art)

Photography taken and/or edited by Greg Le Couteur (Shadow Sounds).
Photography from Sìchuān kindly contributed by Menachem Kuchar.

For our families and our patients.

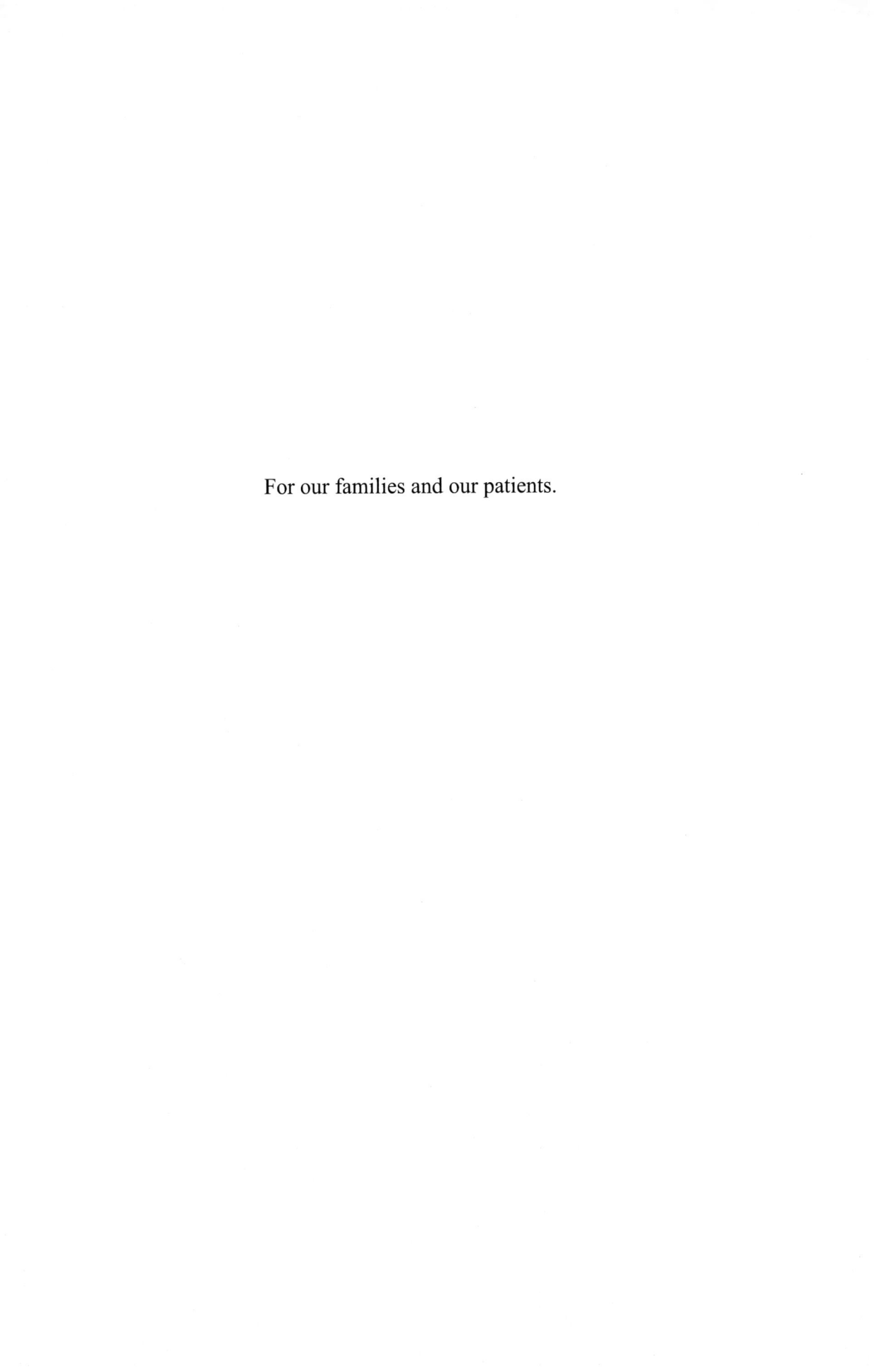

Contents

Acknowledgments	i
Preface	ix
Author's note	xii
Foreword	xiv
Introduction	1
Brief historical perspective	12

Chapter One
    Shí Yīn Fū and the Ledger of Good and Evil   17

Chapter Two
    Clarifying Fundamental Concepts of the Heart   52

Chapter Three
    The Lost Heart   92

Chapter Four
    A Time for Giving and a Time for Taking   118

Chapter Five
    Explaining the 100 Diseases   135

Chapter Six
    I Know Words   148

Chapter Seven
    Tàijí: Without an Apex   165

Chapter Eight
    The Wounded Warrior   182

Chapter Nine
    Revering the 100 Medicines   206

Chapter Ten
    The Concealed Words   215

Conclusion   238

Bibliography   242

Appendix A: 石音夫功過格   248

Appendix B: 說百病崇百药   263

Appendix C: 劉沅: 槐軒全書   271

Index   370

Commentary on the Lost Heart of Medicine   387

Scholar's Notes   390

Acknowledgments

"There is a defining moment in the study of Chinese language
when you realize that the page of text you're looking at is actually the right side up."[1]

Michael Max

When my daughter looks at a sheet of music, she sees and hears the notes. When I look at that same page, all I see are dots and squiggles. So as I sat looking at the prodigious compendium written by Liú Yuán (劉沅) that we were to work through for the composition of this book, I had the same feeling as when I try to help my daughter with her cello.

It has been said that the entirety of historical Chinese medical thought was filtered through the brilliant mind of Zhāng Zhòngjǐng (張仲景), and the result of this distillation was the Shāng Hán Lún (傷寒論).[2] In working with Dr Yaron Seidman I have been amazed at how he can look at these extensive manuscripts and instead of seeing radicals and phonetic components, he is able to synthesize and digest what is at the Heart of the text. The ten volumes of the Huái Xuān (槐軒) philosophy of Liú Yuán (劉沅) have been filtered through the mind of a contemporary sage, and what remains is the pure essence. It is thanks to Dr Seidman that this book exists, and I thank him for allowing me to be a part of the journey.

The defining moment in the evolution of this book came during the Hùnyuán Research Institute's trip to the People's Republic of China in June 2012, to seek out the Qīng dynasty physician, Zhèng Qīnān (鄭欽安). Through studying his lineage we discovered that he was but one of the *thousands* of students of Liú Yuán, the great Master. We were fortunate enough to be able to learn from his great grandson, Master Liú Bǎigǔ (劉伯谷), lineage bearer of the Huái Xuān school of philosophy. The concepts we extrapolate upon are thousands of years old, but in this book we bring them into the present and share their importance and *vitality* for medicine. Therefore, it is important for us to acknowledge here the lineage of thinkers, philosophers and healers that came before, and respect our duty of furthering their work, especially in regards to the practicality of transforming philosophy into practice. Guiding us to all this information was the Huái Xuān Shuāngliú Cultural Association (槐軒雙流文化研習會),

---

[1] H. Huang, *Ten Key Formula Families in Chinese Medicine*, trans. M. Max, Eastland Press, Seattle, 2009, (Translator's foreword), p. xi.

[2] A. Versluys, *Elementary Aspects of Canonical Chinese Medicine,* lecture series, Sydney, October 2012.

administered by some true physicians of the Heart, President Master Liú Chí (劉馳) and Director Master Lǐ Tíngxīn (李廷新). To these men in particular, along with Master Gān Liǎo (甘了) and especially Master Liú Bǎigǔ for so generously giving his time to teach us, we offer our Heartfelt thanks.

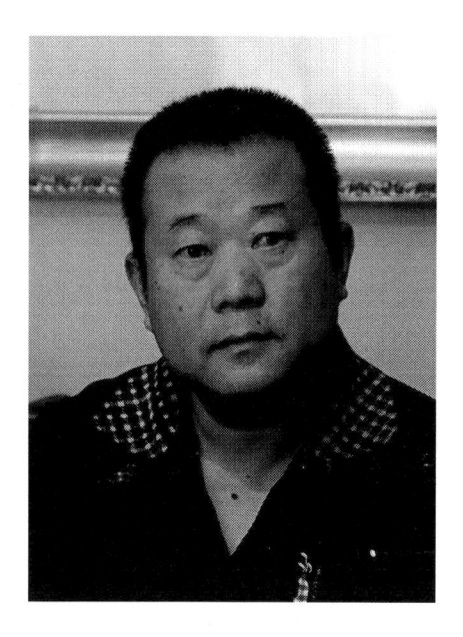

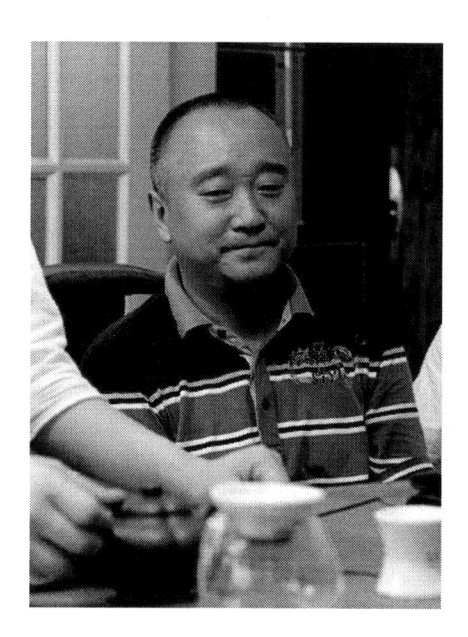

Liú Chí and Lǐ Tíngxīn at the Huái Xuān Shuāngliú Cultural Association.

"A teacher affects eternity;
he can never tell where his influence stops."

Henry Brooks Adams

It is through their assistance, and our insistence, that we were able to visit the burial ground of Liú Yuán and his family. This burial site was moved in the middle of the 20th century due to political issues, and the site had not been maintained since. In order to find his tomb we were given machetes with which we hacked our way out into the fields of Shuāngliú. As the dust settled we realized we had found the *Lost Heart of Medicine*.

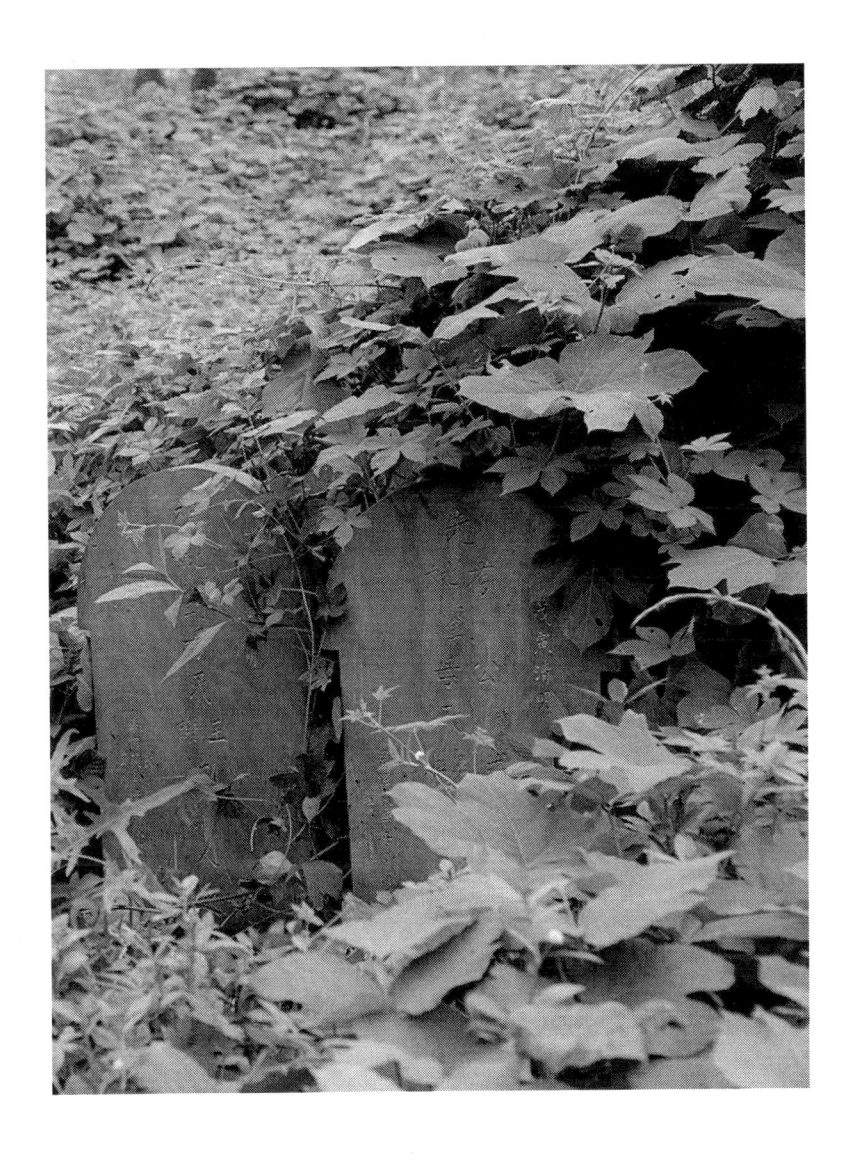

...into the fields of Shuāngliú...

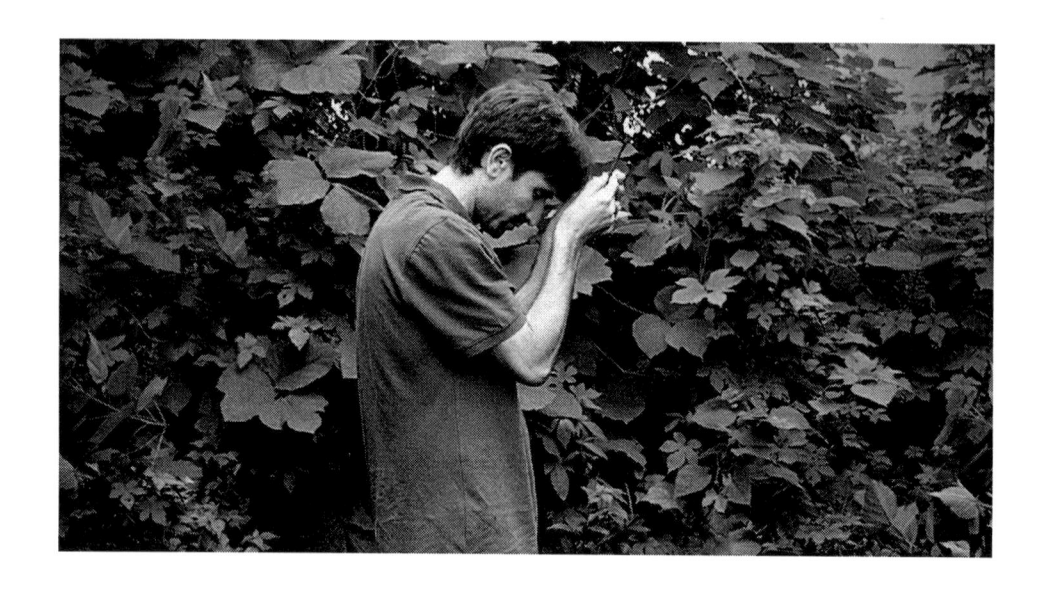

Yaron Seidman paying his respects to the family of lost tombs.

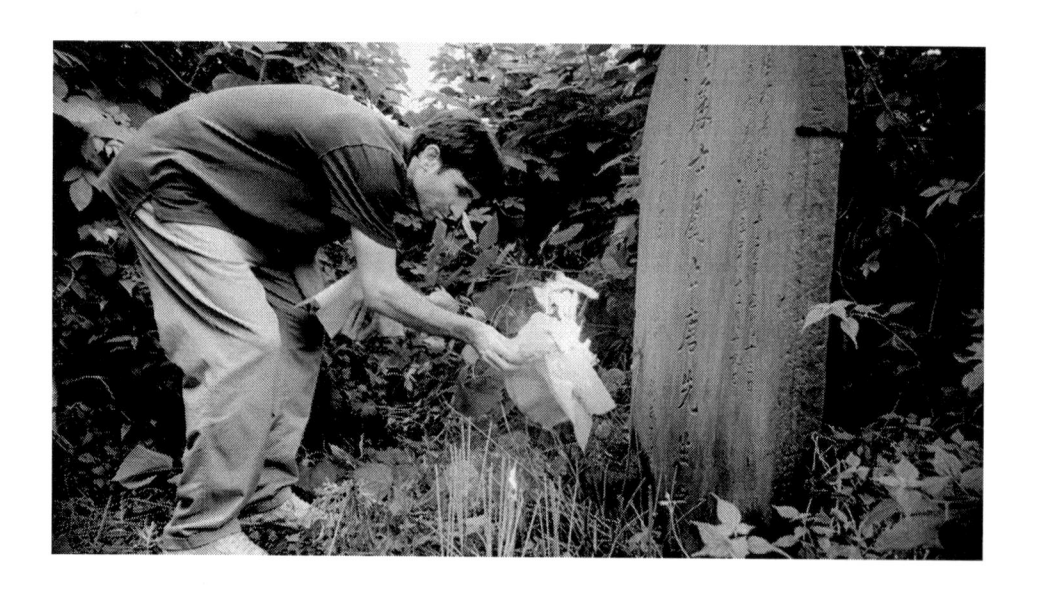

Yaron Seidman burning blank paper money as sign of respect for the deceased.
It is a Chinese custom to burn fake paper money for the deceased to have in Heaven,
however for enlightened persons, who require no material things on Earth or in
Heaven, the custom is to burn blank paper.

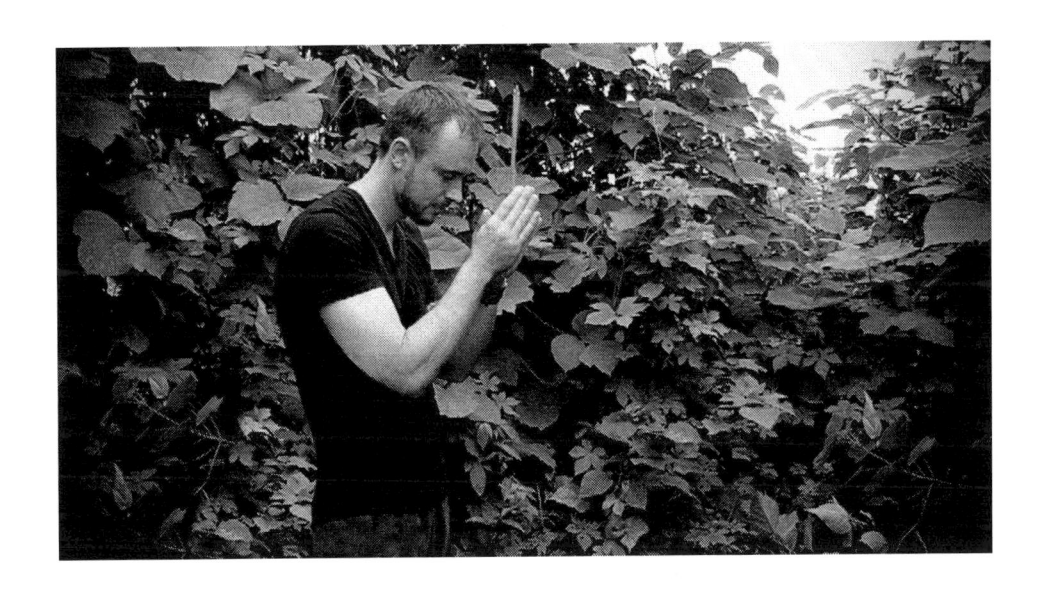

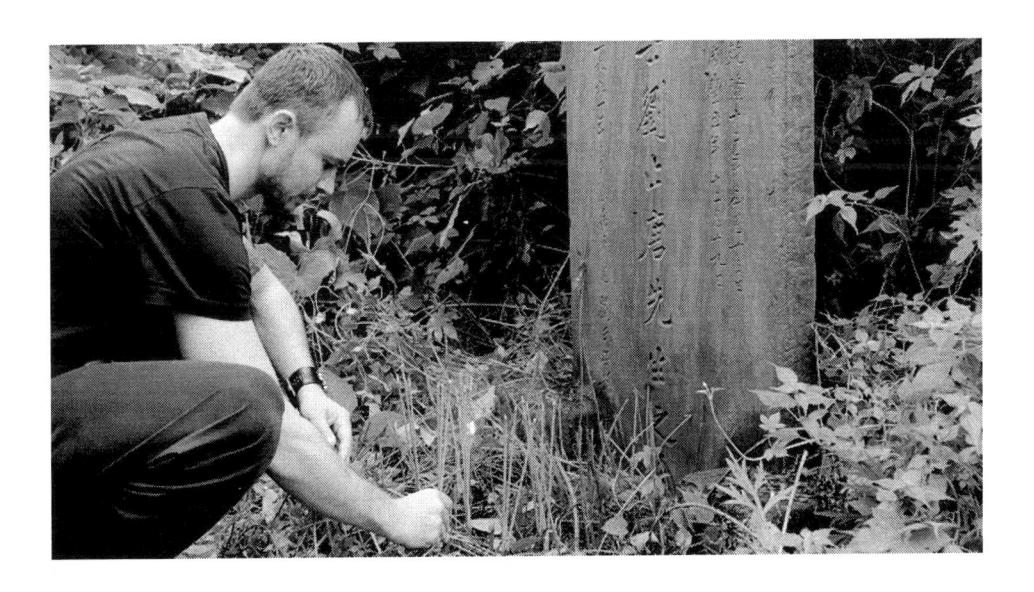

Teja A. Jaensch offering incense in the overgrown field.

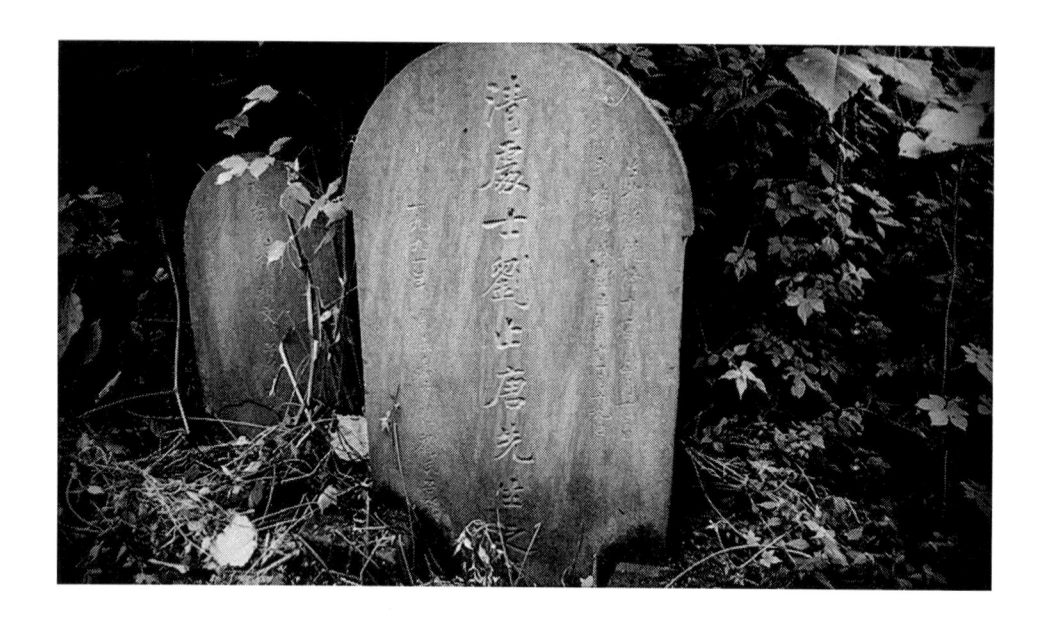

The tombstones of Liú Yuán and his eldest son Liú Bèiwén.

Our deepest gratitude extends to all of those who have contributed to this book. In particular we would like to thank Master Wú Zhōngxián (吳忠賢) for both his beautiful calligraphy on our cover, and the time he took to look over our work and give us feedback. To William R. Morris (PhD), author of *Li Shi-zhen Pulse Studies: An Illustrated Guide*, for his thoughtful contribution to our book in the foreword, we are eternally grateful. To the current Director of the College of Traditional Chinese Medicine and Associate Head of School, (Medical and Molecular Biosciences) at the University of Technology, Sydney, Associate Professor Christopher Zaslawski, we thank you for your constructive critique and analysis. To Master Chén Zhōnghuá for his exquisite calligraphy in our conclusion to this book and for his continued inspiration in helping us find Center.

To Kelly Mitchell, for editing the text at each and every draft, we know it was a labor of love, and we thank you. To Jacinda Jaensch, who tirelessly read over and over the manuscript highlighting any oversights, from the depths of our Hearts, we thank you. To our fellow Hùnyuán

Research Institute colleagues, Tristin McLaren and Alex Kolaczynski, thank you for being a part of this project and for furthering our limited capacities of contemplation. Tristin in particular arranged our impassioned words into legible sentences; this book, Tristin, is more yours than ours and we thank you for your dedication, enthusiasm, professionalism and compassion.

The text took me on a journey, says Robyn Bowcock, mental health nurse and Associate Lecturer at the University of Western Sydney (School of Nursing and Midwifery). Robyn, for your perspective and insight, we thank you. To Master Robert F. Feng, Stuart Rushton, Annika Andersdotter, Peter Schäfer, Sarah Arratoon, Julie Partridge, Anthony Captain, Menachem Kuchar, Denice Finnegan and Debbie Simpson, Julia Tyne, Monica Perez-Pardo and Maria D'Urso; thank you for the time and effort you took to read through our early drafts and offer guidance. To all of our patients who have had to hear us badgering on about Confucius and Mencius over the last year, we thank you for your patience. And to the masterful Evgeny Kissin for his amazing performance of *Mussorgsky: Pictures at an exhibition*, thank you for getting us through those long nights in front of the keyboard with your food for the soul.

Lastly and perhaps most importantly, from both Yaron and myself, we thank our families; our parents, our beautiful wives and wonderful children for supporting and inspiring us. We are sure that this is just the beginning, with many miles to go before we sleep.

Whose woods these are I think I know.
His house is in the village though;
He will not see me stopping here
To watch his woods fill up with snow.

My little horse must think it queer
To stop without a farmhouse near
Between the woods and frozen lake
The darkest evening of the year.

He gives his harness bells a shake
To ask if there is some mistake.
The only other sound's the sweep
Of easy wind and downy flake.

The woods are lovely, dark and deep.
But I have promises to keep,
And miles to go before I sleep,
And miles to go before I sleep.[3]

Robert Frost

---

[3] R. Frost, *Stopping by Woods on a Snowy Evening*, 1923.

Preface

The first book I wrote, I printed and bound myself. It was 1997 and I was finishing my final year of high school. After studying Kung Fu during my adolescent years, I felt I needed to write something to fill a void that existed in my training. The book was called Yì Shén (意神), *Remember the Spirit* (literal translation – the *meaning* of spirit), and was a pleading to myself to seek what was beneath the layers of external movement, behind the kicks and punches.

Later, when my journey began into the study of Chinese medicine, language and culture, I discovered that what I was aiming to be was an Yī Shēng (醫生), a doctor. Literally again, this means someone who *cures life*. Throughout my studies, both in Australia and the People's Republic of China, I found myself continually seeking something to fill the void, just as I had been in my martial arts training. Despite the fact I had, in my opinion, some of the very best educators in the world, I could not help but feel I was lacking in my practice of medicine.

> Clouds drift by deserted city walls,
> Filling the collapsed spaces...
>
> Cheng Man-Ch'ing

Then I was fortunate enough through miraculous circumstances, *in the middle of the road*, to become acquainted with Dr Yaron Seidman, founder of the Hùnyuán Research Institute for Chinese Classics in Connecticut, USA. In this man I found someone who had that same feeling and was walking that same path, yet was already contemplating amongst the mists at the mountain peak as I stood at its foot peering upward. Dr Seidman's approach to medicine and life is to be *clear and yet clearer about virtue*; to continually study and research and question in order to be the best doctor and teacher there can be to his patients and students. Hùnyuán (混元) literally means the *origin of life*.

With this dedication he founded the Hùnyuán Research Institute for Chinese Classics, which is now an international think-tank of like-minded physicians. Over the years of exploring the very foundations of Chinese medicine to such a pedantic point of nailing down the ancestry of every word in our Classics, he has formed a unique understanding and way of describing what it means to be *alive*. Medicine is for the living; it is to heal *life*. So gaining an appreciation for what life is, rather than just trying to understand disease, is vital. To do this, Hùnyuán medicine uses this image to describe the basic processes of living:

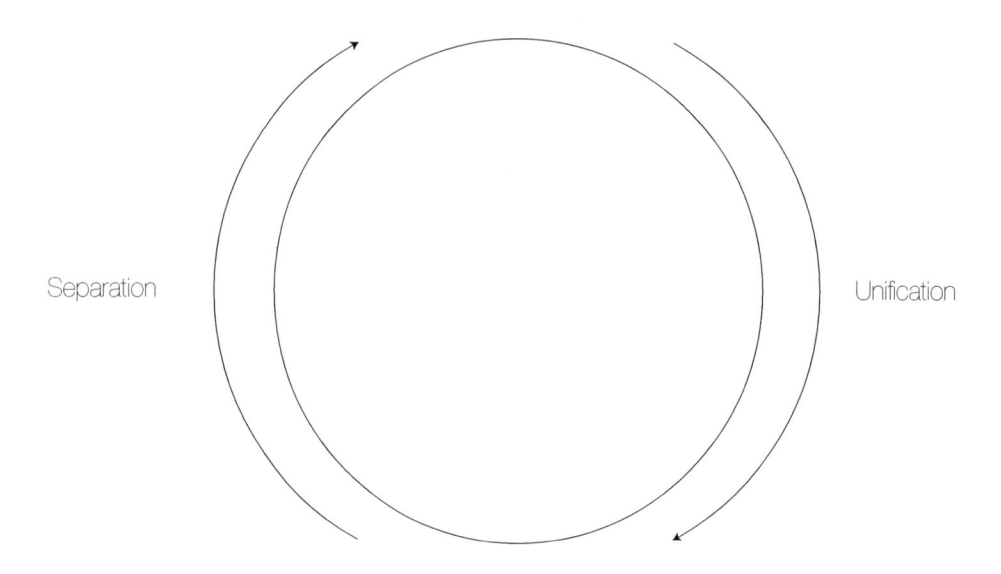

Separation   Unification

If Lǎozǐ (老子) was right and *every journey begins with a first step*, this is and should be, the starting point for any medical understanding and inquiry. This picture articulates the difference between our bodies when we are alive to when we have expired. For now, we could simply define Unification as breathing in and Separation as breathing out. This circulation of respiration is *vital*. The implications for Unification and Separation run very deep and are discussed throughout the introductory chapters in more detail.

Yet as important as this first step is, it is just that, and the journey is long. The primary argument of this book is that we need to constantly dig deeper, constantly seek out the *Lost Heart of Medicine*. Through the works of the Chinese scholar, Liú Yuán, we have found it: it is our *Center*. If we can find this Center then our approach to health and disease, the way we react with our external and internal environments and the way we think and feel about ourselves can change for the better.

It was only at the end of this process of working with Liú Yuán's material, toiling with the translations, that I came to a point of honest realization. When we first started this book we discussed many Confucian ideas with Master Liú Bǎigǔ, such as filial piety, the son respecting the father, self-examination (géwù 格物) and selfishness in particular. I kept badgering the poor fellow to give me the answers that I *wanted* to hear; however, being the sage that he is, he would not budge and just continued repeating the words that I *needed* to hear. It was only whilst grappling with the final chapters of this book a year after he spoke to me, that I finally heard him. Letting go of our *childhood ignorance* is a challenge, for no one more than myself. But there is no escaping it once the process of cultivation has been planted and starts to grow within you. I am no longer a child. I am a man. My life. My choice. The challenge here has been not just to translate philosophical concepts from Chinese to English, but also to translate this internal experience in a way that is accessible to others.

Previously it was common for me to chant the following aphorism: *'The Yijīng (易经) tells us that the only constant is change. Every thing is under the influence of change, so therefore we are either changing for the better, or the alternative'*. Through the process of working on this book, I find myself reveling in the realization that there is something within me, within all of us (not a *thing*) that does not change, that is constant. This constancy is what unites us as doctors, patients, family, friends and strangers. The world needs to focus more on what unites us and less on our preoccupation with division and Separation.

Teja A. Jaensch,
Sydney, Australia
February 2013

Author's note

A long time ago in a remote village in southwestern China, lived an old teacher. To his simple school, a structure with a roof but no walls, came children from all around the countryside. The pupils would wake up at three o'clock in the morning and walk as many as four, five or six hours holding a small lantern in the dark until they reached the little school. There, they would listen to the old teacher for a few hours, then make the long journey home again. Most, if not all of his students came from poor peasant families. The parents wanted their children to go to school but often needed them to stay home and help in the field. As a result the children would only attend the little school one or two days per week, staying home on the other days to help their parents in the fields.

One day the old teacher sat in his school and no pupils showed up; they had all stayed home. 'Maybe there is something lacking in my teaching,' he thought to himself, 'and as a result, my class is empty today. I must find out how to be a better teacher and what it is my students need to know.' He packed a few balls of rice and pickles in a napkin and set off for the mountains. He had heard of an old recluse living amongst the cliffs and valleys and thought that the monk could teach him more about teaching. Across the fields he walked, until he came to a river blocking his way. The current was swift, trying to make him slip; hesitantly he forded the waters. At the end of a long day's journey he finally reached the old recluse.

'I came to ask you about teaching,' he said reverently.

'There is only life that we need to learn about,' the recluse replied. 'And that is it.'

'I would like to learn this,' the teacher continued.

'Life is everywhere and within everything,' said the recluse. 'This is all you need to teach.'

'I think that makes sense,' said the teacher. 'But how do I teach this?'

'Tell your pupils that all they need to do is to love all people and all living things alike. Heaven's life is in everybody and everything. I have meditated here in this cave for fifty years and have realized that life is equally precious in everything the universe created. Looking at this beautiful tree in front of me, I love it as if it were my father. Everywhere, in everything, life is all alike.'

With that, the teacher bowed his head to the ground, thanked the recluse from the bottom of his Heart, left the food he had brought with him as an offering of appreciation and departed. It was already late by the time he reached the riverbank, yet the waters seemed calmer than before, gently caressing him as he made his way across. On the other side, the teacher found a large tree with a vast canopy to cover him. Curling up under its embrace, he fell asleep. In a dream the tree spoke to him.

'I am here to shelter you tonight, but tomorrow after you leave, you are on your own. I cannot go with you and take care of you tomorrow night. For this, I am very sorry.'

'There is no need to be sorry,' the teacher replied in his slumber. 'I am just thankful that you are here tonight.'

The next morning, the teacher thanked the tree again for the shelter it offered and then departed. In the middle of the road he tripped on a stone, fell to the ground and bruised his leg. 'My leg hurts!' he thought, looking at his wound. 'Now that I think of my body, I start realizing that I have one'. Then another thought rippled through him, 'I only have this body because of my father and mother. They created it and now I am here with a bruise. My body travels with me every day of my life. Yesterday's tree is no longer. How can I love the tree the same way I love my parents?'

Sitting next to the stone in the middle of the road, the teacher thanked it for tripping him. As he observed the stone he remembered the time, now many years past, when his parents had passed away and the burial that he had arranged for them. Tears started flowing down his cheeks. 'I love my parents very much,' he thought. 'How can I love a tree the same way? I am like a stone dropping in the middle of the pond, the ripples created expand all the way to the tree by the water's edge.' He realized that the ripples created by this stone were at first small and strong and then they expanded far and wide. The wider and farther the ripples traveled, the weaker and softer they became. In the Center they were very strong, while on the periphery, weak.

'My parents are closest to me, while the tree is far away,' he said aloud. 'I cannot love my parents the same way I love the canopy. While I am thankful for the canopy and the stone, I can tell the difference now!'

Tears came rushing as he remembered his mother and father. Without knowing why, he felt as if he could have helped them more; that he had not done enough in years past.

'I am so thankful to the recluse,' he thought. 'I finally understand what I need to teach my pupils. I need to teach them to keep being *who they are*.'

Yaron Seidman
Connecticut, USA
March 2013

Foreword

> Physician: a person who is skilled in the art of healing.

In this extraordinary book, authors Dr Yaron Seidman and Teja A. Jaensch bring Heart to the physician and the practice of medicine. They facilitate new light through a critical explication of the philosophies contained within the canons of the Huái Xuān. Thus, parting the veil, they provide a glimpse into the nature of medicine.

Hùnyuán Xīnfǎ: The Lost Heart of Medicine will find use by those who wish to understand the Hùnyuán approach to medical practice. It also provides a depth of insight for those who are involved in the deeper study of medicine, resulting in a refinement of our humanity. Seidman and Jaensch employ a traditional path of transmission by elucidating the textual basis of Liú Yuán's deepest thoughts. Rather than a mere recitation of the Classics, the authors hold true to the spirit of Liú Yuán scrutinizing his writings in search of the true principle. Thus, *Hùnyuán Xīnfǎ: The Lost Heart of Medicine* provides discourse which guides the practitioner deeply within to the hidden places.

The authors' approach to the construction of knowledge employs what I call *contemplative hermeneutics*, which adds the notion of contemplative practices to the discipline of studying ancient manuscripts. Specifically, they provide a unique construction of early literature gained by deep contemplation of the works combined with a disciplined analysis of the characters comprising the text. This approach maintains the relevancy and currency of their work.

Given the inspired nature of this book, it feels important to highlight its location in the field of knowledge production. To achieve this, I considered the distinctions between reproductive and creative knowledge. Memorized and repeated, classical passages reproduce previously constructed knowledge. The value of such work increases with the pursuit of accuracy. The divine spark of inspiration, ephemeral and elusive, risks being lost in the reproduction and desire to capture the intent of writers from bygone eras. Careful to the spirit of the word, translators attempt to capture the essence of intent. Contrarily, a work of creative knowledge production seeks depth of insight without the attempt to reproduce the original thought of a given author. In this instance, there is a transcendence of past, future, theory and practice, which gains a presence and luminosity within the current of Heart transmission.

This book received inspiration through the authors' work with Master Liú Bǎigǔ, the great grandson of the Qīng dynasty scholar physician, Liú Yuán. They bring their experience and views as contemporary practitioners to bear upon the problem of knowledge transmission, shining the light of their own Spirits into the inquiry upon the *Lost Heart of Medicine*.

In this effort, the authors explore the term *Xing*, meaning *Natural Character*. Thus, the need to attain Natural Character becomes the principle from which the text receives guidance. With a focus upon an enlightened Heart, the authors point toward a life that comes from Natural Character, a life defined by the continuous rotation of Heaven. Heaven's life and the Natural Character of the human being are one and the same, as above, so below, *the Two are One and the One is Two*. Hence, we explore a path with Heart.

Opening with the story of Shí Yīn Fū, the authors highlight the question of virtue through a fabric of Dàoist, Buddhist and Confucian values. Through this process they create an ethical framework that empowers the physician. In their discovery of the Heart's depths, they pursue the question of life and consequently, medicine.

Aligning with true principle, the practice of Hùnyuán medicine proceeds through continual cyclical motions of Separating returning to Unification. This is accomplished by seeking the source of the universe through Xīnfǎ, which is a path of the Heart. Hùnyuán medicine provides an avenue into life and Heart that alters and empowers the practitioner. Accomplished in part through understanding Separation and return, the cycling of Yīn and Yáng, up-bearing and down-bearing, these deep philosophical foundations of Chinese culture are addressed by drawing upon the essential traits of Confucianism, Dàoism and Buddhism.

Upon reading this book, I am enthused, excited and am falling in love with medicine in a new way. I believe that no matter your level of experience, this book will blow your mind and affect your practice in deep and meaningful ways.

William R. Morris, PhD
Author, *Li Shi-zhen Pulse Studies: An Illustrated Guide*

Introduction

歪門邪道

Wāi Mén Xié Dào

Far too often our perception is obscured by what we see. This is evident in current trends of modern bio-medicine as well as contemporary Chinese Medicine, where the circular thought patterns that traverse the Oriental medical paradigm are replaced by linear Western constructs, which look only at the physical body, the vessel. The reason we use the word *Medicine* in our title and not *Chinese Medicine* is that we are dissolving lines of division. There is only medicine, and it is either effective medicine or defective medicine. Alternative or complementary therapies along with general medical practice are all aimed at the same thing, serving the same purpose: to heal illness, ease suffering and do no harm. Therefore, there is no Chinese Medicine and no Western Medicine, there is just *Medicine*. On occasion we do draw a line and define what we do in our clinics as Hùnyuán medicine, referring to a medical practice based upon continued investigation into the understanding of the living being.

The idiom wāi mén xié dào (歪門邪道), *taking the wrong path leads to the wrong door*, applies here to medicine in all its guises. This issue is equally important for physicians and patients alike. We are all patients at one time or another and too often blindly entrust our health to others as opposed to taking personal responsibility for our well-being. In order for us to reach *true* healing we need a true *principle* to act as our guide. We must first know which is our correct path and then our physicians can assist us along it. As physicians, our role is to facilitate patients on the *appropriate* path out of suffering, rather than appeasing them with what they *want*.

Throughout this book we use the term *Heart*. We capitalize the 'H' to differentiate the word from the anatomical structure and function of the cardiovascular *heart*.[1] According to Hùnyuán medicine it is what is imbued within the Heart, our Center, that makes us *alive*. The core principle of this system is simply to find the truth and then apply it to our medicine accordingly. In the process of seeking this we are confronted by a plethora

---

[1] See the works by Joseph Chilton Pearce for some interesting thoughts on the heart and mind.

of theories, and many of us lose our way. If we are looking for the true principle of life we must not let physical manifestations confuse us. What is the difference between a body that is alive and one that is not? All the physical components can be seen in both. Therefore, our scope of study must be beyond the physical realm, beyond that which we can study with a microscope, beyond the visible. This then leads us into some difficulties, as it is easy to become lost when seeking that which is *not* visible. Consequently, we have to face the problem of wāi mén xié dào.

Seeking that which lies at the deepest level of our being can be daunting and we can easily become entangled in superficialities. These then impact not only ourselves, but our patients, children, students and our family. Hence, this book seeks the *root*, the Lost Heart of Medicine.[2] From a medical perspective, this is of further consequence as our prescriptions *must* be guided by true principle when dealing with the lives of others. People who are in pain and suffering tend to make poor decisions regarding their health, emphasizing the responsibility of the physician *themselves* to seek and adhere to the proper path. Pursuing the depths of the Heart has the potential to reveal insights into the deeper workings of life, thereby opening the way to improving and increasing life, which is the true and proper path of medicine. Hùnyuán scholars are not alone in this pursuit; throughout history many schools of thought and religions have been built upon similar truth-seeking principles.

From these schools we study and distill the information, building upon that which we find to hold truth and discarding that which went astray. Notoriety, the number of loyal students, followers or amount of books published, are not what define a great teacher or school. Being misled by superficial attributes is akin to a sheep being led by a wolf rather than a shepherd. As students, teachers, and physicians it is only through the effort to stop at nothing but truth and clarity that the correct path is revealed, not devotedly following a famous teacher's words, medical paradigm or science. The same must be said of the classical texts of Chinese medicine: though it is customary to give them an honorary status, even these are not above our

---

[2] "The important thing is to seek out the root. Dig beneath the complicated surface of reality. And keep on digging. Then dig even more until you come to the very tip of the root...This is how the world works. The stupid ones can never break free of the apparent complexity. They grope through the darkness, searching for the exit, and die before they are able to comprehend a single thing about the way of the world. They have lost all sense of direction. They might as well be deep in a forest or down in a well...they do not comprehend the fundamental principles." H. Murakami, *The Wind-Up Bird Chronicle*, trans. J. Rubin, Random House, London, 2003, p. 242.

scrutiny.[3,4] By weeding out errors from our minds and practices and through critical thinking, reflection and analysis, we differentiate insight from oversight and rely on more than our good intentions. We choose not to be deafened by what we hear.[5]

> A man whose axe was missing suspected his neighbor's son. The boy walked like a thief, looked like a thief and spoke like a thief. But the man found his axe while he was digging in the valley and the next time he saw his neighbor's son, the boy walked, looked, and spoke like any other child.[6]
>
> Traditional German proverb.

This is achieved by cultivating ourselves using a method called Xīnfǎ (心法), the Heart method. By gaining an understanding of the goodness of our Heart, problems are approached from a perspective of Center. What happens after decades of mistaking the pointing finger for the moon?[7] Unless the error is exposed it is continually transmitted from teacher to student, parent to child, from generation to generation. The error then becomes gospel, beyond question or further inquiry. Therefore, we must exercise gōngfu so we can clearly recognize a problem and then act accordingly to correct it.[8] If we are off by one grain of sand at the beginning of our journey, by its end we are off by a whole beach.

Unschuld tells us that *medicine is a puppet on the string of society.*[9]

---

[3] "An old aphorism explains the phenomenon: 'Accumulated falsehoods become the truth.' The longer—and more sincerely—such stories are repeated, the more convincing they appear." A. L. Schmieg, *Watching Your Back: Chinese Martial Arts and Traditional Medicine*, University of Hawai'i Press, Honolulu, 2005, p. 157.

[4] See the Analects, book fifteen, line 36. "The Master said, 'From a gentleman consistency is expected, but not blind fidelity.'" A. Waley, *Confucius: The Analects*, Wordsworth Editions Limited, Hertfordshire, 1996, p. 107.

[5] See J. Rose, *Music of the Human Heart may hold clues to Healing*, 2005. "If you've got a stiff heartbeat, that means your blood is like 'squirt, squirt.' Not a nice flow...". Please see bibliography for full citation.

[6] C. Feldman & J. Kornfield (eds), *Stories of the Spirit, Stories of the Heart: Parables of the Spiritual Path from Around the World*, Harper Collins, New York, 1991, p. 110.

[7] This analogy is used in Buddhism when the teacher points at the beauty of the moon, yet the student just stares at the finger.

[8] Gōngfu (功夫): Skill, art, training, hard work, labor, effort.

[9] P. Unschuld, *Chinese Medical Ethics and patient/physician relationships in ancient China*, lecture, 15th April 2000, University of Technology, Sydney. "...illustrating how direct experience of the body is inseparable from culture-bound preconceptions and theoretical constructs." V. Lo & M. Stanley-Baker, *Chinese Medicine: Chapter 9 of The Oxford Handbook of The History of Medicine*, M. Jackson (ed), Oxford University Press. Oxford, 2011, p.163.

Indeed, when we study the history of medicine we can see evidence of society's impact time and time again, yet there is no need to continue allowing these factors to influence medicine. The true principle of life is constant and timeless and remains untouched by societal fluctuations. Whilst our specific medicinals and treatments may change over time, the principle remains the same whether from two hundred or two thousand years ago. Becoming distracted and following erroneous paths often leads to unquestioningly following sages, forgetting that sages must be questioned and the sincerity of their Heart and words must be observed. Only then can we differentiate those who guide us along our proper path and those who would lead us astray.[10]

Modern Chinese medicine is a fusion of social and political ideals in the People's Republic of China during the 20th century. Alongside the reformation of the political and social structure, a whole new system of Chinese medicine was developed based on the logistical paradigm of Western medicine. The following quote from the 1977 publication *Creating a New Chinese Medicine and Pharmacology*, should demonstrate these reforms:

> During the Great Proletarian Cultural Revolution, the political consciousness of China's medical workers was raised as they studied seriously Chairman Mao's teachings...In this we were guided by Chairman Mao's philosophical thinking. Chairman Mao taught us: "There can be no differentiation without contrast. There can be no development without differentiation and struggle..."
>
> Chairman Mao said: "Every form of motion contains within itself its own particular contradiction. This particular contradiction constitutes the particular essence which distinguishes one thing from another..." Their mother said with deep feeling: "Chairman Mao takes care of us poor and lower-middle peasants. He saved our family and gave my children eyesight. Chairman Mao's revolutionary line is our life-line, our happiness line."[11]

The role of medicine is to help people, not politics, and it must be based on more than mere ideology. Incorporating the agenda of Máo Zédōng (毛泽东)

---

[10] "Do not believe in anything merely because it is said, nor in traditions because they have been handed down from antiquity...nor in writings by sages because sages wrote them...nor in the mere authority of our teachers and masters. Believe when the writing, doctrine, or saying is corroborated by reason and consciousness." L. Colgrove, 'Theosophy & Initiation' in *The Theosophical Forum*, Theosophical University Press, 1941, April forum.

[11] *Creating a New Chinese Medicine and Pharmacology*, Foreign Language Press, Peking, 1977, pp. 8, 27, 32, 81.

into medicine was evidently questionable. Thus, *all* classical medical literature must be understood from an historical perspective, accounting for the political distortions of the time. In this book, by studying the philosophies of China through the Heart of Liú Yuán, we uncover the *true principle*, a fixed point of reference from which *all* medicine should approach *all* suffering.

The true principle of life is not mysterious, exotic or esoteric; it is simply the truth. Hùnyuán medicine approaches the physical body and health through researching this principle. It is not the physical body that demarcates life and death, but something deeper. It is a cyclical movement between two states: an open state we call *Separation*, and a closed state of *Unification*.

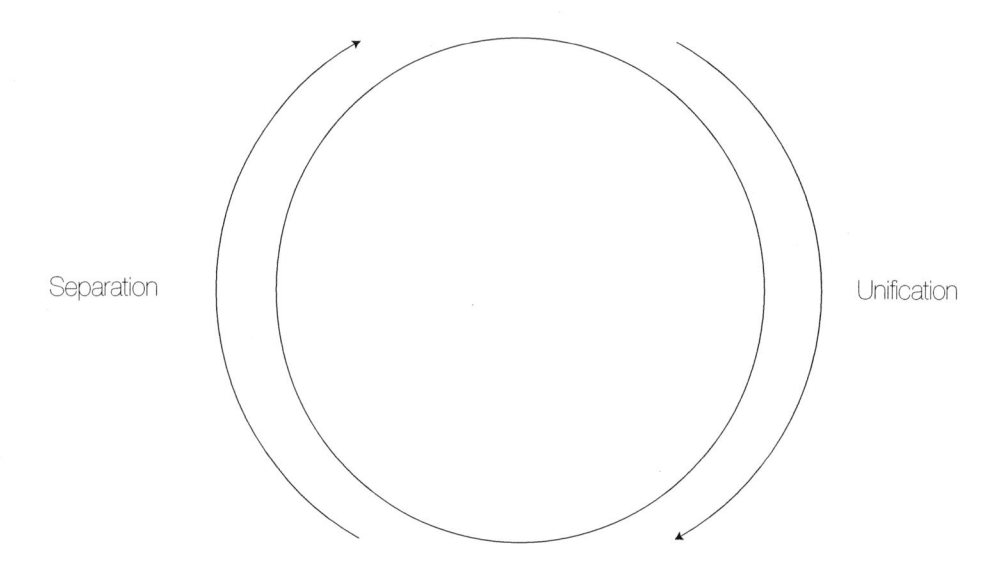

Separation   Unification

A dead body finds itself in a state of complete and constant Unification. It is one with the Earth, like a fallen tree, gradually decomposing. In contrast, to maintain life there must be a cyclical motion from Unification back into Separation. The fact that we sleep and wake up each day is a result of this. So how do we become clear and yet clearer about this principle?[12]

---

[12] "The materialistic image of man, though false at present, tends to build a future in which it becomes true. A self-fulfilling prophecy; a self-accelerating process." Professor of Physics and Anthroposophy, Dr Ernst Katz, via the philosopher Peter Schäfer. Personal communication in possession of the author.

> An Empty sort of mind is valuable for finding pearls and tails and things because it can see what's in front of it. An Overstuffed mind is unable to. While the Clear mind listens to a bird singing, the Stuffed-Full-of-Knowledge-and-Cleverness mind wonders what *kind* of bird is singing. The more Stuffed Up it is, the less it can hear through its own ears and see through its own eyes. Knowledge and Cleverness tend to concern themselves with the wrong sorts of things, and a mind confused by Knowledge, Cleverness, and Abstract Ideas tends to go chasing off after things that don't matter, or that don't even exist, instead of seeing, appreciating, and making use of what is right in front of it.[13]

Day and night, winter and summer, these cycles occur each day and every year. There is constant transformation from one state to the other. These cycles that are present throughout the environment are the same that keep our physical vessel alive. Petals open during the day to accept the warmth and close at night to avoid the cold. For people, being awake to carry out action requires Separation while our deepest state of Unification occurs at night when we sleep. During sleep the eyes close and there is apparent stillness. During the day the body is engaged and moving and the eyes are open.

> And a man said, Speak to us of Self-Knowledge.
> And he answered, saying:
> Your Hearts know in silence the secrets of the days and the nights.[14]
>
> The Prophet

Separation is our engagement with the world, which comes at a cost. To balance the equation, the body must recharge, which is accomplished through Unification. Whilst these are opposing states, they each contain the seed of the other: Yīn and Yáng. At night when we sleep our body is relatively still, but our hearts beat and our lungs breathe. During the day as energy is expended, recharging still takes place through eating, drinking and breathing, by what we see, hear and feel.[15] These sense organs are our *Recharging Instruments* which conduct information *into* the body and Heart

---

[13] B. Hoff, *The Tao of Pooh & The Te of Piglet*, Methuen, London, 1982, p. 158.
[14] K. Gibran, *The Prophet*, 1926, cited from the new illustrated edition, *Kahlil Gibran's The Prophet and The Art of Peace*, Duncan Baird Publishers, London, 2008, p. 95.
[15] The strength of this recharging capacity depends on our health and the *quality* of what we eat and drink, the *quality* of the air that we breathe, and what it is we see, hear and feel. Likewise, the best *quality* of Unification is achieved through sleeping at the *appropriate* time. This is our *relationship* to sleep.

and are represented on the right hand side of the circular diagram below.

"Life enters through the mouth and nose, eyes and ears."

Liú Yuán

To form an understanding of how Hùnyuán medicine approaches treatment, we divide the two broad movements of Unification and Separation into *six segments*. Three of these, related to Unification, guide life into the Center: Yángmíng (阳明), Tàiyīn (太阴) and Shàoyīn (少阴). Those that direct life out of the Center and relate to Separation are Juéyīn (厥阴), Shàoyáng (少阳) and Tàiyáng (太阳).[16] All six segments work together to keep the cycle continuously rotating: circle-ation.

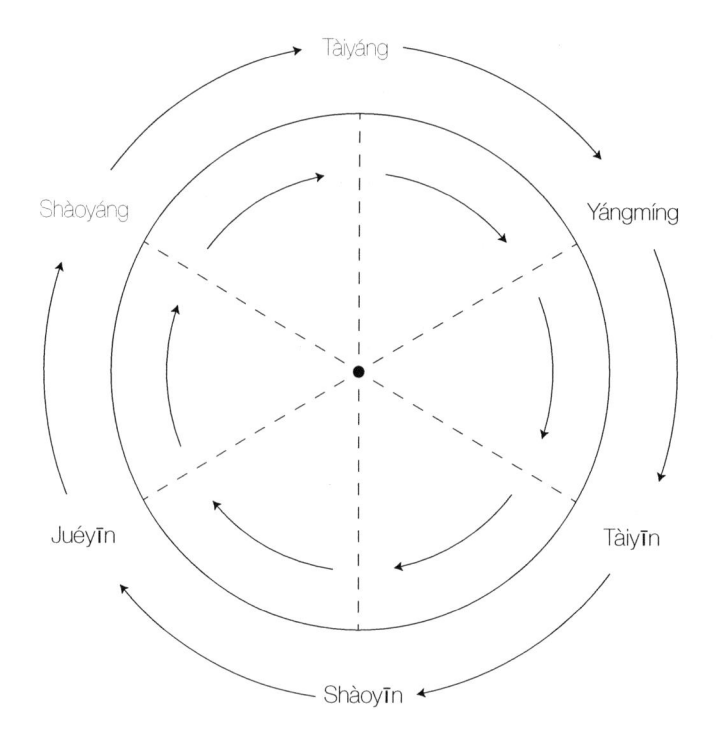

---

[16] While these segments may seem similar to references from the Shāng Hán Lún (伤寒论), they are not synonymous. Hùnyuán medicine understands them as: *Separation Concealing Inward* (Yángmíng), *Concealed Movement* (Tàiyīn), *Unification Instrument* (Shàoyīn). *Concealed Separation Outward* (Juéyīn), *Revealed Separation* (Shàoyáng) and *Separation Instrument* (Tàiyáng). These are the nuts and bolts of treatment with Hùnyuán medicine using acupuncture and herbal therapy. They are included here as an introduction to the *Outer Water* and *Inner Fire Circles*, yet they are not the focus of this book.

Each of these segments is associated with the structural organs of the body: the zàngfǔ (脏腑). Shàoyīn (少阴), the segment at the bottom of the circle, relates to the zàng of the Heart and Kidneys and where we are most connected to nature. This is where Unification occurs, when we are most disconnected from the myriad things of the external world. The top of the circle represents the exterior of the body and the outward movement of Separation where we engage with these myriad things. This segment is referred to as Tàiyáng (太阳), which in turn has a relationship with the fǔ of the Bladder and Small Intestine. Shàoyīn and Tàiyáng are aligned on a vertical axis, revealing a fascinating association between what we can observe externally and our internal realm.

The exterior aspects of our body and life that are associated with Separation are palpable: the skin and hair, the functions of ingestion and elimination and also with the activities we carry out during the day. On the contrary, the concealed events of Unification are not clearly visible. The energy we acquire through our Recharging Instruments during the day is drawn deep into the body via the segments on the right side of the circle to be distilled by Shàoyīn.

In chapter 3 while searching for the Lost Heart, we explore this further, introducing the Outer Water Circle and Inner Fire Circle. Regarding Shàoyīn, the Kidneys are on the Outer Water Circle and the *human* Heart is on the Inner Fire Circle.[17] The organs (zàngfǔ 脏腑) of human Heart and Kidneys unite together to form Shàoyīn.[18] Our task and our skill (our gōngfu) is to contemplate the concealed occurrences of Shàoyīn. With persistent, conscientious reflection, clarity emerges; many illnesses have their root at this level and deeper.

Deeper still, we contemplate how the structures come to life and we use the picture of a *vibrating* thread. The physical vessel's partnership with life, later referred to as the *Heaven principle*, is maintained by this thread. Hence, we call it the One Thread of Life. Finding it inadequate to treat the Kidneys, Shàoyīn, the Qì and blood, or the Five Elements, we utilize these exterior observations of bodily functions as the first step on the journey into the forgotten realm of Center.

沒齒不忘

Mò Chǐ Bù Wàng

'Unforgettable'

---

[17] We introduce and clarify the concept of the human Heart and the Dào Heart in later chapters.

[18] Later this very issue is discussed using the kǎn ☵ trigram of the Yìjīng (易經), Classic of Changes.

Contemplation of this realm requires an entry point and this is the One Thread of Life: a visual representation to guide our minds inward, to matters not of the intellect but of the Heart.[19]

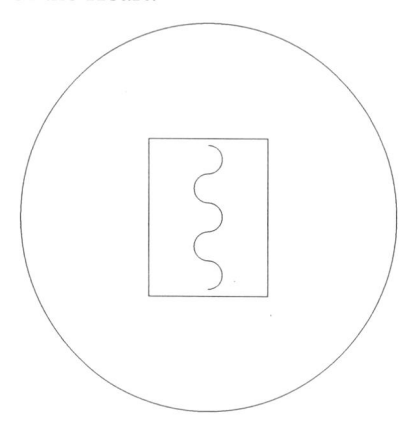

Maintaining life depends only upon the movement of this One Thread. This is all that differentiates the living from the deceased. Western and contemporary Chinese medicine both struggle to understand the root and increasing prevalence of chronic and debilitating disease.

Our good intentions may help heal the snakebite on the surface, yet the venom can remain circulating within.[20] All physicians engage with their craft with the best of intentions, yet these alone are not sufficient. We all need to be governed by a fixed point of reference from which each diagnostic assessment is addressed. The ultimate goal of medicine is to allow the instruments of Separation and Unification to work optimally, thereby reducing the patient's reliance on medicine. Seeking and using this true principle not only governs our pursuits in medicine but also reveals the root of our existence and our relationships.

Humanity's relationship to the world should be a reflection of Center. Often though, we are unstable. It is from our Center that our emotions

---

[19] "Many find it fatuous and downright repugnant to claim that the wonders of the life and the universe are mere reflections of microscopic particles engaged in a pointless dance fully choreographed by the laws of physics. Is it really the case that feelings of joy, sorrow, or boredom are nothing but chemical reactions in the brain–reactions between molecules and atoms that, even more microscopically, are reactions between...vibrating strings?" B. Greene, *The Elegant Universe: Superstrings, Hidden Dimensions, and the Quest for the Ultimate Theory*, Vintage, London, 2000, p. 16. Here is an approach to the same issue but from the perspective of physics, which necessitates further dissection of reality. For our work here in Hùnyuán Xīnfǎ contemplate a different chronology. Our One vibrating Thread is what connects the vessel to Tàijí, allowing for movement, vigorous, subtle and sublime. Our *vibrating strings* of physics are mere reflections of *Heaven principle*.

[20] Referencing the experience of Shí Xīn Dé in chapter 1.

discharge. When moving excessively the One Thread of Life is shaken violently, resulting in psychological and physiological symptoms and patterns.[21] Movement describes and defines the life of the myriad things, from Unification to Separation, from Yīn to Yáng. In our Center, movement is so subtle that it *appears* still. Approaching stillness is a challenge for the active mind, thus we grapple and struggle with finding Center.

Present moment awareness is a state of being which reveals a harmonious, peaceful and subtle movement of the One Thread of Life. To the left of Center is the past; to the right is the future. When we swing busily from one side to the other, reacting habitually to our surroundings, we cease to live in the present. The pendulum of preoccupation with *things* of yesterday and possibilities of tomorrow, whilst beyond our control, begin to define our propriety. Distracted and off Center we start believing that our circumstances excuse us being ignoble.

Emotional reactions fall in line with Unification (our likes) and Separation (our dislikes), which add to the fray. To be (*or not to be...*) Centered is Wúwéi (無為), or the principle of following the path of least resistance. When absorbed in events and words that have already taken place or those yet to eventuate, we fail to act appropriately when action is required. Action only occurs in the present and the ramifications of this can send ripples throughout our lives.

Our life is our set of pottery tools that we use to carve out and shape our existence. These implements were donated by our parents and forebears. When it is time for us to hand these on to our children, if we have been careless and chipped them, we blunt their effectiveness. If we drop our wares and leave shards on the floor, this is our legacy. Our children will then inherit the fruits of our thoughts, decisions and actions, having to clean up (heal) with defective tools.[22]

"The day will come when our children will undo what we so foolishly have done."[23]

---

[21] "...thoughts – just mere thoughts – are as powerful as electric batteries – as good for one as sunlight is, or as bad for one as poison." F. Burnett, *The Secret Garden*, Puffin Books, London, 1911, p. 321. We are blessed by some brilliant literature for young people. For example, *The Secret Garden*, teaches us and our children much about life and our responses to it. Another great example is David Shannon's beautiful story about resilience, *A Bad Case of Stripes*: "Soon everyone was calling out different shapes and colors and poor Camilla was changing faster than you can change channels on a T.V." D. Shannon, *A Bad Case of Stripes*, Scholastic, New York, 1998, p. 7. When one finds cross-cultural references discussing the same issues, especially when separated by time as well as space, it points to something unified.

[22] This is a very real issue. Please refer to C. Arnold, *Effects of Stress Can Persist for Generations: how your grandpa's rough life might make you more anxious*, Scientific America, February 2013. Please see bibliography for full citation.

[23] Edward St John QC, Lake Pedder Committee Inquiry, 1974.

Hùnyuán (混元) means *the origin of the universe*. Xīnfǎ (心法) is *the method of the Heart*: using our Heart to contemplate the origin. For medicine, this will be the origin of disease and suffering. In China, Xīnfǎ is the term used to describe when a teacher or master transmits the *secret* principles. Yet through Xīnfǎ, which is described and defined throughout the following pages, we discover that there is no *secret*. Looking up from our musing, we uncover the *Lost Heart of Medicine*.

Recognition and application of Xīnfǎ starts with the cultivation of goodness, compassion and virtue. Walking with us, step by step on our journey into the Heart of things, is the Qīng (清) dynasty scholar, Liú Yuán (劉沅), who is introduced below in the *Brief Historical Perspective*. Following this we study Liú's interpretation of the Sòng dynasty story, *Shí Yīn Fū and the Ledger of Good and Evil*. People learn best through stories and this particular tale created a shift of consciousness that has rippled through us personally and out into our relationships. By very simple means we can keep account of our virtue. Following this story we work through and extract the precious from Liú's vast compendium of the Huái Xuān (槐軒) philosophy.

> That the practice of Chinese medicine is itself very individualized is often taken for granted and is therefore rarely considered in Western books or schools. However, in the clinic, Chinese medicine is an instrument that each practitioner plays differently, some better than others, and each with an individual predilection for a theoretical or therapeutic style that best suits their individual skills and personality. This breathes life into the tradition of Chinese medicine and allows it to grow.[24]

Whilst true in one sense, medicine *must* be based on a principle that transcends time and space and that transcends *styles*, *theories*, *schools*, and *East or West*. Using the works of Liú Yuán as a springboard for our own contemplation into this timeless principle, reading this book is your doorway to the path of Xīnfǎ, cultivating the *Lost Heart*.[25]

---

[24] Z. T. Liang, *A Qin Bowei Anthology*, trans. C. Chace, Paradigm Publications, Massachusetts, 1997, p. xi.

[25] Schmieg (2005, p. 23) quotes Xúnzǐ: "When men ford rivers, they leave markers in the deep spots." These *markers* are what we are seeking in the works of Liú Yuán.

Brief Historical Perspective

劉沅

Liú Yuán

Liú Yuán (劉沅), also known as Liú Zhǐtáng (劉止唐), was born in Shuāngliú county, Sìchuān (四川雙流), China, in 1767 CE, the 23rd year of Emperor Qián Lóng (乾隆) and died in 1855 CE, the fifth year of the reign of Emperor Xián Fēng (咸豐). One of the Qīng (清) dynasty's greatest scholars, Liú was an educator, religious thinker and medical philosopher whose work has become known as Huái Xuān (槐軒) philosophy.

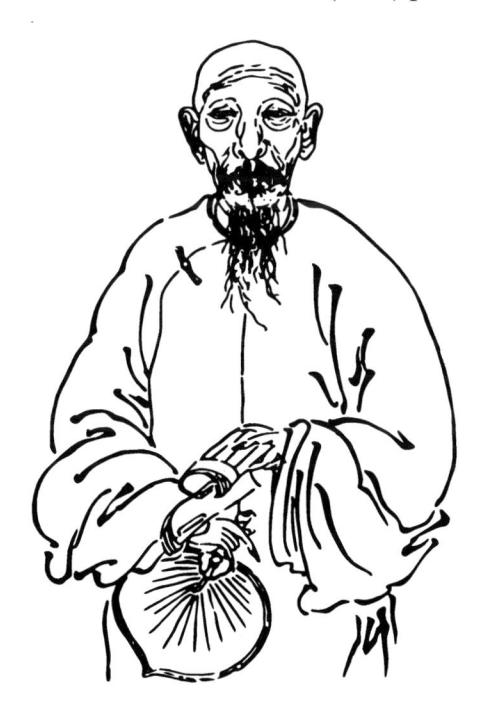

As a youth, Liú studied the Confucian Classics with his father and passed the provincial imperial examination when he was twenty-five years old. At the age of thirty, Liú gave up the pursuit of an official's career and instead stayed at home to care for his aging and ailing mother. This was a difficult time for Liú as, aside from caring for his sick mother, his young son passed away and his own health was declining rapidly. It was during this dark time, *the middle of his road*, that Liú fortuitously met an elderly Dàoist monk named Lǎo Yěyún (老野云).

This old monk saved Liú's life by giving him the key to the majority of his future work: the knowledge that experiencing longevity was not to be found by experimenting with miraculous medicinal substances, an error made by so many well intentioned Dàoists and physicians alike. Rather, that it is only found through benevolence–the cultivation of one's Heart–that we can truly experience longevity. During the eight years that Liú studied with Lǎo Yěyún his health and scholarly capacity improved exponentially and he began to attract many students and followers. From a state of illness in his earlier years, he became healthy and prosperous in his later years and by the time he was sixty he had eight sons born to several wives. His eldest son was Liú Bèiwén (劉棍文).

After his sojourn with the Dàoist, at the age of forty-six, Liú moved to Sìchuān's capital city, Chéngdū (成都). Liú's study was not segregated into a single school of thought, but would research and investigate both ancient and contemporary literature of his time including the three major religious traditions prevalent in China: Buddhism, Dàoism and Confucianism. He was seeking a true principle, something constant and timeless. An advocate of taking the middle road of reason, Liú would not meekly follow or propagate dogma. Through the analysis of *tiān lǐ rén qíng* (天理人情), *the essence of Heaven and human emotions*, he strove to scrutinize everything and would often comprehend difficult issues using an analogy. For example, a mountain may obstruct Water temporarily but in the end Water *will* arrive at its destination. This is due to the inherent *nature* of Water. He uses this analogy to describe our ignorance, our *youthful folly*, which we can flow out of: finding our exit from ignorance.[1] He admired the competence of prior scholars and peers but was not afraid to highlight and then discard their incompetence. Therefore, in the fields of classical literature and medicine, he created his own philosophical doctrine and school, the Huái Xuān Academy.

Delving into his inquiry of the literary Classics with prodigious dedication and sincerity, he gave lectures, taught many students and wrote scholarly works that greatly influenced future generations of philosophers and physicians. One of his students was Zhèng Qīnān (鄭欽安), a noted physician-scholar (1824–1911 CE) who revived classical Chinese medicine at the end of the Qīng dynasty and founded the Fire Spirit School.[2] Liú's style of teaching was to have all his students scrutinize the classical texts

---

[1] This specific example is further elucidated in chapter 8, *The Wounded Warrior*.
[2] Huǒ Shén Pài (火神派). For more on Zhèng Qīnān, please refer to the Hùnyuán Research Institute's scholarly articles.

and contemplate these in relation to their experience of reality. Only then would the pupils congregate and he would hear and answer their difficulties and questions. He instructed one and all to meditate and contemplate from dawn till dusk to nurture their Hearts, preserve their spirits, to improve their health and to strengthen their bodies.

He completely disregarded tuition and allowed students to decide how much he or she could pay according to their family's financial situation. If their family was exceptionally poor they did not have to pay at all as Liú believed that a school should be a place of learning where talent is cultivated, not a place of business. The accomplishments of his students were his gain, not their tuition fees. Because of this and the love that his disciples felt for their learned teacher, the Huái Xuān Academy's achievements were remarkable. Indeed, Liú's influence on academic circles was so extensive that at the end of the Qīng dynasty and the beginning of the Republic, almost all of the great scholars of classical Chinese literature in Sìchuān came from his school. Liú's definitive research was vast and he composed many works, which were later compiled, arranged and printed as *A Comprehensive Volume of Huái Xuān* (槐軒全書) between 1875 and 1908.[3]

In *The History of the Qīng Dynasty* it is stated that disciples of the Huái Xuān Academy numbered several thousand, of whom over one hundred passed the provincial imperial examination, many of whom were recommended to the imperial court as outstanding scholars. It became the largest private academy in Sìchuān involved in the study of classical Chinese literature with over three hundred active students at any given time. Pupils would study in the academy for up to ten years. Over the years the Academy expanded and by the time of Liú's passing it covered more than eight acres, with many teaching halls, pavilions, towers, flower gardens and ornamental hills, all on the shore of the Jǐnjiāng River. Two magnificent stone lions guarded the entrance, standing on either side of a large black door. Inside towered four colossal camphor wood pillars that emitted an enchanting fragrance. Within the main courtyard grew an ancient scholar tree whose many branches and dense foliage clearly demonstrated the contrast between light and shadow. This tree was an immense inspiration to Liú, so much so that his Academy was built around it. The scholar tree is called Huái shù (槐樹) in China.[4]

---

[3] For a list of Liú's extant works, please refer to the end of this historical segment.
[4] Huái Xuān means the canopy of the Huái tree. This tree is also known as the Locust tree or the Japanese Sophora tree, *Sophora japonica*.

After the rise of the Chinese Communist Party in 1949, the Huái Xuān Academy was demolished[5] and in its stead the Jǐnjiāng assembly hall (錦江禮堂) was built in 1958. Gone was the old Huái tree and with it, the Huái Xuān Academy. Despite the loss of their place of learning, Liú's students kept studying and researching the Classics.

In June 2012, the Hùnyuán Research Institute traveled to China and visited Liú's grave in Shuāngliú county. Once a large structure, the tomb was moved in the 1950s and hidden in a field to avoid desecration by the Communist government. The Institute's scholars found his tombstone and those of his immediate family deep in a deserted overgrown field. They burnt incense and paper money showing their respect to his teachings and hoping to follow his insight and scholarship. It was in Shuāngliú in 2012, at the extant Huái Xuān Cultural Association, that we met and studied with eighty-four year old Master Liú Bǎigǔ (劉伯谷), Liú Yuán's great grandson, the Standard Bearer of the Huái Xuān School.

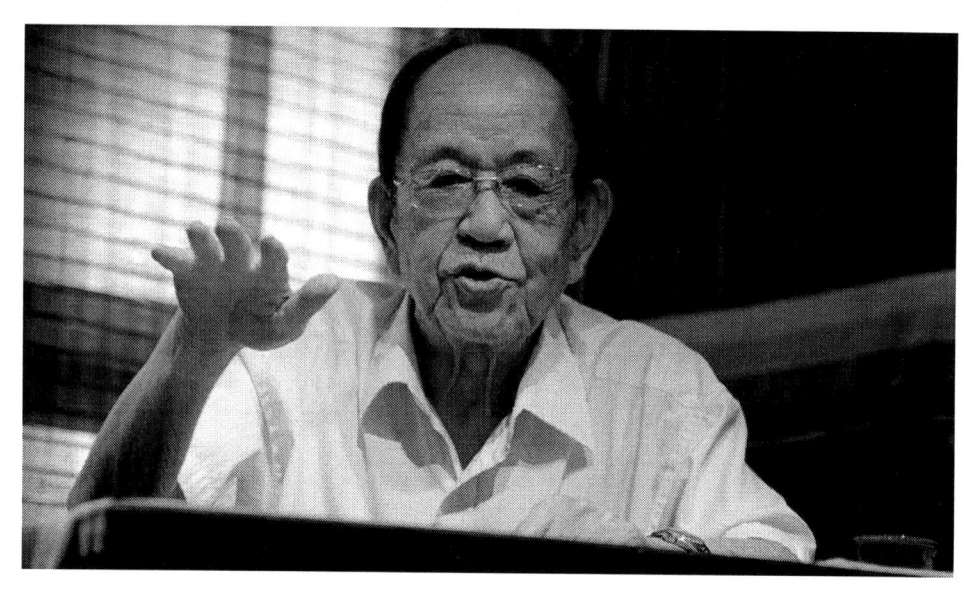

"Mencius said that everyone can be as great as the Yellow Emperor!"

Liú Bǎigǔ, June 2012.[6]

---

[5] "Great spirits have always found violent opposition from mediocrities. The latter cannot understand it when a man does not thoughtlessly submit to hereditary prejudices, but honestly and courageously uses his intelligence and fulfills the duty to express the results of his thought in clear form." Albert Einstein, quoted in New York Times, March 19, 1940.

[6] All quotes throughout this book by this great sage were taken from our lessons with him in 2012.

While most commentators say that Liú Yuán was a Confucian due to his reliance on the Confucian teaching of the Five Cardinal Relationships, when we read his life's work starting with the story of Shí Yīn Fū, we see a man seeking the truth, regardless of where it came from. There were many ideas from the Sòng dynasty that he exposed as erroneous, indifferent to how famous or rich its exponent was. Seeking true principle was the main point of his work, therefore Liú was not interested in romantic pontifications and labeling him a Confucian, Dàoist or Buddhist would be questionable. He was a thinker and a skilled one at that. Through his extensive work commentating on the great written texts and philosophies of China, he was adamant that with the right tools even the lowest peasant could achieve the knowledge and wisdom reached by the sages. Every person, regardless of time, place, culture and heritage, has it in their Heart to reach this point through cultivation. This is the same path those of us investigating Hùnyuán medicine walk, so we journey with Liú Yuán, with his words indented and *italicized*, on the same road throughout the chapters that follow.[7]

"Among book-writing good doctors, there has not been a single perfect man."[8]

---

[7] Liú Yuán's texts can be divided into two main categories:
1. The true meaning of the Classics
2. The philosophy of the Classics
In the first group there are annotations on the Four Books and Six Classics of Confucianism. The Four Books being: the Great Learning Common Explanation (大學恒解), the Doctrine of the Mean Common Explanations (中庸恒解), the Analects Common Explanations (論語恒解), and Mencius Common Explanations (孟子恒解). The Six Classics being: Zhōuyì Common Explanations (周易恒解), the Book of Poetry Common Explanations (詩經恒解), the Book of Historical Documents Common Explanations (尚書恒解), the Three Rites (三禮), the Spring and Autumn Common Explanations (春秋恒解) and the Classic of Filial Piety Common Explanations (孝經恒解). The Three Rites includes the Officials of the Zhōu Common Explanations (周官恒解), the Etiquette Common Explanations (儀禮恒解) and the Book of Rites Common Explanations (禮記恒解). In total there are annotations for twelve Classics. Within the second group, the philosophy of the Classics, there are many texts of which the following are noted: The Master's Questions (子問), the Additional Questions (又問), the Huái Xuān Pledge (槐軒約言), Correcting Errors (正譌), the Customary Speech (俗言) and the Ancient Printing of Great Learning's True Words (大學古本質言).

[8] Minehan quotes Wáng Qīngrèn (王清任), *Yi Lin Gai Cuo: Correcting the Errors in the Forest of Medicine*, trans. Y. Chung, H. Oving, & S. Becker, Blue Poppy Press, Boulder, 2007, p. v.

CHAPTER 1

石音夫功過格

Shí Yīn Fū Gōng Guò Gé

Shí Yīn Fū and the Ledger of Good and Evil

The original author of this story is unknown, but it has been circulating in China since at least the Sòng dynasty over nine hundred years ago. Liú Yuán transcribed his own version and both his and that of the Sòng dynasty have been consulted in the research for this book. The original version had two extra characters in the title, Xǐng Mí (醒迷), which translates to *'waking up from obscurity/confusion'*.[1] Comparing the two, we see that Liú's version seeks truth and practicality; therefore approximately seventy percent of the Buddhist references to spirits, ghosts and demons were omitted. We believe those that remain are suggestive of the religious socio-political climate of his time. In an attempt to avoid his audience becoming mystified by the mysterious, he emphasized and even added themes that alluded to the cultivation of one's Heart. This process of cultivation, in Liú's mind, was something that was independent of religion. There are many embedded meanings within the story and the names of characters also have significance, which we include in footnotes throughout the tale. We let Liú himself introduce his rearranged version of the text with his preface and then we provide our abridged translation.[2]

> *Human nature is all goodness, therefore every person should be good. However, there are cases where it is not such. Being perverted with habits and customs, hiding behind fame and riches, drifting along in comfort, gradually it loses its normal nature. In our nation Dào has long formed. Sages and scholars were teaching the Four Masters and Six Classics, clearly like the Sun and Moon*

---

[1] Therefore the full title reads: 石音夫醒迷功過格.
[2] For our translation of his work, we try to maintain his syntax and the reader will note the absence of intricate descriptions of landscapes and characters. In the hope of making the story clearer, we have made a small alteration to the text by linking together two of the characters, Mr Qián and Shí Xīn Dé.

traveling the sky, like the rivers flowing the Earth. But some common people not yet educated either did not know what goodness ought to be, or that evil had to be dispersed. The original author of 'Shí Yīn Fū and the Ledger of Good and Evil' is unknown. The story's intention is of goodness, and yet within the original text there are many errors. A friend wanted to publish it and asked humble me to write a preface. Goodness and I have nothing in common, but respecting him I dare not to decline his request. I love the fine detail of the story and have weeded out the superfluous and unqualified. This process does not contradict what our forefathers engaged with. I was worried that the reader will not carefully inspect the truth, and would take the wrong path, and the shepherd would lose his sheep. This would disappoint the original author's intention. The knowledgeable can draw forth the lessons.

The era of Dào Guāng Emperor (1821–1851 CE).
The year of Gēngzǐ, two days past the Birthday of the Flowers.
Zhōngguó, Sìchuān, Shuāngliú, Liú Yuán.

Once upon a time there was a beggar who had pursued many avenues to change his circumstances. His maternal guardian had ended her life when her husband had died after being forced into labor in order to repay a debt to a wealthy man. To make his way in the world, before he was a beggar he had tried being a carpenter and put his hand to various other trades, but he never succeeded. So, with no other choice, he went from door to door begging for food and lodgings. One day as he was traveling in the middle of the road, he came across a Dàoist monk, who had just journeyed through Shānxī.

"Dear monk, will you please reveal to me a path for my life so I may have a livelihood?" he asked.

"When you ask this, what do you mean by life?" replied the monk, "Do you mean life and death, or do you mean growing and giving birth to new life, or do you mean the life of commerce? Or rather life within the myriad things of existence?"

"Which way of life out of all of these is the most difficult to follow?" asked the beggar.

"The life of business and commerce is the most difficult," responded the monk.

"Then can you show me this way?" pleaded the beggar.

"At the third or fourth month of each year," began the monk, "the price of rice is very expensive, so buy fifty bundles of rice earlier in the year for less and then sell them later for more. This is how you can make money."

The beggar pondered what the monk had said. "But how can I buy rice when I do not have any money?"

"Well, if you have no capital then this can be very difficult," agreed the monk, "perhaps you can collect firewood in the mountain forests and sell it to people in their villages."

"After doing that type of difficult labor for some time, is it possible to then release myself from the suffering of this hardship?" the beggar asked.

"No," answered the monk, "Not only with the cutting of firewood, but all tradespeople and business people are also prisoners of this suffering without any means to release themselves from its grasp."

"So what is the way to free myself from this suffering?" asked the beggar.

"Only by following life within the myriad things," answered the monk, "taking this path will eventually free you from all suffering."

At this, the beggar shook his head. "If you mean by this not to kill any life, if this is the life of the myriad things," he said, "then this is far too difficult. If I cannot kill chickens and ducks, why would I raise them? If I cannot kill oxen and horses, how can I take their hides and hoofs? If I cannot kill sheep and pigs, how can I make sacrificial offerings? If you mean not to hurt any life then I must not cut the bamboo and trees, so I will not be able to collect firewood or build a house. This is very difficult indeed."

"On the contrary," smiled the monk, "this is in fact a very simple issue. With chickens and ducks, if you do not hurt their eggs or chicks, if you do not waste their lives for nothing and only use the mature animals when you need meat, how can you call it killing? Horses and oxen help people travel and turn the soil and then when they reach old age and die on their own, there is no need to kill them for their hides and hoofs. When bamboo and trees are growing they do not break, but when they are old and soon to fall, this is the appropriate time to cut them. For all the myriad things there is an appropriate time and place."

"If this is the case," said the beggar, "when things are supposed to grow and flourish and be alive and you slaughter them, this is then defined as killing. If they have reached their maturity and are at rest and then you slaughter them, this is not considered killing."

"Indeed so." confirmed the monk. "The ones that are supposed to be alive, flourishing and prospering, they do so through the influence of Heaven and Earth and one should not go against them. Only when Heaven and Earth go into storage can we take from them. In this way, we can use our resources forever and never exhaust them."

Immediately the beggar understood. "Heaven and Earth have the virtue of giving birth and making everything alive. The myriad things have the Heart of reproducing and making future generations. Whenever our conduct follows the principle of Heaven and that of our own Hearts, when we do not go against these but benevolently perform a deed, this becomes a good deed."

"These words you speak have a great destiny," agreed the monk. "However, words alone are not sufficient and you have yet to accumulate enough virtue so it will still be difficult to free yourself from suffering. Use all your Heart to make your actions and affairs truthful and honest. In this way your virtue will gradually become full and complete. Persistently pursue goodness and then life and death will be concealed within you. Only then can you be free." The monk gestured to the beggar, "Kneel down and I will give you a new name."

So the beggar prostrated himself in the middle of the road, bowing his head.

"From now on," commanded the monk in a deep voice, "I will call you Shí Yīn Fū!"[3]

When the beggar, now with his new name, stood up, the Dàoist monk had disappeared.

Shí Yīn Fū fell to the ground again and began to cry.

"My Heart is so often confused, how can I become a good person?"

Slowly, he devised a method to keep himself on track. He went on begging and always asked for yellow and black beans. Eventually he had a bag full of both. Taking the black beans, he tied them to his right side and the yellow beans he tied to his left. Then he made a third bag, and tied it around his neck so it hung on his chest, over his Heart.

Day and night, whenever any small affair of a corrupt Heart entered him or if he committed any crooked deed, Yīn Fū would take a black bean from the bag on his right and put it in the bag over his Heart, thereby making a record of his error. Any good affair he engaged in would yield a yellow bean. After continuing in this way for one hundred days he poured out the contents to see the quantity of his faults and his merits. This was his ledger of good and evil.

In the beginning there were many black beans, but after a year of this training, he only saw yellow ones. In such a way, his Heart gradually began to transform. Becoming more aware of his movements and impact on the world, he would avoid needlessly crushing the soft grass and would not tread on bugs and ants. He made sure he was well concealed whilst defecating and would not tread on melons in the fields, or knock plums off with his hat in the orchards. If he came across another traveler in the middle of the road, he would step aside and let him pass. When women passed by, he would keep his distance and would not leer. If he found a lost item, he would earnestly look for its owner and return it. If it were sunny and hot or raining and cold, he would not blame Heaven. If he would see dangerous and obstructing mountains and rivers, he would not blame the Earth. If people laughed at him or scolded him, he would not return a word and never allow hatred to take hold of his Heart. When he came across strangers he would love and respect them. Yīn Fū continued in this way for two and a half years. His Heart became calm and at peace and his body became vigorous and healthy.

In Shānxī there was a wealthy merchant called Shí Xīn Dé[4] and he had a daughter named Shí Yīn.[5] From childhood she was extremely clever, which made it quite difficult for Xīn Dé to find a suitable husband for her as all her

---

[3] Shí Yīn Fū (石音夫): Rock, Sound of the Heart and Man/Husband, or simply: the husband of Shí Yīn.

[4] Shí Xīn Dé (石心德): Rock, Heart and Virtue.

[5] Shí Yīn (石音): Rock and Sound of the Heart.

suitors could not match her wit. One autumn night while Xīn Dé lay asleep, a spirit came to him in a dream telling him that a man named Shí Yīn Fū would arrive at his house the next day and advised Xīn Dé to take good care of him.

Bemused by his dream, Xīn Dé awoke early. He went out to the front door and swept the entrance, making sure it was in good order for the man who would come today. At midday no one had arrived except a lowly beggar. Thinking very little of beggars, Xīn Dé kept him outside and waited for another arrival. By sunset, however, still no other had arrived. Dejectedly, Xīn Dé went inside where his wife spoke to him sternly, telling him to go and speak to the beggar and offer him lodgings for the night as this beggar may have some good aspects despite his appearance. Xīn Dé agreed and going back outside, he inspected the beggar.

"From your appearance," he said to the beggar, somewhat surprised, "you seem quite calm. Apparently your life is not without joy. How can this be from a beggar in your world of suffering? Please tell me your name and from where it is you have come."

"I am in your honorable presence," said the beggar, "you, the precious host and your precious home and I am imploring you to let me rest here for the night so I dare not speak anything but the truth to you. Humble me; I am a native of Sìchuān. My whole family met disaster when I was an infant but fortunately a kind man called Qián,[6] and his wife fed me and looked after me. They both died before I could learn anything of their ancestry and after I buried them I lent my hand to many trades, but in these I never succeeded. All that was left for me was begging. Some two years ago I met a Dàoist priest who gave me a new name, Shí Yīn Fū." As he said his name he wrote it out on the dusty ground. "I am in your presence, you, the precious host and your precious home."

Hearing this name and seeing the characters written there in the dust, Xīn Dé realized what the spirit had meant in his dream. This man had his last name, and within his name was Shí Yīn, his daughter. Had he not been searching these many years for a husband for her? But why would the spirit recommend a lowly beggar? He must have some virtue from a previous life that brings him here to my door, Xīn Dé thought. Then he made up his mind.

"When I look at you I see such a clever boy and yet from morning till night you are constantly scrounging and begging. Surely this cannot become your lifelong profession? Unless you become a real man, how else will you be able to get some credentials and bring prosperity to your family? You may be happy to float leisurely along like you are for now but in the end you will find that you have wasted your life." Feeling that he had laid

---

6   Qián (錢): Money.

sufficient grounds, Xīn Dé made his proposal. "I have a daughter and I want you to marry her! What do you think?"

"Absolutely not!" cried Yīn Fū, burying his face in his hands. "I am a little person of absolutely no consequence who can hardly take care of himself! How could I ever enjoy your riches and good fortune like a parasite?"

"Nonsense!" laughed Xīn Dé. "This marriage will be a result of all the virtue you have accumulated in previous incarnations. Therefore, how could it be that you do not deserve it? A spirit in my dream foretold this very issue to me last night! My daughter's name is Shí Yīn!"

On hearing this, Yīn Fū raised his head. He finally understood the meaning of his name and why the Dàoist priest had given it to him. He was to become the husband of Shí Yīn, this much was clear. There was no point in arguing. This is where his road had led him. Standing up, he agreed and began living in the Shí family household.

Shí Yīn Fū was very happy to marry Shí Yīn, who was such a kind soul and together they discussed the path of merit and virtue. His happiness was short lived, however, as through living in Xīn Dé's household, he came to see how his father-in-law had become so wealthy. He often observed Xīn Dé using different scales and weights to settle transactions whilst doing business with the peasants and other merchants. When buying goods, he would weigh them on a big scale but then work out his payment on a small scale, thereby buying a kilogram, but giving less. When selling goods, he would use light weights to measure his stock and heavy weights to demand his payment. For many years he had been cheating his clients this way.

Yīn Fū, who by means of his black and yellow beans had already been practicing the cultivation of a good Heart for some time, went to his father-in-law and pleaded with him to change his wicked ways, but Xīn Dé ignored him. Many times he tried to convince him to change but his voice fell upon deaf ears. Nevertheless, Yīn Fū would not give up, until finally Xīn Dé became angry.

"You useless man!" he cursed at his son-in-law. "You never produce anything but words! How can you feed a family with words? Get the hell out of here! Go and live in the village! I don't want you disturbing my hard work any longer!"

In this way, Yīn Fū and his new wife moved out of the family household and went to live in the village nearby.

"My father-in-law has great wealth," he sighed, "but it is all derived from cheating people. Whilst I am grateful for the kindness he showed a beggar, how can I tolerate his stooping so low? We must try somehow to help him change his crooked ways."

For many restless days and nights the couple discussed the problem and eventually decided to go back and try to convince Xīn Dé again.

Unbeknownst to Yīn Fū and Shí Yīn, Xīn Dé's evil doing had already reached its peak. The gods above in Heaven ordered that his house should be destroyed by fire and lightning and that he should be shaken to death by thunder. This would be the penalty for his many crimes.

At this very moment, however, Yīn Fū and Shí Yīn arrived at Xīn Dé's house to plead reason and virtue. Afraid of harming the couple who had such developed benevolence, the gods held back their furious storm.

With all their hearts they wanted to convince Xīn Dé, but when they arrived at the house they were denied. Undeterred, they sat outside for many days. On one cold night, Yīn Fū had a nightmare. "Your father-in-law is evil, and has filled his cup with it," he was told. "Fire, thunder and lightning are coming to destroy him, so you must leave now to save yourselves!"

Waking in a sweat, he saw the ashen face of his wife. She had dreamed the same dream. Without a second's thought they ran into the middle of the road and knelt before Heaven. Yīn Fū prayed aloud with his virtuous Heart.

"Each person brings Heaven's condemnation upon himself. This, we understand, is the way of nature. However, humble me, your servant, I want to turn this around. I must help my father-in-law become a good man. Let me strike a deal! If he does not turn away from evil, I wish to die in his stead."

This sincerity moved the gods, and they agreed to hold back their fury. Xīn Dé, meanwhile, was totally unaware of this. To the contrary, when he saw Yīn Fū in the middle of the street crying to the sky, he thought his son-in-law had gone crazy and still he refused entry. Demons and ghosts came to him that night in his dreams, wanting to drag him down to the King of Hell. He awoke totally terrified and decided it must be due to his cruelty to Yīn Fū and Shí Yīn, so the next day he allowed them to return to the household. As soon as Yīn Fū, with his vast virtue, returned, the ghosts and demons dared not enter. However, this did not mean that the couple was able to change any of Xīn Dé's evil ways.

One day, Xīn Dé was traveling alone. In the middle of the road a large snake lay coiled, blocking his path. Annoyed, he kicked it aside. Little did he know that a demon, seeing that Xīn Dé was alone, had disguised itself as the snake. Twisting around, it struck out and sank its fangs into Xīn Dé's foot. Cursing, he returned home immediately, but as soon as he entered the house and Yīn Fū came to help, the bite stopped hurting.

Continuing on his quest to improve Xīn Dé's character and always performing good deeds, his father-in-law yet again became irritated by Yīn Fū and again told him to leave. As soon as Yīn Fū had left, the ghosts and demons came rushing back inside and made the snake bite hurt severely, making Xīn Dé very sick. His wife sent a message to the village and immediately Yīn Fū and Shí Yīn returned. No sooner were they within his courtyard, the pain eased and Xīn Dé felt well again. "How come as soon as Yīn Fū returns my foot feels so much better?" he asked himself. To test it again, he told them to leave and at once the pain returned. Finally Xīn Dé began to understand.

"Virtuous son-in-law," he pleaded, "please return with Shí Yīn and live with me again!"

"I can return, but only if you change your wicked ways," offered Yīn Fū "If you change the scales and the weights so you never cheat again, then I will come back."

"Are you sure you want me to change these things? These methods have brought great wealth to my household. Why would you want me to change?"

"Whenever people preserve an honest and upright Heart, spirits and ghosts must always conceal themselves. If the Heart is made turbid by cheating, then ghosts must come.[7] This is a true principle. In order to prevent disaster you must stop this evil."

Realizing that the reason his foot felt better was all due to the repeated prayers of his children, he instructed his family to dispose of the scales and weights he used to cheat people with and promised to follow the path of virtue. Pleased, Yīn Fū furthered his advice.

"You must make a banquet and invite all of those you have wronged, all those who owe you money and all those who are suffering or distressed. To those you have cheated, repay them. To those who owe you debts and interest, tell them they are now free of these obligations. To those who are suffering, help them with your wealth. Use yourself as an example and try to convince one and all to become good people."

After his banquet, Xīn Dé practiced what his son-in-law advised for several months. He even began to feel a sense of calmness in his Heart. One day a doctor was traveling by and requested lodgings in his residence. Xīn Dé asked him if he could cure his old snakebite, that would still nag him on occasion when Yīn Fū was absent. Taking some medicine from his bag, the

---

[7] From our perspective, this is a point where one could become distracted, depending on one's religious beliefs or lack thereof. In the martial arts, our demons are always within us. They are our fears, our lack of self-worth, our anger and hatred. Training can help us recognize these. Later we explore this more with the Wounded Warrior, the ghost that is always present, ready to wreak havoc and chaos.

doctor smeared it on the bite and immediately it felt better.[8] Suddenly Xīn Dé came to the conclusion that he had been fooled.

"For these past months I have followed Yīn Fū's advice and have been doing naught but good deeds; now I see that this was a mistake. During a man's life he naturally accrues some good merit, regardless of any slights of hand he may have occasionally committed." In this way, Xīn Dé was gradually able to convince himself that his recovery was not due to his good deeds but rather from the doctor's medicine. Looking sternly upon his son-in-law, he began to think of going back to his old ways.

Shortly thereafter, a Buddhist monk came to the residence looking to receive a rich man's money to assist in the repair of a local bridge. He could not tolerate spending poor people's rice money. Xīn Dé, thinking this a good opportunity to do good with his stolen funds, agreed immediately and the monk happily began the project. In honor of Xīn Dé's generosity, the bridge was named Solitary Goodness Bridge.

Hearing of this, the abbot from a local temple and his disciple came to visit. Named Niàn Hé,[9] the abbot also wanted to spend a rich person's money to repair the upper and lower halls of his temple.

"Surely it matters not if the person is rich or poor," argued his disciple, "just as long as they give what they can from their Hearts? We should not force people, rich or poor, to give away their money." So Niàn Hé sent him off to the village to see what he could collect from the Hearts of the peasantry.

Hearing of the abbot's woes with his dilapidated temple and despite the considerable amount being requested, Xīn Dé was keen to assist and thereby further his good deeds.[10] Niàn Hé was more than happy to accept Xīn Dé's money and returned home to begin work. The disciple came back empty-handed as the peasants had no money to spare. Xīn Dé's contribution was more than enough to finish the repairs, which took almost a year.

Who knew that the abbot Niàn Hé was committing inappropriate actions? Secretly, he had a secluded chamber made at the back of his upper hall, which had a hidden doorway to enter it by, all paid for with Xīn Dé's funds. Therein, he was having an affair with his neighbor's wife. One dark night, his mistress needed to use the bathroom. The temple's toilet was a wooden shack outside with a deep pit covered by two narrow boards upon

---

[8] Here is a clear message Liú sends to both the physicians of his time and indeed ours. You may ease the superficial discomfort, but have you addressed the toxin within?

[9] Niàn Hé (念和): Study Harmony.

[10] "This is what is called 'Qì going together with righteousness and the Dào' and in this state there is no starvation or collapse. This is born out of our accumulated righteousness and cannot be appropriated through random acts of kindness. When one acts below the standard set in their Heart, any uprightness will collapse." Liú Yuán in his commentary on the book of Mencius. Quoted in full in chapter 6.

which to squat. She quietly crept through the upper hall and down through the lower one making her way outside, careful not to be noticed. As the abbot had been too lazy to organize the digging of a new pit the current one was filled with malodorous excrement.

Gingerly squatting in the dark, the mistress began her business. Suddenly there was a loud crack, the boards snapped and into the pit she fell. Wanting to scream but not wanting to be exposed, she writhed in the sticky smelly mess trying to pull herself out. After some time, Niàn Hé became worried and came to investigate. Holding his candle high to see better in the darkness, he found his mistress struggling in the feces. Astonished, the abbot failed to realize that the candle he held aloft was starting to burn the roof, and soon it was ablaze. Quickly he tried to pull her out, but he stumbled and fell in as well. A gust of wind blew, spreading the flames from the toilet roof to the newly finished temple, which also caught fire. The bedraggled couple finally managed to crawl to safety, just as the toilet collapsed. By this time the locals all came running and they found the abbot and his mistress, covered in filth and staring dumbstruck at the temple awash with flames. So intense was the inferno that they were unable to save the temple, which quickly burnt to the ground. Then rain started to fall.

Such a large deluge fell that the rivers became swollen. One bridge, called Solitary Goodness Bridge, was washed away in the flood, despite being newly repaired. Not one piece remained when the waters receded. Xīn Dé, who had just recently paid the last of the construction fees for the temple, was informed of the fire and flood.

"How is this fair?!" he lamented. "I have just lost almost all of my fortune in building costs and materials, all on ventures that have amounted to nothing! What happened to my merit and virtue? I gave it out of the goodness of my Heart and now there is nothing left to show of it!" For days he cried with grief. On hearing of these sorrowful affairs Yīn Fū tried to console his father-in-law.

"All my riches are used up!" Xīn Dé retorted. "All that is left is this house and a small field. Everything else was given to these two catastrophic debacles! My virtuous actions have all been in vain! How can you tell me not to be sad?"

"Dear father-in-law," said Yīn Fū calmly, "in previous years you accumulated such a vast sum of money. How were you to come by this wealth so quickly?"

At this, Xīn Dé stopped weeping and lowered his head. After some time sitting in silence he spoke.

"By means of evil trickery and I can see that trying to create virtue out of this money has been futile." Looking up with hope in his eyes he continued, "Now that it is all lost, this wicked wealth, let us not despair. With what little remains we can still eat and drink. Over time I can regain my fortunes! Then I can fix more bridges and make more temples!"

"This is all well," replied Yīn Fū, "however, you should also do some good deeds."

This made no sense whatsoever to Xīn Dé. "In my son-in-law's world," he thought, "why does he say to do good deeds when that is all I am trying to do with my money? Surely that is meritorious enough? What more must one do?"

Shí Yīn Fū had accumulated virtue for many years already. Not one of his actions or thoughts were without it, and through this he had become enlightened. He was not simply balancing good deeds with bad ones. Everything within him followed his life principle and he could see clearly the myriad things between Heaven and Earth. It was from his Heart that he answered.

"What you are asking is about doing good deeds, but these do not necessarily accumulate merit. This can only be achieved through the cultivation of your Heart."

"Are not good deeds and merit synonymous?" asked Xīn Dé.

"Big and small are not the same, superficial and deep are not the same, heavy and light are not the same. If a person takes something from me and ruins it I do not begrudge him. If he cannot return it then I do not want him to. If someone borrows money from me and then cannot repay it I do not want compensation. However, if I borrow money from somebody then I must return it. I never speak ill of others or give them bad names. Nor do I ruin the good deeds performed by others or promote anger in those around me. We must avoid upsetting family relations, causing parents and children to argue. Do not kill animals without need or let the bad influences of others distract your virtue. In the same way you must not force someone to do something. This is called practicing goodness.

"If you use your money to build roads and temples, print books of sacred texts and carve holy statues, this does appear to have merit, but these deeds do not necessarily free us from our suffering. Devoutly praying to deities is not enough. Good intentions without good actions are meaningless. Good actions without good intentions are likewise void of virtue. If you want to accumulate cultivation the Heart must have gōngfu. You must become an arrow of goodness. Whilst others may not see this goodness, *you* will be able to. If one seed of evil resides others still may not know of it, but *you* will know it is there. When there is nothing but goodness in your Heart, evil cannot grow. When all you can do is good, this is called accumulating virtue and only then can you be free."

"How then," asked Xīn Dé, "do you exercise this gōngfu? What is the first step?"

"This is easy," explained Yīn Fū, "I take three bags. One I fill with black beans and tie it to my right side, another bag I fill with yellow beans and tie it to my left. The final bag I leave empty and hang it on my chest. Whenever your Heart has evil thoughts or you do a bad deed, you take a black bean and put it in the bag over your Heart. When you have a good Heart or do a good deed you place a yellow bean there. Do this for one hundred days and see the balance of your virtue and offenses. In the beginning the offenses are many, then they become half and after a long time the virtues are the only thing that you see. Take this first step earnestly and then the rest of the path becomes clear."

Whilst simple, this idea both terrified and amazed Xīn Dé as he thought back to his many ill deeds and thoughts and how many black beans he would have accumulated so far.

"I see," he sighed. "This is indeed the method of fulfilling our Natural Character which should be naught but goodness.[11] This is the way of studying life. When I was younger I studied all the great books. The principles therein I thought I understood, though despite reading the sage's words, how could I embody the sage's Dào? I was never able to make it my own, make it a part of my body. On hearing your method of determining good from evil, I want to study this. Even if I never succeed I will persevere and die a happy man."

Xīn Dé organized the three bags. He gathered the black and yellow beans and once on this path never again dared to let go. He had to sort out his Heart.

One day as they were walking over a bridge, Xīn Dé noticed a wobbly board. Concerned that it may cause someone to fall, he got a stone and fixed it. Then they continued on their journey. Yīn Fū observed the whole time.

"Father-in-law, why is it that you have yet to take a yellow bean for your good action?"

"Oh, that was such a small issue, how can we say that this is enough for accruing merit?"

"How is this not worth recording as a merit?" Yīn Fū asked. "Not only did you have a good intention, you also translated this into a good action. You made both the first and the second steps!"

"It looks like a small merit," pondered Xīn Dé, "so therefore within it there must also be a small evil. Did not Zǐsī say, '*You must be careful of*

---

[11] Please see the following chapter for Liú's explanation of Natural Character (*Xing* 性) and other terms.

that you do not see and be afraid of what you cannot hear. What you cannot see is hidden. What is not revealed are the fine details, the essence hidden within. This is why the nobleman must be cautious about his solitude'?[12] What one thinks is a good deed may indeed have evil within it, something that we are ignorant of."

Impressed by his progress, Yīn Fū continued to observe his father-in-law and noticed how he began to handle his affairs. One day Xīn Dé was urinating into a river and then he realized that he was polluting the water, so he took a black bean and put it next to his Heart. The next day he saw an ox which had wandered into another man's field and was eating his grain. After restraining the beast, Xīn Dé noticed that it had already devoured a lot of grain, so he dragged it to the farmhouse nearby.

"My ox has eaten much of your grain," he explained to the farmer, "so I would like to give you some of my rice as compensation."

"Why do you say this?" asked the farmer after inspecting the field. "He ate only a little and there is no need to compensate me."

They respectfully departed and Xīn Dé took a yellow bean to record this good affair. Seeing that his father-in-law's skill was developing, Yīn Fū's Heart was filled with joy.

When Xīn Dé returned home, he found a Buddhist monk sitting in lotus position outside his door with his eyes closed. Xīn Dé approached and respectfully greeted him but as he did so the monk leaped up, striking him with a stick.

"Old monk, why are you so angry?" asked the shocked Xīn Dé. "Whatever money I have to give you to build your temple I will give it to you freely. Why would you hit me?"

"To escape Hell," said the monk aloofly, "you must open the road to Life and Death!"

Intrigued, Xīn Dé asked, "What do you mean, *the road to Life and Death?*"

"You have to become a monk of course," explained the monk confidently, "and read the scriptures many times. Only then will you open this road."

"And what do you mean by Hell?" asked Xīn Dé.

"The world of mortals is Hell," stated the monk.

Through his practice of goodness Xīn Dé was already becoming somewhat enlightened. He was not so easily deafened by what he heard and could read the situation well. He smiled at the monk.

"Most honorable guest, how long have you been a monk?"

---

[12] Zǐ Sī (子思): the only grandson of Confucius, alleged teacher of Mencius and who wrote the Zhōng Yōng (中庸) *Doctrine of the Mean*.

"Since I left home to do so. I am not distracted by calculating the years."

"How did you find the path you have been walking?"

"It was as if the great Dào was right in front of my eyes."

"Ah!" exclaimed Xīn Dé delightedly. "Please reveal to me this Dào, which is so clear to you!"

"The mystery of the universe," said the monk shaking his head, "cannot be seen by a common person."

Xīn Dé looked directly into the monk's eyes. "With one look," he said slowly, "I can see the disease of the flesh."

Surprised by this statement, the monk did not know how to respond.

"Your eyes are red," continued Xīn Dé, "which means your Heart is not at ease. Your eyebrows are dry; therefore your Heart has regret, which damages the Qì of the Liver. Within your Heart you hold many thoughts of revenge, which is revealed in your shrunken face and lips."

Terrified, the monk wanted to leave but his legs would not obey him. All he could do was lower his head.

"I see that your Spleen is weak which means you desire alcohol and meat. You resentfully dwell on that which you cannot have. This is not the way a monk reaches contentment. Tell me, where is it that you think that body of yours came from? When you were little and entered the temple you had no choice but to respect the command of your parents. However, when you reached your middle years, this is when your Heart hardened and you separated from your obligation to care for your parents. Monk or not, your first obligation is to care for your father and mother. Hence, due to your neglect, the heavenly Kinship suffered.[13] You retreated into the deep mountains and became a recluse, like the stones and the trees. What kind of merit does that have for humanity? All that is needed is for a man to resolutely cultivate and accumulate virtue; it has nothing to do with becoming a monk. Being or not being a monk is irrelevant."[14]

Still unable to utter a word, the monk looked up at Xīn Dé.

"When I look at your complexion," he continued, "and I hear that you have been trying to cultivate the Dào, it is as Confucius said, '*we can all eat and drink, but few can differentiate the flavors*'.[15] Seldom can we differentiate good from bad."

---

[13] Referring to the *Wǔlún* (五倫): The Five Cardinal Relationships or Kinships of Confucianism, which are: 1. Ruler and subject, *jūnchén* (君臣): 2. Father and son, *fùzǐ* (父子): 3. Elder and younger brother, *xiōngdì* (兄弟): 4. Husband and wife, *fūfù* (夫婦) and 5. Between friends, *péngyǒu* (朋友).

[14] This argument continues today, for example, R. Dawkins, *The God Delusion*, Bantam Press, Great Britain, 2006, pp. 241-267, versus T. Crean, *God is No Delusion: A Refutation of Richard Dawkins*, Ignatius Press, San Francisco, 2007, pp. 95-106.

[15] Quoted from the Zhōng Yōng (中庸) *Doctrine of the Mean*.

When Xīn Dé's speech had finished the monk stood, bowed, and thanked him for his teachings. Head lowered, he left. Suddenly he stopped in the middle of the road and said aloud, "That was the essence of goodness! Had I not met this man today, how could I ever have seen the great mistakes of my life?" In an instant his Heart lost all its hatred and resentment and he let go of all his erroneous thoughts. Realizing the wrong paths he had followed, wandering with his scriptures, he immediately returned to his hometown seeking his parents. Thankfully he discovered that they were still alive, but they had to till the soil arduously to try and survive. In his Heart he was happy and the monk took his parents to his monastery to ask the abbot if they could come and live with him in the temple. This was contrary to the general principle of the temple as a monk must leave his family to allow for total absorption in spiritual training.

"They could work the land," argued the monk, "and I will help them plough the fields. We will grow crops and I will pay rent to the temple and whatever is left I will use to care for my parents. If we are allowed to grow livestock, any money from these will be saved to cover future burial costs so not one penny will have to be spent by the temple."

Initially, the idea disturbed the abbot, but the more he contemplated, his mind began to change. "This disciple of mine has such a strong filial Dào," he thought, "and this relationship between parents and children is indeed a Heavenly kinship. If I do not agree to this how is my disciple to maintain a calm Heart? Even though it is contrary to temple rules how will my disciple ever reach happiness if I refuse him? We are all monks here within these walls but any good we do is nothing compared to that achieved by caring for one's parents."[16]

And so the monk was granted his wish and was able to fulfill his filial duty.[17] Without hesitation, he traveled the path of virtue. He collected alms in the ten directions,[18] repaired neglected paths in the rugged mountains, built bridges and made boats to help others cross the dangerous rivers. He bought animals and set them free, releasing life and gaining good

---

[16] Indeed, Buddhism is not without its own filial code. See for example, E. Yoshikawa, *Musashi*, trans. E. O. Reischauer, Kodansha International, Tokyo, 1971, pp. 709-712, The Sutra on the Great Love of Parents:
"*At this time the Buddha preached the Law as follows:*
'*All ye good men and good women,*
acknowledge your debt for your father's compassion,
Acknowledge your debt for your mother's mercy.
For the life of a human being in this world
Has karma as its basic course, but parents as its immediate means of origin.'"

[17] Here is an example of how Liú Yuán sees the capacity for an individual's goodness to be able to transform anything, even religious rule and reckoning.

[18] Asking for alms gives the giver an opportunity to accrue good karma.

karma in Heaven. He built coffins and buried bones he found on the roadside and collected clothes and food for the poor. When all his money was spent helping others, he invited the masses to help. Not only were his outer actions of merit,[19] but the ledger of merit within his Heart was also attuned to goodness. At night he had no thoughts of desires and during the day he would sit in meditation until he was at peace. He would cleanse his body, then bow four times to the west and burn three cones of incense. After years of practicing this way, he was awakened to the meaning of life. He sat in meditation and suddenly the light of Buddha shone from his third eye, reflecting the brightness within his Heart. His body became light and his spirit opened to the Dào. He had reached enlightenment.

Over the years many people heard about Xīn Dé and his practice of goodness. One such person, a Dàoist monk, thought little of what he heard and decided to go and trick him. Posing as a religious pilgrim seeking alms, he knocked at the door of Xīn Dé.

    Respectfully, Xīn Dé brought a bowl of rice and some tea. Offering these to the Dàoist, the monk took just seven grains of rice and began to leave. As Xīn Dé called him back, the monk leaped upon a table and sat in supposed meditation, and there he sat quietly for three days and nights without speaking, eating or drinking. Xīn Dé was amazed at this monk who was able to sit so still with no sustenance for such a time. Unbeknownst to him, before arriving at his destination the monk had made some small beef balls and kept them hidden in his sleeve. When Xīn Dé was not looking he would sneak some into his mouth.

    "Elder saint, please come and sit with me," offered Xīn Dé politely at the end of these three days. "I, your humble student, realize the benefit of such a great destiny in meeting you. Please offer me some guidance."

    "What is it you seek?" asked the monk as he climbed down from the table and sat next to Xīn Dé. "Do you want the Inner or Outer Elixir?"

    "Please explain the meaning of the Inner Elixir."

    "This secret is not transmitted amongst the Buddhists, just between Dàoists. Transporting Fire and Water within you create a fine mist that spreads to the crown of your head. After doing this for three hundred and sixty five days your body becomes light and you can fly!"

    "And what of the Outer Elixir?"

    "This secret is not transmitted amongst the silversmiths. First you melt lead and make it into mercury and the Elixir comes. Then use fire to turn stone into gold and copper into silver!"

---

[19] These outer actions are referred to in the text as *Gōngdé* (功德).

"And how much must I spend to obtain this privilege?" asked Xīn Dé.

"Just three hundred pieces of silver for one Elixir."

"If I choose to buy it who will collect all these exotic ingredients?"

"We will go together to collect them!" responded the monk.

Xīn Dé observed the Dàoist. A monk such as this should be without desire, his Heart should be happy and at peace and his expression at ease. However, looking at this man, all he could see was a lump of stagnating Qì.

"Old saint," began Xin De, "surely you have brought some of this Elixir with you? Please bring it out so we can use some here and now!"

"No, I do not have any with me..." stammered the surprised monk.

"Since you have obviously been a saint for so long, definitely more than one year, you must have already cultivated this Inner Elixir! We must go outside and you can show me how you fly!"

Becoming increasingly uncomfortable, the Dàoist's agitated face drained of color. He knew that Xīn Dé had discovered him as a fake and had the better of him.

"In our world," Xīn Dé said sternly, "there are only eight small grams of life. There is never enough. Exhausting everything under Heaven, still we are not satisfied. In your previous life you failed to accumulate virtue and now you suffer in misery. If it takes just one year with this Inner Elixir to become the Dào then why are you still here? Here, sitting agitated in my house, I can see that you are without substance, just one cloud of floating Qì. If you cannot even protect your physical body how can you talk of cultivating the Dào? If you can make your own silver with your special skills why do you ask others for money? You and your teacher, studying the Dào by means of this Elixir, surely would have some of this precious substance with you. Even if you yourself cannot conjure it, your teacher would have left you some. In addition, the spirits and saints never departed from loyalty and filial piety. When we cheat our way through life, how is this any way to repay our fathers and mothers? Instead, you have entrusted yourself into a world of unreality. Faking your magic you lie to get money out of your victims. This is a sin against your own Heart that you have created for yourself. What is the possible result of this? Will you not look back upon your life and reflect?"

By this time the Dàoist was sweating from head to foot. He fell to the floor and begged for some guidance. Xīn Dé told him the story of Shí Yīn Fū and how he himself had been able to transform from a cheat into an honest man. Seeing the error of his ways, the Dàoist started crying aloud.

"Tell me why you are crying," said Xīn Dé, softening a little after his stern speech.

"I was never satisfied receiving alms," sobbed the monk, "so began posing as a Dàoist master and selling my Elixirs. I shall regret this for the rest of my life. Hearing your words of goodness, oh how my Heart has broken...Oh, what have I done?!" Still sobbing, he bowed many times to Xīn Dé before backing out of the house and then he quickly departed.

Still shaken by his experience, in the middle of the road the Dàoist came across another monk, though much younger than himself. The youth stopped him.

"The Buddhist path is such a difficult one to follow," he groaned, kneeling before the Dàoist. "I would rather now follow that of the Dào. I implore you Shīfu,[20] to teach me the way!"

"When I was a child," said the Dàoist sadly, "like you I also became a monk seeking to cultivate my Dào. How was I to know that I was being led astray? Erring repeatedly I have walked the wrong path. Luckily, a kind person taught me this lesson: regardless of which religion you follow they all have the same foundations. Following filial piety, loving your brothers and sisters, being loyal and trustworthy, only doing the right things, being respectful to nature, following the right etiquette, being honest and humble, these traits encompass Heaven's palace.

"The Dàoist recluse does not have loyalty and righteousness, but rather selfishly hides away in his hermitage. In my life so far I have failed in my cultivation. Coming into this world and living this life and failing to cultivate myself for the next, what fate awaits me in the future? Am I going to be a person or a rat?! I must go back to my family and exhaust my obligation to my parents. Only by fulfilling my filial Dào can I truly know myself."

The young Buddhist stood up, thinking.

"My Buddhist Shīfu took me in when I was orphaned as a baby," he said after some time. "He fed and clothed me, kept me warm and educated me for many years. He never sought assistance from anyone. One day though, I suddenly left him and the temple. It was with a hardened Heart that I abandoned him and have never returned. My hardened Heart...this is my self-inflicted sin. Surely I must be offending Heaven! What kind of Hell am I sinking to?"[21]

This unexpected meeting with the Dàoist had allowed the young Buddhist to find his good Heart and realize Heaven's principle. Now anxious to see his Shīfu again, he thanked the Dàoist and hurriedly returned home. It

---

[20] Shīfu (師傅): Master, someone that is highly accomplished in their field of expertise.
[21] Here we see filial piety expressed not only to one's parents. Mòzǐ (墨子), a Warring States Period philosopher (475–220 BCE) taught that we should love everyone's parents as our own.

had been six long years and when he knelt before his Shīfu their tears fell like rain. Onlookers also cried when they heard of the young monk's return. Once again, there was a rejuvenated feeling in the temple. Later, when the young monk had to leave on a trip, he would explain it to his Shīfu first and always set a return date. After many years of cultivating himself he awakened to the Natural Character of life and he eventually became a great Zen master.

After his lesson and scolding by Xīn Dé, the Dàoist monk returned home, seeking his family. Shocked, he discovered that all his relatives had died in an epidemic. On questioning the locals, he learned that his grandfather had used trickery to harm others and thereby ruined any credit the family had in Heaven. Then disaster had struck.

With nothing left the Dàoist went looking for a quiet place to record his ledger of good and evil. He avoided pernicious pathways and never cheated in dark rooms. As he started to accumulate virtue through his meritorious deeds he began repairing himself and also helped others to do likewise. One such person was a young man named Bái Yù Kāi.[22]

With a compassionate Heart he dealt with animals, looked after orphans, took pity on widows and was always respectful to the elderly. He was thankful when kindness was afforded him but would immediately forgive any who resented him. Never mocking the sages, he would not use goodness to promote evil or shift blame onto the blameless. Not ever letting go of what was proper he would never wear a wicked Heart inwardly and then display it as goodness outwardly. He never deluded people with false doctrines and was always respectful to the divine. He would not use a kitchen stove to light incense and would not use dirty firewood to cook his food. By only benefiting the myriad things, he was able to cultivate goodness and prosperity, thus earning positive karma for his next life.

Early each morning he would calm his spirit and adjust his Qì. He would use seven lanterns and burn seven cones of incense, then bow seventy-two times to the north. With a sincere Heart he would recite the sutras and resolutely he would study and write poetry. After many years on this path of saving himself and others he became clear about life in the depths of his Heart. He knew the destiny of his future generations and eventually he reached the status of an immortal.

Why would one have to be a monk in order to cultivate oneself? Movement and stillness are the same for all of us and when we pursue a Heart with a clear conscience, then the whole country blossoms. Indeed, the impact of goodness can travel like the wind. Unfortunately, the opposite is

---

[22] Bái Yù Kāi (白玉開): White Jade Opening.

also true.

There was a young man who had, despite his arduous studies, never managed to become an official. These lengthy studies, however, had taught him the need to cultivate his actions. In search of a teacher he and his parents left on a journey. In the middle of the road they came across a Dàoist monk and the young man asked him for guidance and discipleship.

"What is your name, young man?" asked the Dàoist.

"Me, the little person, I am called Bái Yù Kāi."

"You should know, Yù Kāi, that in cultivating our actions we must have an eternal Heart."

"I understand this Dào," responded the youth.

The Dàoist monk could see that this young man's Heart was already filled with goodness. Desperately he wanted to help him avoid treacherous paths of erroneous doctrines, the likes of which he himself had so foolishly traveled. "I shall put him to the test," he thought.

"In Dàoism, the Five Kinships are considered most important, especially regarding the kinship we have with our parents. Only by honoring this can we truly achieve greatness in the afterlife. As a Dàoist, we seek the Inner Elixir. By transporting Water and Fire we raise a fine mist to our head. To return our true Qì to the origin we use an arrow to penetrate the nine heavy drums and the yellow lady enters our bed chamber, then the three personalities join into one. Mysterious theory after mysterious theory.

"When you practice this you become one with the Dào, but this the common person cannot do. When we seek the External Elixir we burn lead and smelt mercury, gathering true Earth and mixing it with ice and coal. Using the spirit of the bāguà[23] we write special documents to Heaven and the Lí palace.[24] The Heaven trigram can smelt out this Elixir using Fire to make copper into silver, stone into gold. Administering this transforms the body into the Dào and we become a Heavenly immortal. Discussing these immortals with all their powers, even amongst them, there are only a few who can create these Elixirs. Often the saints themselves could not achieve it so why then would a commoner be able to? This is truly a gōngfu, it must come from one's Heart and when the Heart flower opens, naturally one is clever without end."

"Please explain further," encouraged Yù Kāi.

"Disciple!" yelled the Dàoist, laying his trap. "Pick up your stuff, we are leaving now!"

---

[23] Bāguà (八卦) are the eight trigrams of the Yìjīng (易經), the Classic of Changes. Please see the following chapter for more information on these.

[24] Lígōng (離宮): Lí is the Fire trigram ☲, implying a palace where Fire is used to smelt elixirs.

"Where are we going?"
"We will travel to Zhōngnán mountain!"[25]
"How far is it?"
"It is at the end of the world and we must walk for five years."
"And when will we return?"
"Never!"
"In this case," said Yù Kāi, "I cannot follow you."
"So you do not want to be one with the Dào?" challenged the Dàoist.
"My parents are still here. How can I go forever and not come back to them?"
"Fine!" yelled the Dàoist, leaping up and striking Yù Kāi on the head.

When Yù Kāi awoke he found his parents by his side, weeping in the middle of the road with aching hearts. He had lost a teacher. But then they found a note written on his chest.

"Above your Heart there is a rock and below it is virtue. If you practice this for a long time this will be your Dào," the Dàoist had written. This was a riddle pointing the youth to a real teacher of goodness.[26] As he trusted the Dàoist, from that moment on Yù Kāi decided that he would follow these instructions to the best of his ability. But where was he to start? He must not listen to any words but these written on his chest and not follow any stray schools of thought, but from his Heart practice this gōngfu. So with his parents, they continued their travels.

One day, they reached a Buddhist temple, where they saw the abbot cursing one of his disciples, laying insults on the disciple's father and mother. Hitting him for not preparing the midday meal in time, the abbot spoke like a scoundrel. Despite the fact that the Buddhist cannon clearly states the importance of filial piety, brotherly and sisterly love, loyalty, propriety, trustworthiness, honesty and humility, the abbot's behavior was not in accordance with this. Therefore Yù Kāi readily realized that this was not the right path to follow and that nothing useful could be learned here.

Growing older and wearier his parents could not continue their travels with Yù Kāi, so they all returned to their hometown and he continued to accumulate good deeds and cultivate his Heart. A few years later his

---

[25] Zhōngnánshān (终南山): A mountain near Xīān (西安), capital city of Shānxī (山西), hometown of Shí Xīn Dé. In the context here it also refers to the end of the south mountain, pointing to the end of the world.

[26] If we remember the name Shí Xīn Dé (石心德) means *Rock, Heart, and Virtue*. On one side of the Heart is a rock and on the other side is virtue. In traditional Chinese, characters are written from top to bottom, hence the rock is above the Heart while virtue is below.

parents passed away peacefully and Yù Kāi buried them appropriately. Since he no longer had any family bonds he left once again in search of the Dào. For many months he walked yet observed not one person acting without selfishness or greed, fear or hatred.

Once he came across a vegetarian monk and stayed with him for some months, until the monk lost his wooden fish drum[27] and began cursing those around him, yelling that they would die without offspring. Yù Kāi could see that initially from the outside there appeared to be some goodness here, but on the inside things were far too brutal. Clearly, this was also not a place where one could cultivate oneself.

Some time later, in the middle of the road, Yù Kāi heard about a man who practiced goodness, named Shí Xīn Dé. Whilst pondering this name and the riddle left by the Dàoist monk, he found his way to Xīn Dé's residence where he was well received and treated as an honored visitor.

"Dear guest," said Xīn Dé politely, "I can see that your expression is pure and your movements extraordinary. You must be on the path of cultivating your Heart, seeking the immortals."

"Your disciple is Bái Yù Kāi," responded the youth, following etiquette. "I do not mind traveling vast distances in order to better cultivate myself."

Finding this young man to be honest and sincere, Xīn Dé asked him to stay in his home and introduced him to Shí Yīn Fū. Yù Kāi observed these men and saw that they spoke and acted without a trace of selfishness or wrongdoing, so he was happy to stay and discuss goodness. These three people worked together in cultivating themselves and in time, Yù Kāi was equally as skilful as his hosts.

Not wanting to leave but also not wanting to burden his hosts, Yù Kāi opened an herbal medicine clinic nearby and began treating the sick. Even those without any money he would treat equally respectfully and give the best medicines. Through his virtue his medicine became divine. No matter if the disease were small or big, as soon as he gave his medicine it would be cured.[28] Xīn Dé and Yīn Fū watched Yù Kāi, observing his transformation into pure goodness with nothing contrary to benevolence. This filled them with great joy.

One day, as the three scholars Yù Kāi, Xīn Dé and Yīn Fū all sat together discussing matters of the Heart, a visitor was announced. This guest had traveled for many days in order to speak with Yù Kāi, whose reputation had

---

[27] The Wooden fish drum, or *Mùyú* (木魚), is an instrument commonly used whilst reading Buddhist sutras, mantras or sacred texts.
[28] Refer to Master Gān Liǎo's discussion in chapter 5, where he articulates how the physician transfers their own merit to their patients.

become great. He had arduously studied astrology, geography, the three doctrines and nine schools and as a Confucian, he knew everything concerning human affairs.

Yù Kāi greeted the traveler as an honored guest and brought him to sit with Xīn Dé and Yīn Fū. Observing propriety they first drank some fine tea and, as was appropriate, Yù Kāi opened the conversation.

"Distinguished guest, may I bother you with making an inquiry of your first and last name?"

"Me, the little brother," answered the guest, "my last name is Lǐ and my first name is Yuán Liàng.[29] Having traveled all throughout the nine provinces, I came to hear of this residence where true cultivation is practiced. Hence, I am in your presence ready to receive your deep teachings."

From hearing just this one sentence, Yù Kāi could tell from the sound of his voice that this man had sadly been walking an incorrect path. To further test his assumption he arranged a banquet and graciously hosted his guest, serving wine three times as was the custom. Feeling relaxed, Yuán Liàng opened a conversation that did not follow the propriety of a guest.

"People who study the Dào," he began gregariously, "all have a great destiny to meet their teacher who will guide them in the right way. For example, Jiāng Tàigōng met Yuánshǐ, Sūn Bìn met Guǐ Gǔzǐ, Hán Xiāngzǐ met Lǚ Dòngbīn, Zhāng Zǐfáng met Huáng Shígōng.[30] Through their greatness we still hear their stories today: thereby they have achieved immortality! They had great luck in finding the truth which led to their successes."

"Yuán Liàng," said Yù Kāi, his suspicions confirmed, "why do you mention these occurrences? These historical figures you mention knew nothing of accumulating cultivation or meeting a true teacher. Zhāng Zǐfáng was an assistant to the king, so it was through his position that he benefited and became famous. Although Sūn Bìn did meet Guǐ Gǔzǐ, he selfishly thought only of fame so did not receive fruit in the afterlife and his life's work was lost.[31] Today's people practice a little goodness and feel like they have accumulated great merit, but immediately they find it is all gone.

---

[29] Lǐ Yuán Liàng (李原亮): Peach, Origin, Bright.

[30] Jiāng Tàigōng (薑太公), Yuánshǐ (元始), Sūn Bìn (孫臏), Guǐ Gǔzǐ (鬼穀子), Hán Xiāngzǐ (韓湘子), Lǚ Dòngbīn (呂洞賓), Zhāng Zǐfáng (張子房) and Huáng Shígōng (黃石公). All these characters are real historical players in early Chinese history.

[31] There is a fascinating history between Sūn Bìn and Guǐ Gǔzǐ. Briefly, Sūn Bìn, suggested descendant of the famed author of the Sūnzǐ Bīngfǎ (孫子兵法): *The Art of War*, Sūnzǐ (孫子), was mentored in military strategy by the recluse Guǐ Gǔzǐ. Sūn Bìn was eventually betrayed and tried for treason. His face was tattooed and his kneecaps were removed rendering him handicapped. In 1972 an archaeological excavation recovered his main treatise: *Sūn Bìn Bīngfǎ* (孫臏兵法).

Admiring the saints rather than contemplating their own Hearts, unavoidably they are led astray. My Heart is like the sages' Hearts and because of that, the sages are like me. The results of our efforts are the same. Why then should we look for distracting stories? How is it that you forgo your own Heart in place of theirs? Looking within, you will see that your Heart is the same as the saints."

Yuán Liàng realized he had spoken out of turn, thereby revealing his faults. He did not dare speak any more stray words as the man before him had a deep understanding and awareness of life.

"Dear sir," he asked softly, "how do you practice this, the art of the sages' Heart?"

"Filial piety, brotherly and sisterly love, loyalty, trustworthiness, propriety, honesty and humility," stated Yù Kāi. "These are the structural roots of each of the three doctrines. In all the religious texts nothing is taught but these words. It is only through following these words that we can cultivate ourselves into enlightenment. Your Heart then becomes bright and you can distinguish the path of life and death, you can see your own vibration and when your time has come to an end. When you go forth seeing this Natural Character and use the doctrines to teach the people the right and wrong paths, this truly has merit. Instead of being bewildered by the visible we engage with the invisible."

"I would like to ask about the Three Destinies,"[32] said Yuán Liàng. "It is often said that these must merge in order to study the Dào."

"These Three Destinies are how we cultivate the Dào. It is how we practice the Dào," confirmed Yù Kāi. "The way to do this is simple. Firstly, if there is no rain or the sun fails to shine, do not resent Heaven. If too much rain falls or the sun shines relentlessly, do not resent Heaven. If your clothes are torn and there is not enough food to eat, then do not blame Heaven. Whatever the affair, if it does not succeed, then do not resent Heaven. This is tying in with Heaven's destiny.

"Secondly, if the mountains are too high to scale or rivers too wide to forge, then do not resent the Earth. If the channels and ditches dug for irrigating the crops block your way and slow your journey, do not resent the Earth. If the soil is barren and your crops fail, do not resent the Earth. Whatever the situation, if it does not succeed do not blame the Earth. This is tying in with the destiny of the Earth.

"Thirdly, if someone is rich whilst you are poor, do not resent Man. If someone is superior and you are inferior, do not resent Man. If someone is strong whilst you are weak, do not resent Man. This is tying in with the human destiny and is how we cultivate the Dào."

án (三緣): Three destinies or fates.

"What of doing good deeds. Does this bring merit and virtue?"

"This we do not separate into big and small," replied Xīn Dé, taking over from Yù Kāi as he remembered the time when he had asked the same question. "Rich or poor, each must do according to their ability. When a family is wealthy and supports its distant relatives, assists hungry neighbors and friends, builds bridges and roads and prints the holy texts, these are outward deeds that must have their seed in an honest Heart. If you do good in order to score merit and then boast of your own virtue, this is not in accord with the Dào. When times get tough you will see that suddenly your Heart changes and you no longer want to be virtuous. If we have accumulated many evil deeds throughout our lives, a few meritorious actions do not equate to goodness and we will find it difficult to become the Dào."

"The great Dào," continued Yù Kāi, "is not in some far off lofty place. It is not all about thinking and being theosophical; it is about the true principles that are practical issues. No magic is needed. As long as one follows one's Heart and the principles of Heaven by fulfilling one's duty to their parents then there is no need for endless theories. If a poor person nurtures his parents and buries them with great fanfare, this is overdoing it. If a rich person buries his parents in a neglectful manner, this is insufficient. Neither of these follows filial piety. Each must do according to his means. When following these true principles what is left to think about? Our thoughts can unfortunately lead us astray. Intellectualism without a root in the true principle takes us far from virtue."

"In the past I have contemplated many wrong schools," said Yuán Liàng, becoming enlightened, "and have followed incorrect pathways and strange thoughts. Now I realize that the Dào is not far from man, however man makes it so.[33] When we try to reach it, the more we grapple with the plethora of philosophies and the more we distance ourselves from the Dào. This clear principle must transform into action, not just empty thoughts."

Making his way to leave, he thanked his honorable hosts. Reaching for the door, he turned and asked what his first step should be.

"Take a bag of black beans and tie them to your right side. Take a bag of yellow beans and tie them to your left..."

Yuán Liàng left the three scholars and began his own ledger of good and evil. On his journey home, in the middle of the road he came across two officials escorting a criminal. On closer inspection this captive was a family friend from his hometown.

---

[33] This concept is expressed by Confucius in the Zhōngyōng (中庸): dào bù yuǎn rén, rén zhī wèi dào (道不遠人, 人之爲道): *The Dào is not far from mankind. When pursuing a Dào which is far from them, this cannot be considered the Dào.*

"Sirs, may I please ask where are you taking this man?"

"To the city of Fēngdū," replied one of the guards.[34]

"What is it he is charged with?"

"His thirteen offenses are listed here." The other guard brought forward a tablet for Yuán Liàng to read, who studied it in detail. Then the guards continued on their way with the prisoner.

It was over a week later when Yuán Liàng arrived home, only to find no one there. A neighbor told him that his family had gone to the residence of Zhāng Xiùzhī[35] to celebrate his fortieth birthday. This news startled Yuán Liàng, as this was the man he had seen not ten days before being escorted as a criminal. How could he be at home celebrating his birthday? With haste he went seeking his family. Arriving at Xiùzhī's house he found a huge banquet prepared with many guests happily laughing. Sure enough, there was Xiùzhī drinking merrily.

"I must be losing my mind!" thought Yuán Liàng. "How can he be here and not in jail? This must be a ghost, an apparition! Seeing this must surely mean that my life's destiny is exhausted and soon I shall die."

"In the middle of the road," he said addressing the crowd, "just a week past, I witnessed my friend Xiùzhī being escorted by two officials to the city of Fēngdū, facing charges on thirteen offenses!" This silenced the partygoers who stood in shock, listening as these offenses were narrated.

"One, he disrespected his father and spoke ill of his mother. Two, he was harsh to his family whilst being kind to others. Three, he secretly entered the widow's inner chamber. Four, he plotted to steal money. Five, he envied the success of others and ruined their affairs. Six, he obstructed the road so that others would trip. Seven, when the ox would not follow, he slaughtered it. Eight, if the fruit did not ripen in time, he poisoned the trees. Nine, when there was no wood for him to gather, he set fire to the mountain. Ten, he made false accusations then boasted about money and women. Eleven, he fabricated slander to give others bad names. Twelve, he ruined nests and eggs and built traps to kill unnecessarily. Thirteen, he followed his wife's word whilst ignoring that of his mother."[36]

Everyone turned to Xiùzhī expectantly, mouths agape.

"These people that I have supposedly harmed," he retorted, "they themselves are yet to report me. So how is it that you, Yuán Liàng, who I have never offended, came here to expose me? It is not as if I have offended Heaven and Earth."

---

[34] Fēngdū (酆都): Famous *necropolis* in the Chóngqìng (崇慶) municipality.

[35] Zhāng Xiùzhī (張秀芝): Open up, charmingly, creeping grass.

[36] These are evil doings of the human Heart, which, depending on society and culture may be considered acceptable or not. Nonetheless, offenses of the Heart are timeless; even if accepted by the society around you, they are still evil doings.

"Have you failed to realize," Yuán Liàng returned, "that Heaven and Earth give birth to fathers and mothers who give birth to sons and daughters? Our Heaven and Earth are imbued with this kindness. The spring discharges, the summer grows, the autumn gathers and the winter stores. It is the same with parents who first nurture the child in the womb within and then raise the child in the outer world. Heaven has rain and dew, wind and sun, which all labor with the Earth. It is like the labor of the mother and father working with their sons and daughters. Teaching them sincerity, they laugh and cry with them. When you hurt someone's son or daughter you hurt the parents, whose Hearts then ache. Therefore you hurt and injure that which belongs to Heaven and Earth. How is it that Heaven and Earth would not retaliate? It is the demons within your Heart that have reported you!"

Xiùzhī stumbled away from his guests and then collapsed in the middle of his courtyard. The shocked onlookers heard him bellow like a bull thirteen times. Suddenly blood spurted from all the orifices of his head and he died. Startled, everyone wondered if the real man had been taken to jail and this, a demon posing in his stead? On hearing this list of evils and seeing Xiùzhī's ghastly demise, everyone looked into their own Hearts and saw their own evils. Diligently they strove to change themselves and soon the whole village followed Yuán Liàng in his cultivation.

One person transmitted it to ten, these ten then transmitted it to one hundred more and the wind of goodness blew away the evil. Through his practice of goodness Yuán Liàng transformed himself, his family and relatives, his village and everyone he met in the middle of the road. By being compassionate to their children, by respecting their siblings and parents, by being honest with their spouse and in-laws, soon his small influence became a large one. By observing their intentions and actions everyone was able to transform him or herself similarly. For many years the village exuded goodness and when he was eighty years old, Yuán Liàng passed away peacefully.

There was a large movement of people from all across the countryside who traveled to be seen by the renowned physician, Bái Yù Kāi. This doctor's every action was solely executed to benefit others. Through his years of cultivation his Heart was filled with light and he felt a boundless capacity for kindness, almost to a supernatural state. The myriad things were so clear to him, he could sense when his bond to this world was diminishing. As his time drew near he visited his old friend, Xīn Dé, to say goodbye and to thank him for his guidance. Xīn Dé's accomplishments were great, however Yù Kāi knew that earlier in life he had been wicked with the scales and weights. Despite his goodness, these prior evils would have to be accounted for at some time in Hell. During his visit the old scholars discussed many things and before leaving, Yù Kāi warned Xīn Dé of what was to come. Walking away, the old doctor found a quiet orchard and sat peacefully in meditation.

The news that Yù Kāi had passed away reached Xīn Dé first and he went to collect the body. After giving his friend an honorable burial Xīn Dé sat contemplating what peril awaited him. Thinking back on all his wrongdoing, one issue in particular ate away at him. A poor family had owed him money and had then been unable to repay him. Being before his awakening to the path of righteousness he saw no problem with taking the husband as a slave and forcing arduous labor upon him as repayment. What he did not know was that the wife, so distraught at the lack of food and at the abundance of suffering, had taken her own life. So vexed by this world her spirit did not scatter but took the form of a small boy, who made his way into Xīn Dé's residence as a servant. For many years this ghostly youth had bided his time.

As Xīn Dé sat in contemplation reflecting on his life, a traveling doctor came to pay his respects. Asking to stay a while and rest, the doctor was shown to a private room where he could sleep and a young male servant brought him some tea. The next day this same servant found the doctor dead.

"My master has killed someone!" cried the youth, running out into the street.

People gathered to hear the story. But why would Xīn Dé do such a thing?

"For money!" the boy lied.

There were some who believed the story and wanted to report this affair immediately. Others were not so easily convinced, knowing that Xīn Dé had transformed himself and now had great virtue and no need for money. Why would Xīn Dé now kill for coins?

"I saw him poison this man!" exclaimed the accuser, "and when the poison worked too slowly, he took up a stick and beat him to death!"

Afraid of their own role in the drama and, if the issue was not reported quickly they might be tried as accomplices to the crime, the villagers went to the local official.

"They say the doctor died in your house," accused the official when he approached Xīn Dé.

"No!" defended Xīn Dé, mistakenly thinking that they were talking about his friend, Yù Kāi. "The doctor did not die in my house!"

Xīn Dé had not even heard of the recent passing of his visitor and was shocked when his relatives reported him missing. The house was searched but no body was found.

Immediately, Xīn Dé was shackled in the square and beaten forty times. Thick ropes were tightened until both his legs snapped. Close to death, he fainted. Immersing him in icy water failed to revive him. Xīn Dé was then thrown into a dark cell. If he were to wake he would face the judge and his death. As his body lay in that dark damp room, his spirit was whisked away to face the judge in Hell.

"Because of your evil and for those you have hurt, you will be put to death!" decreed the fiery judge, "and for the next three incarnations you will be born as an ox!"

Xīn Dé lay prostrate and cried for forgiveness. Seeing a spark of goodness in this man the judge asked for the ledger of good and evil to be brought forward. At first he frowned, but as he read on his expression changed.

"I see that you have transformed your evil into goodness for many years now. You have already received punishment in the Earthly realm so let this settle the matter. Your past errors are forgiven. Now leave and never return to this place!"

Xīn Dé sat up in the darkness and called out, surprising the guards. He requested an audience with the district magistrate.

"Your honor, who is it that accuses me of my crime? How is it that there was no investigation before punishment was dealt?"

The young servant boy was brought forward and he told of where he had seen Xīn Dé hide the body, but when they dug up the shallow grave they found the remains of someone long passed. Obviously this could not be the body of someone recently deceased. Little did they know that these bones belonged to a poor woman who had killed herself years ago.

"The servant boy must die for his slander!" demanded the magistrate. "Let there be no forgiveness for him!"

Broken and beaten, Xīn Dé knew he had erred many times in his life and that this was an opportunity for him to save a life and end this enmity. Otherwise, this hatred may never resolve but echo on into the future.

"Your honor is correct in following the laws of Heaven and Earth and thereby punishing those who have committed a crime. You cannot, however, blame the boy. He was accepted as a servant when he was only a child and I have worked him too hard. This is just a child merely wanting to retaliate. He is still so young and this is his first and only offense. Please show him mercy!"

Hearing Xīn Dé's request surprised the magistrate. This man who had been so wronged was now proving his great virtue.

"As for the law," began the magistrate, "a slave who hurts his master should be dismembered and killed. The clear thoughts and good virtue of this man, Shí Xīn Dé, shows us that no permanent harm has been done. From now on the law will be amended. Only if a servant takes the life of his master shall he too be executed."

It was in this way that one man's cultivation was able to affect the highest level of law and therefore the entire country. All the villagers returned to their homes, ashamed at having been so quick to blame a man after hearing some slanderous words. They had played their part in this error and were therefore also due for punishment. Yet Xīn Dé had not reacted in anger but had saved them all.[37]

Throughout this and afterward during Xīn Dé's recovery, the whole family stuck together and remained harmonious. Xīn Dé had by this time a son and Yīn Fū had two children. Because husbands and wives loved and respected each other and never gossiped or back-stabbed but rather developed their good character and virtue, they had shown their children these same traits. Always respecting their elders, the children were polite to their teachers and studied hard. They never fought amongst themselves and never lied. Therefore this goodness, which started with Yīn Fū, was propagated down the generations. Not just within their own family, their neighbors saw how they raised their children and how they passed their exams and made it into official positions, becoming examples of goodness. Soon the ledger of good and evil was in everyone's Hearts, treading only the true path.

By this time Yīn Fū and Xīn Dé had lived long lives and they knew that their time of passing was drawing close. As part of their preparations they encouraged their children to continue with the method of cultivating goodness and to pass this on to their own children. Wearing smiles on their faces the two men died peacefully. It is said that beautiful clear music and fragrant scents permeated the air for hours afterward.

The future generations of these two men acted like their forefathers and many entered the imperial levels of government becoming virtuous public servants. Even today their goodness continues to impact the people, country and government, all being transformed by goodness.

---

[37] In the original Sòng dynasty version, the whole village is put to death for the part they played.

Liú Yuán's conclusion.

Shí Yīn Fū was a beggar without a single penny, but through his sincere Heart he eventually gained wealth. Xīn Dé gained his money through cheating and was soon to be struck down by thunder and lightning, but through the efforts of his son-in-law, he was able to turn his Heart around and returned to goodness. He was able to change misfortune into fortune, reaching longevity.

That is why we do not discuss rich or poor. We only discuss good actions, sincere Hearts and fulfilling Heaven's will. But how can it be Heaven's way for good people to be poor and hungry, whilst evil people are wealthy? In truth, this issue is not due to Heaven, or rather, it is a superficial view of Heaven. In our world there are some who do not believe in goodness; arbitrarily, they take rash actions and so become wealthy. This is due to the accumulated virtue gained by their predecessors. Through the hard work of their forebears, their accumulated virtue and good deeds, so it is that these future generations reap some benefit. However, if our rash actions and thoughts lead us astray and we do not repent, all this accumulated virtue gifted to us from our ancestors is worn down and frittered away. Eventually we will encounter disaster regardless of our money. In Heaven there is not one small mistake forgotten, everything is calculated on our ledger.

Look for example at the Zhōu family,[38] who founded the dynasty of the same name.[39] For many generations, their virtue was great, with many sages coming forth in those eight hundred years. When the Qín took over violently,[40] the Zhōu family were not massacred but lived into their eighties and nineties without disease, dying in peace. However, if you look at those who did evil, like Cáocāo[41] at the end of the Hàn dynasty, or Sī Mǎyì[42] whose grandson founded the Jìn dynasty, their forebears had virtue, so thereby they arrived at power, but the affairs they

---

[38] Zhōujiā (周家).
[39] Zhōu dynasty (1100 BCE–230 BCE).
[40] Qín dynasty (221–207 BCE).
[41] Cáocāo (曹操), (155–220 CE): A famous statesman, general, poet and warlord at the end of the Hàn dynasty (206 BCE–220 CE).
[42] Sīmǎ Yì (司馬懿), (179–251 CE): A warlord under Cáocāo, and grandfather of Sīmǎ Yán (司馬炎), founder of the Jìn dynasties (265–420 CE).

themselves undertook were bad. Their children, although born into this same position of power, ended up being overthrown and their dynasty came to a short and bloody end. A whole generation was massacred due to this. This issue is even more prevalent amongst the common people. How many of us continue our traits of evil through our children?

Seeking fame and fortune is the normal state of the human being; however, we must conform to Heaven's principles in our thoughts and actions and whatever fame and fortune comes will be in accordance with the natural responses of Heaven and Earth. Wealth will come not when one seeks it, but when one's deeds reflect Heaven. We are not trying to do anything but to follow Heaven. Living like this means that our children will attain goodness, and fame and riches will come naturally. They will not have to suffer due to our evil.

Rather than looking after Heaven's goodness, we deceive ourselves by staring at our gains. Therefore, the fortunes of our children and grand children will be severed and they will be born as oxen and horses. So who wins and loses in the battle between greediness and goodness? Greed often leads to a short-term gain whilst goodness leads to eternal gain.

Often, due to poverty, children enter the school of unreality and become monks in order to get enough food to eat. However, if a child willingly leaves their parents as a means to earning more money, what kind of misery is that? As an adult, if our parents are still alive, we must look after them to fulfill our filial piety. One should know that amongst the sages of the three religions–Dàoism, Buddhism and Confucianism–all are loyal and filial. This should always be the case, monk or not. Only then can you burn incense and read the scriptures without these being empty actions.

When discussing filial piety, not only does this refer to one's own father and mother, but is related rather to all our relatives and elders, especially our in-laws. In the family, the parents are the main figures; whomever they love must love them in return. In our country, the Emperor is the main figure; whomever he loves must love him in return. However, today we are in a state of confusion. If only we could act like Shí Yīn Fū, then we would be good citizens of our country. More so, if we can take this goodness and virtue and transmit it to our children and teach them that they too can become as virtuous as sages, become the pillars of society, how is this not the greatest loyalty we could show our country? And in return each thought of the rulers, officials and the Emperor himself should not be cruel to their people. This then, would be loyalty to the extreme.

Hùnyuán analysis and discussion.

Concerned that people would mistake the pointing finger for the moon, Liú wanted his contemporaries (including us) to avoid concerning themselves with deities, demons and incense, instead turning inward to focus on the empty chalice within our chests, which we can fill with clarity or confusion. As Liú pointed out numerous times throughout this story, finding clarity in our Heart requires not only study or meditation but practical application of the goodness we find there, which we call Xīnfǎ.

The phrase *in the middle of the road* is repeated throughout the story and indeed, we are always in the middle of our own paths. As such it is easy to lose our way and step onto the wrong path at any time, mistaking our good intentions for true goodness. For instance, one does not achieve goodness by simply sitting in a temple of faith each day, as it is irrelevant to what is happening within the Heart. Cultivating true goodness in the Heart can be done regardless of time or place.

As humans we develop selfishness as a result of the need to sustain ourselves. Without inner cultivation it is easy to become lost in the labyrinth of selfishness, losing sight of the correct balance of Separating and Unifying, living and recharging, giving and taking. Accepting the challenge to cultivate goodness within us requires training, or gōngfu, which does not come naturally. For physicians, as witnessed in the example of Yù Kāi's clinic, without cultivating inner virtue our herbs are merely roots and leaves and our needles just metal, the Heart of our medicine is Lost along with our own.

Though it may at first appear that we do this work for our own benefit, cultivating ourselves inevitably affects others; it is not only disease that spreads. Yīn Fū's story reveals the effects of the ripples that extend to others, both positively and negatively. As teachers, doctors, parents and community members, the effect of our actions is often far-reaching and if we become consumed with fame or fortune, this can have a harmful momentum. Acquiring a yellow or black bean is not as simple as deciding whether a deed was good or bad: we must know where the thought came from and why the action was carried out. Only then can we scrutinize whether a deed was deserving of a yellow or black bean.

Liú's true message is the call for inner cultivation, for developing goodness within our own Heart because it is according to natural principle, not for fear of consequences from external factors. This is also the Heart of this book. The challenge to undertake this work is great and the reward is also great. With that in mind, we encourage the reader to return to the story of Shí Yīn Fū after completion of the remaining chapters, for many hidden meanings are likely to reveal themselves.

> And one of the elders of the city said,
> Speak to us of Good and Evil.
> And he answered:
> Of the good in you I can speak, but not of the evil.
> For what is evil but good tortured by its own hunger and thirst?[43]
>
> The Prophet

---

[43] Gibran, 2008, p. 113.

CHAPTER 2

心法基本概念

Xīn Fǎ Jī Běn Gài Niàn

Clarifying Fundamental Concepts of the Heart

"Woke up in the heart of a river.
I chose swimming up the stream.
Even though with every stroke the current pushed me backwards.
Tirelessly I went searching for the source..."[1]

Yaron Seidman

This chapter contains noteworthy sections from the first two books within volume one of Liú Yuán's ten-volume compendium. The first book includes his commentary on the Great Learning, or *Dà Xué* (大学), a text written after Confucius had died, yet is considered one of the Four Books of Confucianism.[2] It is a collection of Confucian teachings accompanied with commentary from Zēng Zǐ (曾子), a disciple of Confucius. The second is Liú's commentary on the Doctrine of the Mean, or *Zhōng Yōng* (中庸), the Confucian guide to maintaining inner and outer harmony. From Liú's discussions, we seek the fundamental ideas that permeate his teachings and understanding of life. This then becomes the framework of our approach to medicine. First, we must deconstruct the language of Liú Yuán, looking at the tenets of his philosophy from every angle.

---

[1] Y. Seidman, *A Voyage Through Humanity: Poems of the Heart. Up the River*, Hunyuan Taiji Academy Inc, USA, 2002, p. 16.

[2] The Four Books (四書): The Great Learning (大学), the Doctrine of the Mean (中庸), The Analects (論語) and the book of Mencius (孟子), were selected by the Confucian scholar Zhū Xī (1130–1200 CE) during the Sòng dynasty. The founder of Neo-Confucianism separated them from the Five Classics, giving them a special importance.

"When considering the Four Great Books of China, learning the Analects and the Book of Mencius requires little contemplation; however the Great Learning and the Doctrine of the Mean require a certain investigation of the Heart to garner their truth. The Great Learning explains the problem facing the human Heart and ways to remedy it, while the Doctrine of the Mean teaches why these phenomenon exist and why the remedy must be so. The classical books teach us how to become good ourselves, not how to lecture other people that they need to be good. In Huái Xuān we use four words to describe this: 成己成人 *chéng jǐ chéng rén*, meaning to first cultivate oneself, and then cultivate others. Once cultivated, our goodness ripples outwards into the world."

Liú Bǎigǔ

To bring the teachings of Liú Yuán into contemporary consciousness we need to learn his language. When you look at this picture below, what do you see?

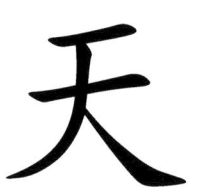

天

It is a picture: brush strokes. This picture does not have a definition but rather it implies a meaning. This image (tiān) is commonly translated as *Heaven*. The problem is that as soon as we write the word *Heaven*, the reader is already on a journey into their pre-existing opinions and beliefs of what the word Heaven means. These can be either positive or negative narratives that lead us into our steadfast beliefs and attitudes. In the process of translating Liú's work we had to constantly remind ourselves of this and we, in turn, urge you to avoid this dilemma.[3]

---

[3] "You confuse my understanding with a maze of words; speak one certain truth so I may achieve what is good." *The Bhagavad-Gita: Krishna's Counsel in Time of War*, trans. B. S. Miller, Columbia University Press, New York, 1986, p. 41.

A big tough samurai once went to see a little monk. "Monk," he said, in a voice accustomed to instant obedience, "Teach me about heaven and hell!"

The monk looked up at this mighty warrior and replied with utter disdain, "Teach you about heaven and hell? I couldn't teach you about anything. You're dirty. You smell. Your blade is rusty. You're a disgrace, an embarrassment to the samurai class. Get out of my sight. I can't stand you."

The samurai was furious. He shook, got all red in the face and was speechless with rage. He pulled out his sword and raised it above him, preparing to slay the monk.

"That's hell," said the monk softly.

The samurai was overwhelmed. The compassion and surrender of this little man who had offered his life to give this teaching to show him hell! He slowly put down his sword, filled with gratitude and suddenly peaceful.

"And that's heaven," said the monk softly.[4]

Zen story.

To truly develop an understanding of life we begin with the traditional way of learning, following the deepest thoughts of wise masters such as Liú Yuán in the texts they left behind. It is not our purpose here to learn the Confucian texts in detail. We simply need to contemplate Liú's inner process of understanding life through studying his commentary of them. Liú does not simply believe in the Classics and take them as gospel. Instead he scrutinizes every word in search of a true principle. Our journey is to find this principle and make this truth our own.

We begin studying Liú's text with a passage discussing appropriate Center. Earlier in the text we introduced the concept of One Thread of Life, the vibrating line that connects life to our vessel through our Center. This concept is similar to what Liú refers to as Natural Character. To further identify with this idea, we can apply the image of a scale.

前途未卜

Qián Tú Wèi Bǔ

'Hanging in the balance.'

---

[4] Feldman & Kornfield (eds), 1991, p. 296.

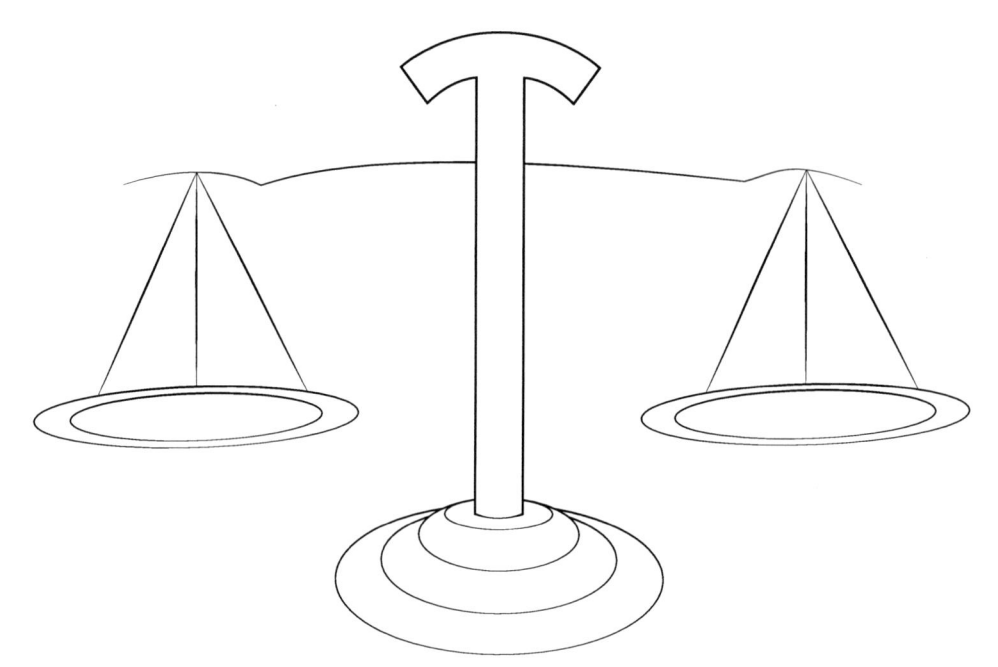

Verily you are suspended like scales between your sorrow and your joy.
Only when you are empty are you at a standstill and balanced.
When the treasure-keeper lifts you to weigh his gold and his silver,
needs must your joy or your sorrow rise or fall.[5]

The Prophet

The central column of this scale represents Center (zhōng 中), Natural Character (Xìng 性), and virtue (dé 德). When the scale is uneven this indicates a change from a static state to one of motion, referred to in the quotes below as *Heart movement* or *discharging from the Heart*.[6] Returning the scale to an even state is called *recovering Natural Character*. Whilst our Center is constantly imbued with Natural Character, when we are out of balance, we tilt the scale, lose our connection to Heaven and perish faster. In other words, our lifespan shortens.

Chū shēng rù sǐ (出生入死): *Through life we enter death.*[7]

---

[5] Gibran, 2008, p. 60.
[6] Xīnzhī fādòng (心之發動).
[7] Dào Dé Jīng (道德經), chapter 50.

To guide us through these important terms and ideas we use subheadings followed by a discussion of the topic. Liú's work is cited in footnotes throughout with indications to the page and slide numbers of the original text.[8] Please keep in mind that this chapter is an introduction to a new set of terms and a new language: the ABCs of the Heart. Whilst not quite as entertaining as the story of the yellow and black beans, it is a vital part of our investigation, building our foundation to understanding and applying Xīnfǎ.

On finding and losing our appropriate Center.

The human being is the Heart of Heaven and Earth and Natural Character is the principle of Heaven and Earth within the human being. In Pre-Heaven there is goodness without evil, however, when in the Post-Heaven, the Natural Character follows the emotions and starts to shift away from Center. It is not through our physical form that we have this disorganization,[9] but rather we tilt through learning and acquiring bad habits. This we must be very cautious about.[10]

Within this first quote there are a number of terms that require discussion. When Liú says that in a *Pre-Heaven* state there is only goodness, he is referring to the time before birth. The fetus inside the womb has no selfish desires. It is only after the baby is born that it begins to develop selfishness and through our lack of understanding of the true principle we foster bad habits and inappropriate lifestyles. Habits, either good or bad, are passed down through generations, from parent to child, teacher to student. Our first teachers are our parents, the Heaven and Earth of the human being and so fathers and mothers are given their own space for discussion below.

---

[8] "We must be leery of reading our own contemporary philosophical doctrines into an ancient teaching." H. Fingarette, *Confucius: The Secular as Sacred*, Waveland Press Inc, Illinois, 1971, p. 15. Therefore, please use the original Chinese text, attached in the appendices, to scrutinize and contemplate our work.

[9] Translated here as *physical form* is the term qìzhì (氣質), which also can be worded as the energy within our material substance, or as mannerism, trait or personality.

[10] Great Learning commentary, p. 9-1.

"...either using one's powers to walk the Way or being too weak, *without power*, and of going crookedly nowhere, falling or weaving about pointlessly in the quest of the mirages of profit, advantage and personal comfort."[11]

On Heaven and Earth.

The notion of Heaven was introduced in the story of Shí Yīn Fū. According to Liú Yuán and our research in Hùnyuán medicine, Heaven is a word embodying the circulation of the Sun and Moon as well as the void of the cosmos. Through being able to observe their movements we can see how we are intimately connected with and reliant upon these forces. Heaven Yáng is the Sun, whilst Heaven Yīn is the Moon, both of which shine or reflect light upon the Earth. The term Heaven can be divided into two subcategories: Pre-Heaven and Post-Heaven, which we elaborate on below. Life manifests on the soil of the Earth through its connection to Heaven and the myriad interactions of Fire and Water.[12]

On the conditions before and after birth: Pre-Heaven and Post-Heaven.

In the Great Learning the Master talks only of the Heart, never mentioning Natural Character. Why is this so? What the Confucian calls Heart is actually synonymous with Natural Character. The Heart has both Pre-Heaven and Post-Heaven, being the difference between the time before birth and after birth. The Pre-Heaven Heart is Natural Character; therefore Mencius says a person's Natural Character is all goodness[13]

---

[11] Fingarette, 1971, p. 21. See pp. 18-36 for more on this interesting discussion of the Legalist school of ancient China, as well as how early translators of Chinese texts were mostly missionaries who tended to translate within their bias.

[12] "Then something began pushing things up out of the soil and making things out of nothing. One day things weren't there and another they were..."What is it?" "It's something. It can't be nothing! I don't know its name, so I call it Magic...Sometimes since I've been in the garden I've looked up through the trees at the sky and I have had a strange feeling of being happy as if something were pushing and drawing in my chest making me breathe fast. Magic is always pushing and drawing and making things out of nothing. Everything is made out of Magic...So it must be all around us...in all places...If you keep calling it to come to you and help you, it will get to be part of you..." (Burnett, 1911, pp. 272-273).

[13] Mencius or Mèngzǐ (孟子), renowned Confucian philosopher (372–289 BCE).

whilst the Post-Heaven Heart is shackled to the physical body and its requirements. Within Natural Character there is Yīn, which are the seven emotions.[14] Accordingly, there is a human Heart and a Dào Heart.[15] The generations following Gàozǐ,[16] especially the schools influenced by Zen Buddhism, followed his ideas rather than those of Confucius and Mencius. In the Great Learning, an upright Heart and sincere intentions–both issues of Post-Heaven–are discussed, whilst Natural Character is not, but these terms point towards recovering one's Natural Character from the Pre-Heaven.

It is only in the Doctrine of the Mean that it is stated: Heaven's decree is called Natural Character. Following this, it says that only under Heaven can absolute sincerity exhaust itself, and Mencius says that only by using the Heart to its fullest can one know about Natural Character. These are synonymous with the references in the Great Learning to sincere intention and an upright Heart. Preserving the Heart and nurturing Natural Character is called serving Heaven, an extreme accomplishment achieved through sincere intentions and an upright Heart. According to the times and customs, the sage and the virtuous talk about this in different ways. In order to penetrate different times and generations without conflict and express the principle that the human Heart is obscured, they used these varied descriptions. However, without putting these truths into practice and only pursuing it in the world of words and text, this is how discord and misunderstanding arise.[17]

Here, Liú brings to light two concerns. The first is terminology and the true meaning behind words. The second concern is the need to reach beyond studying and contemplating by carrying out *actions* in order to retain the true meaning of words. It is not enough to discuss sincere intention, upright Heart or Natural Character, the intent of the words shift, based on time, society and culture. One scholar uses sincere intentions, another says Natural Character, but the essence is the same and they transcend time. Yet the true meanings of words are vulnerable, tending to lose themselves in the mists of time and history. As Liú concludes in this passage it is by putting

---

[14] Qīqíng dòngér (七情動而): *The seven emotions move.* These emotions are discussed further below.
[15] Rén xīn dào xīn (人心道心).
[16] The philosopher Gàozǐ (告子), contemporary of Mencius during the Warring States period (420–350 BCE).
[17] Great Learning commentary, p. 14-1.

these truths into practice as demonstrated by Shí Yīn Fū, that the meanings transcend time regardless of the words applied. When the principle is understood and practiced then a new awareness is awakened within. By sorting good from bad, we cease arguing about semantics.

> *We are born and live because of the Center received from Heaven and Earth. This Center of connectedness is called the ultimate pureness of life. Tàijí is Heaven's Center and this is what humankind attains.[18] This is our virtue. Before birth we call this Pre-Heaven, which at its core is pure and complete. Therefore, Mencius says that whilst our Natural Character is all goodness, after we are born and have to rely upon our physical form, immediately we have desires, likes and dislikes which are constantly tied to things outside us. These desires lead inward to our origin, and so the virtue we naturally have from Pre-Heaven becomes shackled and perishes daily. The sage's many teachings were all directed at the student attaining this principle of completing Heaven through the skill of recovering their Natural Character.[19]*

Before birth, a fetus is in a Pre-Heaven state: Heart and Natural Character are united, with Center received from Heaven into a single, upright Heart. This is the pure and complete Heart. After birth, we acquire post-Heaven desires and so Heart and Natural Character separate into two. The Heart follows our desires and physical needs on the exterior while Natural Character is buried deep inside Center, obscured by our pursuit and preoccupation with material needs. Once buried in material affairs, the methods of cultivating Natural Character are lost and thus it perishes faster than it should. Being in the earthly realm, meeting our physical needs is a requirement to sustain life; however we must do this with an eye always toward nurturing Natural Character. Hùnyuán medicine has an image to clarify the post-Heaven aspects of Heart and Natural Character:

---

[18] Tàijí (太極) ☯, is the source of all things. This image is flawed according to Liú Yuán, who sees Tàijí as this O. It is through our work in cultivating ourselves that we reach to this principle. Tàijí is discussed in detail later.
[19] Great Learning commentary, p. 18-1.

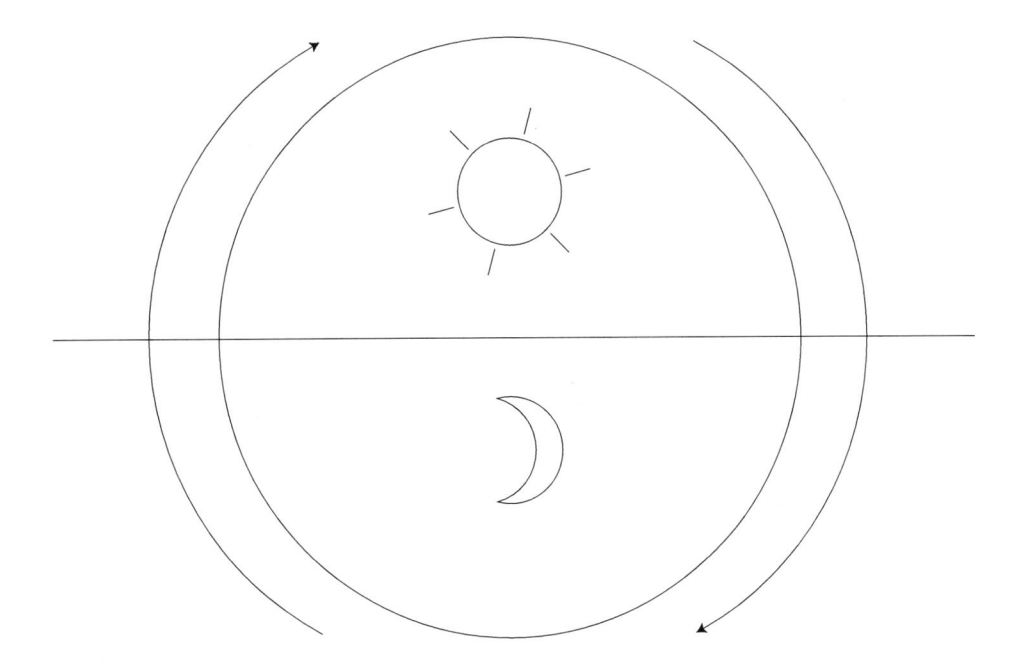

The connection of our physical body to the outside world is represented in the top half of the circle, the time of Separation, an upward and outward movement. Following the progression down the right side we move inward toward Center. This naturally occurs in the afternoon and evening as we slow down and prepare for sleep, but we can also encourage inward movement with cultivation activities during the day, provided that they are based on sincere intentions and appropriate actions.

> *Repeatedly, the Classics explain that if you have the intention of cultivating your morals[20] you must first make your Heart upright. How could it be that the intention is not the Heart? Intention and uprightness is the Heart. But sincerity and uprightness, are they not the same? It is through the daily practice of sincere intentions that gradually selfishness diminishes and the good upright Heart increases. The Heart that does not discharge emotions does not slant towards evil. This evil is only present in the Post-Heaven Heart and is the Yīn in the midst of Yáng, the emotions in the midst of Heaven's principle.[21]*

---

[20] Xiūshēn (修身): To cultivate one's moral character.
[21] This concept of *Yīn in the midst of Yáng* is seen in the ☲ lí (離) trigram, which is used as a symbol for the Inner Fire Circle.

> *The body receives life from the father and mother and then it is born. Is this anything different to what we get from Heaven and Earth? No, they are the same. The pure nature of Pre-Heaven is tied down within the physical material of Post-Heaven, and so it loses its completeness. If our character, held within our body, contracts bad habits, it starts to slant away from goodness. Day by day these habits sink deeper and deeper within us, becoming our dominant features. In this way, the principle of Heaven evaporates. So what is it then to cultivate ourselves? It is simply through sincere intention and appropriate action. However, even if we discharge sincerity and strictly nurture our Center, if we do not reach this principle of Heaven deep within our Hearts we will fail to separate ourselves from material accumulations, and so fail to unite with our Hearts and thereby have emotions like anger.[22]*

We need our physical form in order to live, which we do by desiring things that are outside of ourselves. However, the more we desire the more discontentment we experience and the further we separate from Center. Anger, hatred, sorrow and fear lock felicity and tranquility away in a dark maze.[23] Without true principle we cannot see that we require more than physical attachments to sustain a healthy life; we become confounded by the myriad things, further inhibiting our ability to unite the pure goodness within our Hearts. In the story of Shí Yīn Fū, Liú explains the two levels necessary for sorting out our Hearts: sincere intentions and appropriate actions. Only when these two elements combine is a yellow bean merited.

> *And so knowing that Natural Character is Heaven's principle, before our birth the Heart is one with Natural Character. As soon as we are born, our Heart separates from this and the seven emotions start their movement. So easy it is to become confused. We must recover our Natural Character and thereby return to the mandate of Heaven.[24] Confucius and Mencius explain this issue thoroughly in the Doctrine of the Mean.[25]*

---

[22] Great Learning commentary, p. 34-1.
[23] "Hatred is like a long, dark shadow. In most cases, not even the person it falls upon knows where it comes from. It is like a two-edged sword. When you cut the other person, you cut yourself. The more violently you hack at the other person, the more violently you hack at yourself. It can often be fatal. But it is not easy to dispose of...It is very dangerous. Once it has taken root in your heart, hatred is the most difficult thing in the world to eradicate." (Murakami, 2003, p. 312).
[24] Tiānmìng (天命): Mandate of Heaven, fate, destiny, one's life span.
[25] Doctrine of the Mean commentary, p. 106-2.

Confucius and Mencius, the founding fathers of Confucianism, use the trigrams from the Yìjīng[26] to further explain Pre-Heaven and Post-Heaven.[27] A trigram is a set of three lines, either solid (Yáng) or broken (Yīn).[28] There are eight ways these three lines can be combined, resulting in the eight trigrams, or the bāguà.[29] Liú uses these images to deepen our understanding and we have added the images where necessary to assist our study.

> *It is only the kǎn Water ☵ trigram that relates to the living Heart and we can learn much from studying it.[30] Before the Separation of Heaven and Earth, the Heaven was pure Yáng ☰ and the Earth was pure Yīn ☷, which was connected to Tàijí ○. This is the one origin, the state of pure Yáng and pure Yīn.[31] This place of pure oneness is our Pre-Heaven, the source of our Natural Character and life. As soon as Heaven and Earth start to separate, the three solid lines ☰ become pregnant with a broken line in the middle ☲, giving birth to the lí Fire trigram. Opposing this, the pure Yīn lines of kūn Earth ☷ become pregnant with a Yáng line ☵ and we have the kǎn Water trigram. Yīn amidst Yáng and Yáng amidst Yīn: this is all connected to Tàijí, which makes creation and transformation possible.*
>
> *It is in the Post-Heaven where the emotions flip from Yīn to Yáng and Yáng to Yīn, relating to the qián ☰ and kūn ☷ trigrams, which reveal their characteristics of the Sun and Moon. The seed of Pre-Heaven lies within the Center of the human body in the Post-Heaven. In order for Tàijí to become complete within the human vessel, the Pre-Heaven Natural Character from qián ☰ must enter into kūn ☷ to form the kǎn ☵, so Yáng is concealed therein. Thereafter, the Post-Heaven Yīn is brought to life and so we have disturbances of the emotions and our reliance on material substances. This is the natural state we find ourselves in, so recovering the Natural Character does not come to us easily but requires skill and dedication. The grand Qì of the Pre-Heaven reveals itself in our true sincerity and this is entirely the one principle of purity we must follow. Being calm*

---

[26] Yìjīng (易經): The Classic of Changes.
[27] For more on the Yìjīng specifically, please see: Z. Wu *Seeking the Spirit of the Book of Change: 8 Days to Mastering a Shamanic Yijing (I Ching) Prediction System*, Singing Dragon, London, 2009.
[28] Guà (卦): Trigram.
[29] The bāguà (八卦): ☰ qián (乾), ☱ duì (兌), ☲ lí (離), ☳ zhèn (震), ☴ xùn (巽), ☵ kǎn (坎), ☶ gèn (艮) and ☷ kūn (坤).
[30] Therefore, the destination of Heaven Yáng in our body.
[31] Yī yuán (一元): One origin, univariate, only variant.

and still, we see the myriad thoughts in the midst of the vast abyss.

One moment of stillness and Heaven and Earth are quiet and compliant, standing mysteriously. With one movement the ten thousand virtues are all appropriate within the void of the vast abyss. And so Heaven and Earth start their transformation, emerging and spreading like arteries throughout the universe.[32]

Liú analyzes the beginning and source of life through the study of duality. Yīn and Yáng merge and combine to form the myriad things, but their combinations are not infinite. They are definite and can be reflected upon by observing the formations of the trigrams. As we read in the passage above, investigating the interplay of the Sun and Moon, one can discern how pure Yáng ☰ and pure Yīn ☷ merge to form Fire ☲ and Water ☵. Liú suggests that it is only this last trigram, the kǎn ☵ trigram, which equates to the Dào Heart, the principle of life within us.

The principle of the kǎn ☵ trigram is the central focus and tenet of Hùnyuán medicine. By using the term *Center* to articulate the placement of Heaven principle within the body, we mean the Center of every single living cell. This may cause a conflict for our linear mindsets as we are suggesting Heaven principle is in the middle and at the same time everywhere. To study this whole we make some divisions, easing linear constructs into a curve. Separating the living physical body into the Outer Water Circle and the Dào Heart in the Center of the Inner Fire Circle, we make One into Two. This is not to suggest that one is more important than the other, for the learning curve of careful contemplation merges the Two into One.

> What is acceptable is acceptable; what is not acceptable is not acceptable. A path is formed by walking on it. A thing has a name because of its being called something. Why is it like this? Because it is! Why is it not like that? Because it is not! Everything has its own nature and its own function. Nothing is without nature or function...They are all one in Tao. When there is separation, there is coming together. When there is coming together, there is separation. All things may become one, whatever their state of being... Realization of one's true nature is happiness. When one reaches happiness, one is close to perfection. So one stops, yet does not know that one stops. This is Tao.[33]

---

[32] Doctrine of the Mean commentary, p. 122-1.
[33] Zhuāngzǐ quoted in G. Feng, & J. English, *Chuang Tsu: Inner Chapters, A Companion Volume to the Tao Te Ching*, Amber Lotus Publishing, Portland, 1974, p. 30. Zhuāngzǐ (莊子) was a Dàoist author and scholar (369–286 BCE).

Heaven Yáng is the solid line in the kǎn Water ☵ trigram, which is representative of the entirety of life in physical living material (the broken Yīn lines) in the Outer Water and Inner Fire Circles. Liú explains that in kǎn ☵, the Tàijí principle from Heaven ☰ enters the vessel ☵ to become complete, or alive in each and every cell. Comparing this to the Fire ☲ trigram, the broken Yīn line represents the body's dependency on earthly physical material for survival. Therefore, the Water ☵ trigram is a summary of the living vessel which is encased in Yīn, yet imbued with Yáng. The Fire ☲ trigram has Yīn in the midst of our movement, revealing how overt and exaggerated attachments to the external world divide and conquer the Heaven principle within us. In Hùnyuán medicine, the Water ☵ trigram, with Pre-Heaven Yáng concealed within Post-Heaven Yīn, is the key to understanding life and how to nurture it with medicinals, food, fluids and lifestyle choices. Equally, as shown here by Liú, it is also the key to opening the door to understanding *cultivation of the Heart*.

The suffix *pre-* is easy to misinterpret as it usually implies something that came before. Whilst this is not entirely incorrect it is nonetheless not correct enough. *Pre-* in this context does not refer to the *past* but to the seed of Heaven concealed within, the seed of life. We must nurture this seed and cultivate it into a strong and sturdy tree, thereby fostering a stable Center.[34] Confused and distracted by Post-Heaven affairs and selfishness we habitually neglect that which is most vital, the seed of goodness within our Center.

As we will cover in great depth throughout the later chapters of this book, the wearing down and corruption of this seed leads to ill health as the life within our Center diminishes. The method of curing such diseases is to increase Yáng within Yīn, bringing more life into the physical vessel, as depicted in the kǎn trigram ☵. Strengthening the connection of our pre-Heaven Yáng to nourish our seed is not an easy task, Illustrated by Shí Yīn Fū, it requires dedication to sorting good from evil within the ledger of our Heart. Only then can we remedy diseases of this level.

---

[34] "When we reached the place he was aiming for, he began making holes in the ground with his rod, putting an acorn in each and then covering it up again. He was planting oak trees. I asked him if the land was his. He said it wasn't. Did he know the owner? No, he didn't... He wasn't interested in who they were. And so, with great care, he planted his hundred acorns." J. Giono, (trans. Bray, B.) (1996) *The Man Who Planted Trees*. The Harvill Press. London. p.16.

"When in the womb, everybody is the same. The Heart, pure. After birth, social influences and other external factors shape our Heart into *good* or *bad*. Therefore, the Center of cultivation is the teaching of goodness, kindness and compassion. This then spreads out into society as a positive influence, eventually eradicating evil from the world."

Liú Bǎigǔ

What cannot be seen often leads to erroneous paths.

From the Sòng dynasty onwards[35] the Confucians surmised that the human Heart is Natural Character, forgetting that there are two hearts: the human Heart and the Dào Heart. This confusion comes out of the influence of Zen Buddhism. The human Heart can nurture one's Natural Character, but it is not Natural Character. And so through many years of guarding the Heart they reached a clever understanding of cultivating, organizing and ruling the country; however they could never actualize this understanding and they failed to practice its real skill.[36]

Liú would teach the Confucian, just as he did the Buddhist and Dàoist scholars[37] and so to refer to him as a *Confucian* would be an injustice. He was a thinker in his own right. Teaching here as he did through the story of Shí Yīn Fū, Liú postulates that whilst guarding one's Post-Heaven Heart with meditation can achieve some sense of peace, it alone cannot bring the goodness of the Pre-Heaven Dào Heart into practice in the real world. And if this goodness is not brought into practice in day-to-day life, it is as if the skill we are after does not exist at all. Endless hours of meditation are spent in vain.[38]

---

[35] 960–1279 CE. This was a time in China when Confucianism was being revived, after a lengthy decline in popularity during the Táng dynasty when Buddhism was flourishing. This period of revival is commonly referred to as the Neo-Confucian era.

[36] Great Learning commentary, p. 13-1-2, discussing the problems within Neo-Confucianism.

[37] "...the cross-fertilization and fusion of quite different lines of philosophic thought in China in the age of the 'Philosophers' quickly gave a different cast to what Confucius was saying...*All* our texts and readings are irremediably infected with interpretation, commentary, editorial selection and sheer ideological skullduggery." (Fingarette, 1972, p. x).

[38] We discuss the importance of meditation later, but it is a tool to be used to shape ourselves into goodness. A tool, not a temple.

Zen Buddhists who guard their Hearts have erred in believing that the Post-Heaven Heart is Natural Character. They know the spirit through nurturing their void and emptiness. However, they have missed and neglected the concept of perception. Although they restrain their Heart so it is without movement, stilling the motions of the Heart is not the one and only practice that recovers the connection to the Pre-Heaven. Many undertakings of the myriad things between Heaven and Earth are truly beyond comprehension. How could the common people know that the monks–and what they propagate–is actually following the ideas of philosopher Gào? They have followed an erroneous path, mistaking what Mencius meant when he said, 'Do not move the Heart'.[39]

Regarding Dǒng Zhòngshū[40] *and his work, he proposed that Five Elements complete the Five aspects of Natural Character. In this he erred in his thinking, as the Five aspects of our Natural Character are in reality only one, as the Five Elements are only one Tàijí.*[41]

Hùnyuán medicine agrees with this principle and indeed, it is the basis behind the cliché of treating the body as a whole. The more we separate life, the more we lose sight of the root, leaving holes in our thoughts and actions. Medicine becomes specialized, with each area of the body divided up into pieces. For example, the dermatologist examines the skin, the gynecologist studies the female reproductive system, the surgeon learns to cut and stitch tissue. The psychologist observes the mind, the neurologist treats the brain and the gastroenterologist assesses the intestines, while the podiatrist observes the feet. Imagine if all these specialties approached illness from the same point of Center... *in every different shade and description of what we can see, they are all the diffusion of the one origin...*

---

[39] Great Learning commentary, p. 21-1.
[40] Dǒng Zhòngshū (董仲舒) (179–104 BCE), philosopher and proposed author of the extant *Luxuriant Dew of the Spring and Autumn Annals* (Chūnqiū Fánlù 春秋繁露), influential in establishing Confucianism as the standard system of values of the former Han dynasty, specifically in regard to the Five Elements and their relationship to politics.
[41] Doctrine of the Mean commentary, p. 55-2.

After the Three Dynasties,[42] the Confucian did not understand nurturing the Qì,[43] the yellow caps[44] were inhaling the new and exhaling the old, and they were all in chaos. Yes, they may have been following the seeds cast by the virtuous sages, but the seed was broken and the entry-level skill was not understood. The one origin of Heaven and Earth gives birth to the myriad things and this principle is held in the midst of Tàijí, merging it with the Qì. We call it movement, yet there is no movement; we call it stillness, yet there is no stillness.

The place where the Qì is moving is where we can see the principle. However, in every different shade and description of what we can see, they are all the diffusion of the one origin. The human body is no different. It has Qì and after that it has a physical body, which at its root is nothing but the Natural Character of Heaven. The root of the vast energy of the universe[45] is in Heaven and Earth and it dominates my body. This is the origin of Natural Character and life. This origin is not what the Dàoists nurture as they focus only on the Post-Heaven Qì. Rather, the origin of the principle lies in the Confucian rules of benevolence, righteousness, propriety, knowledge and trustworthiness, which are used to polish the unpolished aspect of our Qì.[46] Happiness, anger, sadness and joy: they all reveal a discharging of our origin and a spreading of Natural Character, the manifestation of Qì.

If this Qì that makes us alive can find its root in Heaven, making our character nothing but goodness, then our Center becomes harmonious. If we fail to love our parents to the extreme then we cannot say that our emotions have uprightness. The sage nurtures his body through his harmonious Center and so he merges with Heaven and Earth. He made common his uprightness and his brightness spread out, so the actions and applications he undertook were a reflection of Heaven and

---

[42] The Xià (夏), Shāng (商) and Zhōu (周) dynasties. For more on this see Seidman's scholarly articles on ancient Chinese History on the Hunyuan Research Institute's website and T. A. Jaensch, "'..deep beneath the layers...' - TCM history in the Shang & Zhou eras", 2001.

[43] Yǎngqì (養氣): Nurturing the Qì.

[44] Huángguān (黃冠), referring to the Dàoist priest who would wear yellow hats.

[45] Hàorán zhīqì (浩然之氣): The expansive vital energy.

[46] "...born into the world...with the potentiality to be shaped into a truly human form. There is, to begin with, the raw stuff, the raw material. This must be...shaped and controlled...[by] 'cutting, filing, chiseling and polishing'... [which] if it is well done...he will walk straight upon the Way." (Fingarette, 1971, p. 21).

Earth. Without discharging his Qì violently he supported his will, so the pure principle was thereby preserved. This is the beginners' entry-level training to the school of virtue, where our will and Qì becomes like pure spirit. If one wants to be noble, this is the path of recovering our Natural Character as if on a military campaign, requiring long-term sacrifice and effort.[47]

Finding the true Heaven principle in our Hearts is a mission we started early in the book with Shí Yīn Fū. The quality of our relationships, along with the degree to which we are enamored upon external objects, reflects our connection to the Heaven principle within our Heart. Sorting good and bad from our Center is like a military campaign. It requires long-term study, dedication and contemplation, scrutiny of thoughts, feelings, actions and behaviors, all directed at reaching to and recovering the Heaven principle within. This is the art of recovering life.

Discussing Qì.

Another word or character with particular significance to Chinese medicine appears in the preceding quote by Liú. *Qì,* often transcribed as *Ch'i* in Wade Giles' romanization of Mandarin, is not a word describing an object; rather it is a concept, an observation, part of the dichotomy of reality, the playground of Yīn and Yáng.

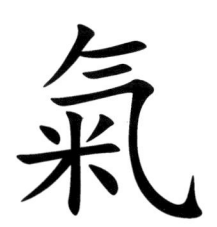

氣

Qì belongs to Chinese culture more so than to its language. When saying an object *has* Qì, it helps the speaker express what is in their Heart and not just what they see. For example, Liú may say *the Qì of Heaven and Earth*, which is contemplation from his Heart. Qì in this context means the principle that Heaven and Earth reveal, yet cannot be seen with the eyes. The word *Qì,*

---

[47] Doctrine of the Mean commentary, p. 127-2.

however, can also mean anything that cannot effectively be translated into English. Intention will transform the meaning. For example, the Qì of a person could mean their attitude, life, level of energy, mannerisms and so on. Hence the definition of Qì requires elucidation by the speaker.

> "When Chinese thinkers are unwilling or unable to fix the quality of an energetic phenomenon, the character *qi* (氣) inevitably flows from their brushes."[48]

Hùnyuán avoids the use of the word Qì, as its use often signifies a vague understanding...*I do not know what to say, so I will say Qì*...Medicine should not contain mystery: what we contemplate with our Heart we express with our words.

On the Seven Emotions and the Myriad Things.

The seven emotions (qīqíng 七情) are outward movements from our human Heart and form how the body can separate. The myriad things, meaning everything around us in the outer material world, are observed and sensed through our Recharging Instruments. Our reactions to these stimuli will be based on our resilience and self-esteem, or the discharging of the Inner Fire Circle.

The seven emotions as taught by Liú Yuán are:

Xǐ	喜	Happiness, joy, pleasure or delight.
Nù	怒	Fury, anger, irritability or frustration.
Āi	哀	Sorrow, sadness, grief, pity or lamentation.
Jù	惧	Fear, worry, fright, shock or anxiety.
Ài	爱	Love, affection, fondness or liking.
Wù	恶	Hatred, loathing, despising, disliking or slandering.
Yù	欲	Brooding, wishing, desiring or obsessing.

---

[48] M. Porkert, *The Theoretical Foundations of Chinese Medicine: Systems of Correspondence*, Massachusetts Institute of Technology Press, Cambridge, 1974.

On the issue of the Father and Mother.

In June 2012, Master Liú Bǎigǔ spoke at length about the importance of respecting one's parents and honoring our responsibilities to them. Likewise, parents should nurture their children. And that is it. When these relationships are not conducted according to true principle we must correct our actions and words to mend them. In the narrow sense, filial piety is the act of children respecting their parents as well as helping their parents become sincere, such as is demonstrated by Shí Yīn Fū in convincing his father-in-law to reform his corrupt business dealings. Thus, part of self-cultivation is showing compassion and kindness towards our mother and father: this is a foundational step toward returning to our Natural Character. As this understanding is gradually established our Natural Character begins to spread, positively influencing those around us, our family, community, patients, and so on. Parents are analogous to Heaven and Earth and each contributes to our existence and so the filial duty of each of us is to be thankful, through words and actions, for our life.

> *To complete all affairs under Heaven requires us to know when to stop with knowledge[49] and sort out our selfishness.[50] Under Heaven there are numerous clever people widely trying to serve it; however they do not follow the principle of cultivating the body and nurturing Natural Character and how these translate into practical applications. Without this practicability, one can never be clear and knowledgeable about virtue. Ultimate goodness is the foundation of cultivating the Heart and nurturing Natural Character. The vast principle of Heaven and Earth is without name, so we call it Tàijí.*
>
> *Tàijí is the Center of Heaven and Earth and the same is true for the human body. Confucius says the school of righteousness is accomplished by preserving the Dào through nurturing Natural Character. The human body, filled with flesh and blood, the Heart and its knowledge, is similar to all other living things; however, the divinity within us is only in our Center, the Tàijí. This Center is the origin of our life, or rather it*

---

[49] Zhīzhǐ (知止). See also Lǎo Zǐ's (老子) Dào Dé Jīng (道德經), chapter 32, line 8: "Zhīzhǐ, suǒyǐ bù dài" (知止所以不殆): *Knowing when to stop, therefore one avoids peril*. Knowing when to stop means reaching the extreme of it, a place where you cannot advance any further.

[50] Géwù (格物) can be understood in two ways: the Neo-Confucianist view of the term *rationally contemplating natural phenomena*, whilst the Huái Xuān school sees it as *sorting out our selfishness*, which is a step deeper. I sort out my Heart first in order to be clearer in my understanding of all phenomena around me.

is through the pureness of Heavens' decree that we have the lives we live. We are given all the elements of our body from our parents and so it is that we are born. In reality, their gift is the upright principle of Heaven, and so we are born.[51]

If there is no Heaven and Earth, there is no father and mother and so how could I exist? Even with Heaven and Earth, if there is no father and mother, how could I exist? To be created, I must have a father and a mother. Therefore you can see that Heaven and Earth, and father and mother, are one and the same thing. And so before birth, we receive the Center of Heaven and Earth, containing the vastness of true principle, and after birth this original Qì scatters and the principle separates from our Center. To understand the void[52] our orifices that can accomplish this–the apertures of the divine–must not accumulate selfishness and desires. Then the only place we stop is at ultimate goodness. We know we have arrived when we return our vision and bring back our hearing, looking and listening inwards. We become crystal clear about virtue. This is where our Natural Character and life join into one, Heaven and Earth are harmonious together and in this way we return to pure Oneness and reach our Center.[53]

Upon reaching true goodness, the myriad aspects of ourselves unite into *Tàijí*. In a state of oneness, clarity emerges: one observes the harmony of Center as the orifices naturally sort the pure from the impure. Liú explains repeatedly that *reaching oneness* is not merely a philosophical idea, that it requires the practical application of sorting good and evil within ourselves and adhering to correct actions. Through this differentiation of yellow and black beans we develop the ability to see the divide we have created between the human Heart and the Dào Heart, and then bring them back to oneness.

---

[51] Modern medicine asserts that we inherit genes from our parents. Liú clearly distinguishes the gift of physical components from our Xìng. We are more than the mingling of a sperm and an egg.
[52] Xūmíng (虚明): To understand the divine, or void.
[53] Great Learning commentary, p. 20-2.

The myriad things have one origin.[54] *Within the Yìjīng, the qián* ☰ *Heaven and kūn* ☷ *Earth trigrams are considered to be the father and mother who give birth to the three girls and three boys, making up the eight trigrams. The rotations of Heaven's creation and mother nature bring kǎn* ☵ *Water and lí* ☲ *Fire into existence, which become the pivot of life. If you continue to separate this, you have the Five Elements. If you further scatter it, you have the myriad things. This principle cannot be exhausted with words. The human body, being a part of the myriad things, is imbued with Heaven and Earth and so within it is the command of Heaven. Its essence is outstanding. It is the dull-minded who separates human beings from the myriad things.*

Confucius tells us that one Yīn and one Yáng together is called Dào.[55] *Dào finds its root in Heaven and Earth. Heaven and Earth are the father and mother of the human being and this is the true root of our Natural Character and our life. The principle of Yīn and Yáng runs very deep. Parents are the Heaven and Earth of receiving life. If one wants to complete the Dào, then they must make their body sincere. The mother and father are the womb of life. Within the relationship of mother and father, and towards them, the Qì must be completely virtuous. Heaven and Earth* is *husband and wife. Understanding this allows our potential to reach the extreme. How can we know this method?*[56]

To serve Heaven and Earth is to serve one's father and mother. This is the one principle that penetrates everything.[57]

One cannot but cultivate oneself. Cultivating it is in the Dào. Dào is the principle of Heaven and that is the end of the matter. Heaven's principle only appears through a benevolent Heart and every single human being has this capacity. To cultivate Dào, one uses their benevolent Heart, pushing it towards the myriad

---

[54] See Lǎozǐ's (老子) Dào Dé Jīng (道德經) chapter 42:
Dào shēng yī, yī shēng èr, èr shēng sān, sān shēng wàn wù (道生一,一生二,二生三,三生萬物).
"The Dào gives birth to One, One gives birth to Two,
Two gives birth to Three, Three gives birth to the myriad things."

[55] *Yī yīn yī yáng zhī wèi dào* (一陰一陽之謂道), from the *Xì Cí Zhuàn Shàng* (繫辭傳上 The First Appended Comments).

[56] Doctrine of the Mean commentary, p. 66-1-2.

[57] Doctrine of the Mean commentary, p. 72-2.

things. Benevolence is revealed in its application and is achieved by avoiding the idea that Heaven's principle is unsatisfactory. Mankind attains their Natural Character by understanding Heaven's principle of endless creation. What makes a person a human being? It is through compassion, kindness, concern, sympathy and empathy, all of which are shown first to one's parents and then are spread outwards to others. Therefore, loving our parents is the greatest form of benevolence. They are from where my body came, and the Center of my body is full of Heaven's goodness. Without parents, how could I have come into existence? If I fail to love my parents, how can I be considered a human being?[58]

Contemplating the term *Géwù* (格物)–the process of weeding out our selfishness and good from bad–is the first step on the path of self-cultivation.[59] Once a person has worked on himself or herself, only then can they make a positive impact on their family, patients, community and country.[60] To be cultivated means that before we think of ourselves we must think of our parents, as they are our connection to the One Origin and, in a practical way, they are our origin. In addition, what does selfishness and selflessness mean? This is a challenging topic and we engage it from varying angles throughout this book. Thus far we can define *selfishness* as not acting with pure goodness and not acting in accordance with Heaven's principle. This relates to how we behave within every aspect of our lives and indeed it starts with our relationship to our parents. *Selflessness* is the most basic building block of human Natural Character.

Liú Yuán explores Natural Character through our relationships with those around us, therefore placing an emphasis on the Five Cardinal Relationships.[61]

---

[58] Doctrine of the Mean commentary, p. 82-1-2.
[59] Qiān lǐ zhī xíng, shǐ yú zú xià (千里之行始於足下), *The thousand mile journey starts with a single step...*from Lǎozǐ's (老子) Dào Dé Jīng (道德經), chapter 64.
[60] Like in Shí Yīn Fū's example, this idea of the individual's actions or inactions affecting more than just themselves is not only emphasized in Confucian thought, but see also Chapter 54 of the Lǎozǐ's (老子) Dào Dé Jīng (道德經).
[61] The *Wǔlún* (五倫): The Five Cardinal Relationships or Kinships of Confucianism, which are: 1. Ruler and subject, *jūnchén* (君臣): 2. Father and son, *fùzǐ* (父子): 3. Elder and younger brother, *xiōngdì* (兄弟): 4. Husband and wife, *fūfù* (夫婦) and 5. Between friends, *péngyǒu* (朋友).

"The Five Cardinal Relationships are integral aspects of our daily life, from morning till evening. Yet, even though common and reachable, the reality is that by practicing them daily, you can indeed reach miraculous levels. A person who practices the Heart method does not require herbal tonics to maintain their health. Practicing cultivation is a tonic for the Heart."

Liú Bǎigǔ

Added to these is our relationship with nature. What is the true principle of Heaven in each and every action? Killing an animal for sport is an example of pure selfishness, in total discord with Heaven's principle. However, killing an animal when they are mature in order to feed one's family, this is not selfishness. Looking through this lens of Liú Yuán's conscience is a process of discovery for us when considering our relationships. We see that customs and culture are not truth and only Heaven's principle penetrates everything and is timeless.

More on *Géwù* (格物) and Selfishness.

This is the focal point of Liú Bǎigǔ's teaching on how to become a *good* person and he offers these five steps as a guide:

格物	(géwù)	is to remove all selfishness by observing inner phenomena, desires and emotions.
致知	(zhìzhī)	is reaching knowledge, which manifests instantaneously after the removal of selfishness.
誠意	(chéngyì)	is sincerity, which is our knowledge naturally reflecting our goodness.[62]
正心	(zhēngxīn)	is the Upright Heart, every thought and deed conforms to the principle of Heaven and Earth.
修身	(xiūshēn)	is the cultivated body, in life every thought and deed conforms to the sage.

---

[62] According to Liú Bǎigǔ, sincerity and the absence of selfishness are where the Heart of utter innocence 赤子之心 *chì zǐ zhī xīn*, finds itself; the Heart of the baby within a mother's womb, one of complete pureness.

The most important step on any journey is the first, and here it is géwù.[63] The final two chapters of this book challenge the beliefs we cling to about ourselves, and propose a more compassionate future.

On the similarity of things: the myriad things come from the one creation.

So often we misunderstand virtue and what the sages demonstrated and taught. We need only desire to cultivate ourselves from within and from without. We must understand this and then understand it yet again, thereby transforming the awkwardness of our existence. Dwelling entirely on this understanding of the divine, one can remove our hidden desires for external things. When this principle is clear and is used to guard the Heart, it shines forth and can be seen by all under Heaven. The Natural Character of all people under Heaven is the same as my own, yet our circumstances are all different.[64] The student talks loftily about life, researching widely in the Classics; however, they struggle to put this into practice. They cannot overcome their emotions. Everybody knows that in the marketplace there is no such thing as complete goodness. The student needs to study in peace in order to find the virtue within, otherwise they find themselves leaning to one side or the other. Then they can push and propagate this to external things. Over time they transform the plethora of human emotions and reach towards the principle of unity.[65]

Whatever finds itself before our ears and eyes in any affair has its own principle that needs to be explored to the extreme. The hawk flies and the fish leaps. They naturally attain their Natural Character as a reflection of Heaven. They each have their appropriate flying and leaping and without thought they can fly to the Heavens or dive to the abyss. The hawk does not know of Heaven, yet it flies and reaches to it. The fish does not know how deep the abyss is and yet it leaps. The hawk in Heaven and the

---

[63] In the Great Learning there are eight steps, including those described above, along with 齊家(qíjiā) and 治國(zhìguó), which together form the idiom *to regulate the family and rule the state* and 平天下(píng tiānxià), meaning *to bring peace to all under Heaven*.

[64] "The *shifu-tuer* [master and student] relationship is between equals, although not equivalents." (Schmieg, 2005, p. 40).

[65] Great Learning commentary, p. 16-1.

fish in the abyss: each one reaches its natural place and each relies on its own innate wisdom. In all things that circulate between Heaven and Earth, all can do this naturally. Seeing this in everything, from the Emperor to the commoners, each should fulfill their Dào. Each should put their Dào into practice.[66]

Everything in nature, including humans, has an innate ability to accomplish its purpose. Unfortunately, selfishness obscures this from us, hiding the true nature of the human being which Liú calls *benevolence*. While culture and customs continually transform themselves, the goodness principle of Heaven is continuous, the same today as it was two thousand years ago. Human Natural Character, when pure and unobstructed, naturally displays *proper* behavior toward parents, sons and daughters, husband and wife, brothers and sisters, neighbors and friends. The appropriateness of behavior is like the leaping fish and soaring hawk. Yet the human Heart is often clouded and this impairs our understanding of Natural Character. Liú Yuán reveals to us how to clear the cloud and fog.

On before and after Heaven: exploring Natural Character, *Xìng* (性).

When the sage taught the many types of propriety, he only desired that his student would attain the one complete principle, the need to recover his Natural Character...by completing his skill of understanding the root and branches, from beginning to end, he can find his enlightened Heart. This is Heaven's decree. Natural Character is the life that comes from Heaven.[67]

Heaven's decree[68] *is Natural Character; it is one and the same thing, the life force that comes from Heaven, which produces and rotates endlessly.*[69]

The fact that the human being is alive attests to the original principle of the universe. The constancy of Heaven decides and dominates incessantly. Mankind attains life from Heaven and what he attains we call Natural Character. Heaven's life and the Natural Character of the human being is one and the same. The

---

[66] Doctrine of the Mean commentary, p. 65-2.
[67] Great Learning commentary, p. 18-1-2.
[68] Tiān zhī mìng (天之命).
[69] Doctrine of the Mean commentary, p. 55-1.

two are one and the one is two.[70]

When we talk about emotions such as happiness, anger, sadness, fear and joy, by regulating these we find the root of Natural Character. Our root is our harmonious Center, which cannot be seen. However, we know its state by viewing the emotions. If the emotions have yet to discharge and one is clear and calm, this is the beginning of preserving the Center. This is the principle. Without exception, our Natural Character should emulate this. Reaching a harmonious Center allows Heaven and Earth to stand in their proper position, giving birth to the myriad things. When written here in words and sentences, it can become disconnected; yet when contemplated within the Heart, we can see the principle. Then we can recover the beginning of Heaven's decree.[71]

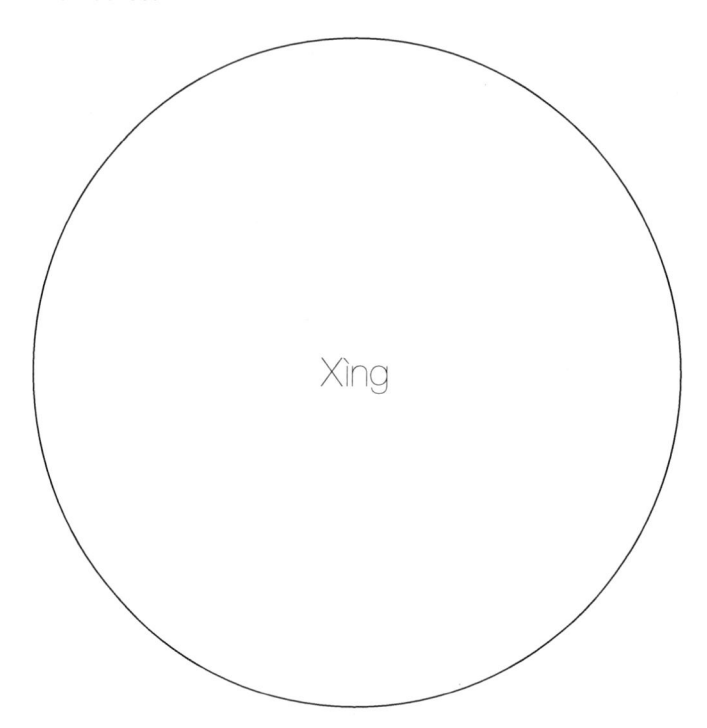

Our *Center* is in the middle of the Hùnyuán circle, which is linked to the physical vessel via Shàoyīn. In the very Heart of the circle is our Natural Character. Our emotions discharge from this Center within us, creating

---

[70] Doctrine of the Mean commentary, p. 53-2.
[71] Doctrine of the Mean commentary, p. 56-1.

movement.[72] We require this movement to maintain life; however, too often it moves excessively, tipping the scale away and askew from Natural Character. Instead, the goal should be to attain balance and only discharge emotions necessary for life, not to give up life. For example, if analyzing infertility, when we are in our proper position–our Center–then the body can more easily deal with the process of creating a new life. Writing or reading about these issues is not what achieves this outcome; one must contemplate them deeply and put them into action. Even the most studious scholars do not automatically arrive at enlightenment. The recognition of Center comes from within, an investigation beyond external phenomena.

> *It is said that Heaven and mankind do not have two different principles, but are one and the same. When the human Heart moves, it connects to Heaven's Heart. Heaven cannot be seen, however the spirit that comes from Heaven can be.[73] This spirit is a mirror of Heaven within our Heart, but it cannot be measured and we know not what it thinks. When a thought comes, often one guards against it as if afraid to be at fault. The spirit has no physical form or sound, therefore reaching absolute subtlety, reflecting the divine.[74]*

As a result of our exposure to Post-Heaven influences our emotional reactions mask our Natural Character. Being closer to the surface, our emotions are more readily experienced and it takes diligence to find our Center. Once a memory or thought arises, an emotion is discharged in response and so we strive to immediately return to Center. We still the scales and restore balance.

> *The human body first has Qì and then a physical body. These two components together are similar to Heaven's principle. What is peculiar about the human being is that we come out as male and female. This division is dark and obscure and it further obscures the Natural Character. The Qì that arrives in the morning, at birth, is shackled to perishing and the mind is fettered with greed. This greed is naturally imbued within all the Hearts of humankind.[75]*

---

[72] Discussed in the introduction as the One Thread of Life.
[73] The word *spirit* is another noun/verb/adjective that could cause us to form roadblocks in our mind. We would define Liú's meaning here as *being alive, as is Heaven's principle.*
[74] Doctrine of the Mean commentary, p. 70-2.
[75] Doctrine of the Mean commentary, p. 97-2.

Mankind is a matrix of energy and physical material and a division of male and female. Yet these divisions distract us from the true nature of the human being, which is identical regardless of gender, appearance and circumstance.[76] The world can be divided innumerably and we can spend eternity breaking apart reality, looking at years, months, weeks, days, hours, minutes, seconds, milliseconds...and never see the full picture. Gazing at the dancing leaves rather than the sturdy roots. To divide is to misplace the Dào. Regarding Natural Character, distinguishing male and female is an example of separating the principle of Oneness into Two, but in truth, the Two are One.

> "The human body contains the Heaven principle, and originally there are no male and female Hearts in the Pre-Heaven; however when the Qì forms, there is thick and thin, clear and turbid."
>
> Liú Yuán

Natural Character is not the *temperament* of a person, though a phlegmatic or sanguine personality reveals the state of their Inner Fire Circle and how the emotions and desires discharge from Center. Liú's teachings explain that Natural Character relates to the Heaven principle in the Center of the human being, which is pure goodness. Hereafter, Natural Character will be referred to as Xìng, using Liú's language to avoid confusion with the English definition of *character*.

> *...we talk of the five aspects of Xìng: benevolence, righteousness, propriety, knowledge and trustworthiness...*[77]

---

[76] This is clearly demonstrated in the fact that human virtue is not defined by gender as a girl or a boy love their parents the same way. Regarding Chinese medicine, "All medicine traditions have dealt with sick women as well as sick men, but not all have had a gynecology. At its base gynecology deals with medical disorders perceived and designated as gendered: that is, pathologies afflicting women alone, or taking different forms in males and females...the concept of 'gynecology' is fully laden with the understandings of biomedicine...the structural language of anatomy as a specialty dealing with the pathologies of women's reproductive organ..." C. Furth, *A Flourishing Yin: Gender in China's Medical History: 960-1665*, University of California Press, Berkeley, 1999, p. 59.

[77] See chapter 3 for the full quote.

On discussing the Heart, Xīn (心).

Anatomically, the heart is an essential organ that pumps, or is pumped by the blood.[78] Being the Center of the cardiovascular system, it is vital; yet when investigating Xīnfǎ, we need to focus on what the living body contains, a *Heart*. *This* is the Heart that Hùnyuán medicine seeks, the vibrating line therein being our connection and connectedness to life.

> *The human being receives their Center Qì[79] from Heaven and Earth in order for life to imbue the hundred bones of the body. All generations–past, present and future–inherently have the grounds for absolute goodness within them. However, it is not within the Qì and blood of the physical vessel that our Xìng of Heaven is contained.[80] After we are born, our knowledge starts to open, and our Center of absolute goodness is disturbed by the seven emotions. In order to have a clear and yet clearer understanding of virtue,[81] first we are required to put the Heart at ease.*
>
> *Without worries it can find itself in its proper place, stopping where it is supposed to be. Once the Heart is harmonious, it is preserved and the Xìng is nurtured. Therefore, the true Dào is to stop only at absolute goodness.[82] If one neglects this, the selfishness of our flesh, blood and bones, leads desires from the outside into one's Heart. When the Heart is indecisive, randomly coming and going, then one slants away from virtue daily. How does one enter this orchard and pick the fruit? How does one know where to stop?[83]*

---

[78] "When the heart begins to function, it enhances the blood's momentum with spiraling impulses." R. Marinelli, B. Fuerst, H. Zee, A. McGinn, & W. Marinelli, *The Heart is not a Pump: A Refutation of the Pressure Propulsion Premise of Heart Function*, Frontier Perspectives, the Journal of Frontier Sciences at Temple University, Philadelphia, Fall-Winter issue, Volume 5, number 1, 1995.

[79] Zhōngqì (中氣).

[80] The physical body and the flesh and blood are impermanent, temporary, whilst the principle is timeless. Therefore, focusing medicine on just the physical body is inherently flawed; one may as well just do autopsies.

[81] The phrase Liú uses here is *míng míng dé* (明明德): To be clear and yet clear again about virtue, or rather, to be *crystal clear* about virtue.

[82] Zhǐwū zhìshàn (止於至善).

[83] Great Learning commentary, p. 16-1-2.

Heaven is not contained in blood or Qì, but in our Center, which is absolute goodness. This is our ultimate stopping point. While we need the Qì and blood along with exterior attachments and the movement of emotions to live, these same necessities are also the cause of our decline. Hence, we must always come back to Center, to Xìng. Defining the nature of this work with words is difficult.[84] Instead of using sentences to define the terms we must grind the idea back and forth, allowing it to penetrate deeper, until gradually an understanding grows in our Heart. Only when truth is felt by the Heart and not heard by the mind[85] do words have their meaning apportioned.

> *The place where the Heart starts moving and discharging is called intention. The Heart becomes appropriately upright when intention becomes sincere. Thus, the Classics talk about cultivating one's morals by making the Heart upright. So how does one separate the Heart from intention? With any thought that comes, we should love goodness and hate evil. Knowing this as our only stopping place, this is the root of the Heart. It contains within it the application of divinity, which one cannot be without: the divine is inherent within us all.*
>
> *As soon as we are born, however, our flesh and blood and our bond to the outside world creates the myriad desires and we often do not know where to stop in order to nurture our origin. Through sincere intention we become cautious of our Heart's movement. The selfishness attached to our body and things outside of us harms us inside. Our Heart fails to maintain uprightness as exterior distracts us.*
>
> *In Pre-Heaven, our Xìng is the foundation of our Heart. As soon as we are born and our Qì and blood must survive in the Post-Heaven, our Pre-Heaven perceptions start to shift with the disturbances of the seven emotions. We are thankful to our physical body for without it we cannot be born, but it also gives us anger. The human body contains the Heaven principle and originally there are no male and female Hearts in the Pre-Heaven; however, when the Qì forms, there is thick and thin, clear and turbid. Some have goodness and others less so. To be clear and yet clearer about virtue means that someone is clear about their Pre-Heaven Xìng, and that is it.*

---

[84] See Lǎozǐ's (老子) Dào Dé Jīng (道德經) chapter 56: zhī zhě bù yán, yán zhě bù zhī (知者不言, 言者不知), *Those who know do not speak, those who speak do not know.*

[85] Whilst the Dào may not be far from us, we make it so with our minds, endlessly lost in thoughts.

> *Xìng is the body of the Heart while the Heart is the application of Xìng. They are interdependent. However, Xìng originally has no action while the Heart has understanding and is enlivened within. This liveliness creates movement and goes astray, becoming false and complicated. Through this, the Qì that comes at the beginning–at birth–is fettered with greed. Practicing sincere intention enables us to restrain the Post-Heaven movements of the Heart; thereby we prevent our lucid mind from being nurtured. Our Xìng is clear about divine matters and is upright, whilst the Heart ensnared with the physical body creates disturbances in this clarity.[86] If the Heart is not upright, how can morality be cultivated? And so Zēngzǐ emphasized that within the body the seven emotions lean us away from Center; therefore, without the skill of an upright Heart there can be no internal cultivation. In order to pursue this method of examining oneself and controlling the Heart, one must reach a harmonious Center and through much effort the Heart ceases to discharge selfishness. Shedding its selfishness, the Heart becomes enlightened and listens to the commands of Heaven.[87]*

Our sincere intention is different from our desires; indeed, it can restrain those that lead us astray. Cultivation of the Heart, Xīnfǎ, is a method to free ourselves from outer attachments and desires which, when internalized, cause illness of the body and mind.[88] Our first step is to recognize that we must work on ourselves constantly. This is the path Shí Yīn Fū trod and we too can start discovering our lost Heart. This initial spark of sincerity must be nurtured; otherwise we remain debating words and arguing with our mind.

> *Intention is the Heart. Separating this, the Heart is the root and the intention is the place from where it discharges. Sincere intention is the root of the absolute Heart, which controls discharging movements. We must be cautious of this movement if we wish to complete Heaven's principle; therefore, Zēngzǐ*

---

[86] Upright meaning appropriate. Our Xìng is innately appropriate regardless of circumstance.
[87] Great Learning commentary, p. 35-1-2.
[88] "All that we are is the result of what we have thought: we are formed and molded by our thoughts. Those whose minds are shaped by selfish thoughts cause misery when they speak or act. Sorrows roll over them as the wheels of a cart roll over the tracks of the bullock that draws it." E. Eknath, *Dhammapada: Buddhas zentrale Lehren*, trans. P. Kobbe, Random House/Goldman, Munich, 2006.

clarified the principle of the upright Heart. The Heart of the Dào has principle: the Heart of the human has desires. If one desires to have a pure Heart, then one must have Dào Heart without that of the human. Without knowing how to stop only at this point of sincere intention, how are we to reach the Xìng of Heaven? At its core, the human Heart is nothing but the Dào's Heart, which is filled with pure principle and can penetrate the stars.[89]

Whilst understanding our inner realm may be a formidable task, with diligence one can see beyond ordinary perception. After starting on this path Xīn Dé could see the poor inner conditions of the monk who had failed to regard his parents appropriately and both he and Shí Yīn Fū knew their time and place in the world. Their ceaseless efforts of self-cultivation allowed them to observe with their Hearts and they developed an awareness beyond the common experience.

The high level disciples of Buddha and Lǎozǐ widely construct metaphors that people rarely understand, saying that it cannot be taught to the absent-minded and absurd. The inferior students are even more negative with their words, cheating and bragging with their lies. Would they just heed the joyful words about the Sun and Moon, about qián ☰ and kūn ☷ !

When Heaven and Earth had yet to differentiate the Sun and the Moon, existence was without physical appearance. The oneness of Yīn and Yáng had yet to divide and all was connected to Tàijí. When Separation began, the Sun and Moon gained their physical forms and true Yīn and Yáng began their transformation. As soon as there is movement, it gives birth to Yáng; as soon as there is stillness, it gives birth to Yīn, all mediated via the Sun and Moon. In the midst of movement there is stillness, in the midst of stillness there is movement. And so the Sun and Moon nimbly give birth to nature. The divine within the human Heart is connected to this creation. The Heart Yáng has essence and is pregnant with Yīn in Pre-Heaven. In the Post-Heaven, our Yīn physical vessel cannot be without Heaven's Yáng.

It is the principle of Pre-Heaven Xìng residing within the vast energy of the universe, through which we can recover a Heart of pure oneness. And so life is possible and life is

---

[89] Great Learning commentary, p. 35-2 to 36-1.

complete. The Xìng is complete and so life is resolute. The Yáng aspect of Xìng is bright and evident and so it holds in its arms the glory of the Sun, shining without exhaustion. The Yīn aspect of Xìng continues endlessly, truly containing the essence of the Moon, circulating and shining over us again and again. So how was it that the sage came to know the spirit of transformation of the myriad things? Without pattern and out of confusion, after looking at the many components of the physical body, he saw the divinity of the Sun and Moon and their alternating brightness. Through the skills of preserving the Heart, nurturing life and Xìng and following Heaven, through advanced study of these we can understand that the union of Heaven and Earth are one.[90]

True to the nature of Chinese philosophy we continue our journey deeper into the subject matter. Like making bread, we must knead the dough before we can bake it. Our body comes to life when the vessel acquires Heaven Yáng. Facilitating this are our *Recharging Instruments:* a connection between our structure and the Dào. Our ears carry sound into us, our mouth accepts flavors, our nose gathers air, our eyes absorb colors and images, our skin accepts warmth, light, and touch, all of which dissolve into our Center. These pathways of information lead in from the outer world and down via the right side of the Hùnyuán circle, avenues for Heaven Yáng to be absorbed, concealed and integrated into the flesh and blood. As such, our physical body provides residence for Pre-Heaven's Xìng.

And so anything that is outside of the body is all distant, while the primary thing within the body is the Heart. The myriad affairs of existence find their root within the Heart, revealing the closeness of distance. Sincerity, uprightness and cultivation: these steps must be urgently performed. Wind is an instrument of Heaven and Earth that expresses itself and is easily seen. For the human being, this equates to the Will. Mencius called it the vast energy of the universe, absolute greatness and strength, directly reaching at nurturing and not harming. Human life receives the absolute principle of Heaven and Earth through the mouth and nose, not knowledge or intellect; it is the Qì of qián ☰, Heaven's origin that we receive. Xìng is distributed to the body, relying on the vast Qì of the universe, which is Heaven's command.[91]

---

[90] Doctrine of the Mean commentary, p. 117-2 to 118-1.
[91] Doctrine of the Mean commentary, p. 127-2.

Heaven's command is the qián ☰ principle within us, the One Vibrating Thread, our Dào Heart. Being alive means constant movement, yet within the Dào Heart this movement is so subtle and refined that it *appears* still. This is seemingly the void in our Center as our perception of subtlety is stunted. Xīnfǎ seeks this apparent stillness within movement, what Liú Yuán calls *observing the subtle*.[92] When we observe movement, this is the *human* Heart. When we observe the subtle, this is the *Dào* Heart.[93] Both are the foundation of our existence. The Dào Heart is contained within the Concealed Circle, the realm of Tàijí, a true circle with no beginning or end.[94] Thus, when contemplating *constant movement* that never reaches an Apex, it has the appearance of stillness. Finding ourselves in the maze of the myriad things, the human Heart can only recognize movement that has an alpha and an omega. Therefore, we struggle to grasp the principle of Tàijí with our intellects; yet when we do, this is called an *upright Heart*. The human Heart is tranquil, reflecting its origin. There is no movement, just rotation.

> "Do not move! Rotate!"
>
> Chén Zhōnghuá

Heaven Yáng enters the body through the Recharging Instruments and Unification, ultimately reaching and nurturing the true principle in our Center, thereby promoting life. Continually contemplating Center is an important aspect of our cultivation process, especially for those of us practicing medicine.

On the concept of Center, Zhōng (中).

We must only stop at virtue, which is absolute goodness. How does Heaven do this? And how can mankind also achieve it? The answer is found within the Heart. There is a Dào Heart and a human Heart. If one wants to quiet the human Heart and have only the pure Dào Heart, one must have the skill of movement and stillness. Stillness is the root of movement and in the

---

[92] Absolute stillness is death, which is brought about prematurely by excessive movement. More on *Observing the Subtle* in chapter 8.

[93] "...as for Heaven and the Sage, their only virtue consists in their never allowing themselves to be restricted or blocked...a virtue that, almost by definition, depends on the ability to maintain at all times the position of *centrality* (zhong)..." F. Jullien, *In Praise of Blandness: Proceeding from Chinese Thought and Aesthetics*, trans. P. M. Varsano, Zone Books, New York, 2008, p. 49.

[94] These thoughts are taken further in chapter 7, *Tàijí: Without an Apex*.

> *Doctrine of the Mean, the concept of a harmonious Center is discussed at length. If there is no Center, there is no harmony. Without harmony, there is no Center. Man absorbs the uprightness of Heaven and Earth. The purity of Pre-Heaven is absolute goodness, as is that of Heaven and Earth. This is where we receive our Center. When we nurture the non-discharging of the Heart in the Post-Heaven, this is the same Center.*[95]

Our Center is connected to Pre-Heaven, and is the energy source of the Post-Heaven, as long as our emotions are stable. Striving for calmness, stillness and humility is a step toward creating a harmonious Center. Using our previous analogy of the set of scales, when the scale is balanced, this is harmonious. The Center cannot exist for long without harmony and so we must bring our emotions back into line.

> *Without seeking absolute goodness in everything outside of our body we cannot nurture and preserve the inner body and the Heart. Therefore, when we embrace evil our Center is in chaos.*[96]

> *If what was not yet discharged is instead embraced and contained within and one does not have even the finest thread of selfishness, then this is called Center. Center is the deepest part of the body: one cannot see it. However, what is contained in the root of this Center is the accumulation of the myriad true principles. This is the grand foundation of all under Heaven. When the root is in the Center, then one has a natural disposition to be good, and from here we take action. The Center is where all the emotions discharge from. When the principle regulates the myriad affairs, this is called harmonious, reaching the Dào under Heaven."*[97]

For many who seek this path, discovering the Center and Heart is uncharted territory. For more still, the process is never even considered, floating through life until the last day. In traditional cultures all over the world, scholars buried themselves in ancient scriptures searching for better words, unaware that the deepest knowledge comes from within.

---

[95] Great Learning commentary, p. 19-2.
[96] Great Learning commentary, p. 20-2.
[97] Doctrine of the Mean commentary, p. 54-1.

On Absolute Sincerity, *Zhìchéng* (至誠).

And so despite the vastness of Heaven and Earth, there is only this one absolute sincerity.[98] The human being, even though relatively small, is also just this one thing. Indeed, all of the myriad things follow this principle of absolute sincerity. What comes out of Heaven we call Tàijí and what comes out of man we call Xìng. The names are different, however, in reality they are synonymous. A person who has absolute sincerity has a Xìng similar to that of Heaven and Earth.

This issue contains the truth and it can develop and grow the myriad things. Mencius advises to directly nurture upon the grand energy of the universe contained between Heaven and Earth. Confucius says the admirable join with the virtue of Heaven and Earth, joining with the brightness of the Sun and Moon; with the spirit it understands good and bad fortunes. There is Pre-Heaven, which exists without conflict, while the Post-Heaven receives the seasons and this essence grows the myriad things.[99]

On self-cultivation and goodness.

Earlier generations did not know virtue and that virtue is the Xìng of Heaven's decree. They emptily clutched at learning with cleverness which unavoidably makes it difficult to cultivate morals, organize the family, control the country and make all under Heaven peaceful. After the time of Confucius, people read the texts and seemingly understood. However, they missed the principle, so how could they run the country? They did not realize that one must not stop until they have reached absolute goodness, which is preserving the Heart and the practical side of our Xìng. The words of Confucius fell upon blind eyes and deaf ears and people never pieced together his many texts, linking all the concepts. One must learn it and handle every aspect of every affair in the proper manner.[100]

---

[98] Zhìchéng (至誠).
[99] Doctrine of the Mean commentary, p. 103-1.
[100] Great Learning commentary, p. 22-2.

Studying the Classics for the sake of the Classics has never resulted in sincerity, uprightness or true knowledge. Time and time again throughout the history of China we find stories of those who, despite learning from the Classics, still went against Heaven's principle and suffered for doing so, lost in the realm of the myriad things. Thus, Liú points out that simply reading and memorizing ancient texts is not sufficient: one must reach the principle of the matter. Only then does one come to understand that the text itself is of no significance. It is only through grasping the principle that truth is found.

> *And so a person must have the knowledge of Heaven in their thoughts. Heaven is where true principle arises and when mankind attains it they become virtuous. Attaining this principle, then we know the Dào: knowing Heaven and therefore knowing humanity. Knowing humanity aids one with one's own cultivation. This all comes down to the Five Cardinal Relationships: ruler and subjects, father and son, husband and wife, brothers and sisters and friends.[101] These five are merged with Heaven and with mankind. Friendly feelings are connected between us: all things relate to each other. Neither the knowledgeable nor the dull-minded fall outside of these relationships. This is reaching the Dào under Heaven.[102]*

> *And so each person receives this goodness, yet each has their own slanting away from their Center. Like being simple and unadorned, respectful, frugal, benevolent, honest, compassionate; all these qualities are different in each person. These qualities are all virtuous. If you attain one of these you are a high level scholar. If you master all of them you are a person full of goodness.[103] Some people attain Qì, which is pure–copious goodness and sparse evil–and to this they add study, thereby transforming whatever evil there is and not indulging it. They gather goodness and bring it back to their Center: this is virtue. Absolute virtue, which encompasses the ideas of benevolence, righteousness, propriety and music, can be difficult*

---

[101] *Father and son.* Traditionally in China, daughters would marry and move to their husband's family household; hence, they could not stay with the parents like their brothers would. This social circumstance then defined Confucian values. It is not that daughters were ignored; as they would eventually have to leave, the relationship between the father and son was emphasized. For our purposes, the relationship would read *Parents and children.*

[102] Doctrine of the Mean commentary, p. 82-2 to 83-1.

[103] Shànrén (善人): A philanthropist, charitable, good-doer.

to attain.[104] Everyone achieves according to their individual capacity, putting what they can into practice. The mouth should not overflow with words that are inappropriate, the body should not commit inappropriate actions and then goodness Qì[105] becomes resolute and overflows with the Heart.[106]

Although one may feel alone on the path to discovering goodness, those choosing to follow it share the road with individuals like Liú Yuán and Liú Bǎigǔ. All who seek Center harmony, from the novice to the Master, become one and the same, following the same Dào.

On Water and Earth, Sun and Moon, energy and body, Pre- and Post-Heaven.

Earth is the amalgamation of Water and soil joining together creating form, so Water flows within the Earth. This is the only thing we can call peace and calm. Regarding the issue of Water and Earth, movement and stillness share the same root. Water and Earth are not easy to explain. Earth is not just soil, but rather Water and soil joined together. When we observe the physical Earth, it is actually Water and soil that we see. However, in Pre-Heaven Water floats and serves as Yáng, whilst Earth congeals and serves as Yīn. This is the rubbing and tossing of Heaven and Earth in Pre-Heaven. In the Post-Heaven, Water carries Qì in order to move; the Earth contains essence and has the ability to create. This is Heaven and Earth forming the material world.[107]

The living vessel materially is a marriage of Earth (the binding structure) and Water (the visible liquid circulation of blood and fluids), yet it is the formless that governs our interaction with the material world. The formless is the principle of Heaven and the cycles of the Sun and the Moon. Earth is the still body, Water is the moving energy, Heaven is what drives it all, the source of mankind.

---

[104] Music in ancient times was used to create harmony between people.
[105] Shànqì (善氣).
[106] Doctrine of the Mean commentary, p. 103-2 to 104-1.
[107] Doctrine of the Mean commentary, p. 116-1 and 117-1.

On concluding terms and definitions.

Therefore, a noble person has virtue and finds no fault when examining their Heart. With the movement of every thought they must add caution, cherishing the absence of evil inside their Will. If there is something the noble person still cannot reach, it is within the issue of being human. If there is something they cannot see, it is within the Heart.[108]

To *know words* means knowing the one origin of the myriad things. The myriad words are the paints and pastels. All of our study into the Heart of medicine reveals two components of understanding.

一 The principle of our Center, our fixed point of reference, is approached with the following words: One Thread of Life, stillness, Heaven's Principle, Pre-Heaven, Natural Character, Xìng, Dào Heart, Tàijí and Wújí, Concealed Circle, 三 and ○.

二 The principle of our relationships, the continual movements of the external world, are approached with the following words: Qì, Yīn and Yáng, Shàoyīn and the other segments, Unification and Separation, Fire and Water, Sun and Moon, Inner Fire and Outer Water Circles, the seven emotions, internal and external diseases, zàngfǔ, Post-Heaven and the myriad things of the material world.

None of 二 can in and of themselves be the truth. This is our training space, our research academy where we diligently pursue our purpose: to be an honest reflection of 一. It is through our relationships (the Five Cardinal Relationships in Confucian teachings, as discussed later) that we reveal our strength of Xìng and where we find the Lost Heart of Medicine.

In the end, one may find solace in studying virtue, the myriad terms and hypotheses and yet there are still miles to go before we sleep. Beyond understanding goodness, we must scrutinize the intentions of the Heart, the desires that enter and provoke movement and the emotions that discharge and perish in the exterior. These are the gifts that grant us life and also cause our demise. The foundations and definitions from the passages in this section will assist our practical explorations in the remaining chapters as we try to comprehend what is actually *in* our Hearts as physicians.

---

[108] Doctrine of the Mean commentary, p. 128-1.

One night the ship foundered in a storm. The scholar anxiously watched the crashing waves and held tightly to the mast. The sailor approached the scholar and asked him, "Have you, my good man, by any chance studied swimology?" In puzzlement, the scholar could only shake his head. "That really is too bad," said the sailor. "You have wasted your whole life, for the ship is sinking."[109]

Buddhist story

---

[109] Feldman & Kornfield, (eds) (1991) p. 252.

CHAPTER 3

損心

Sǔn Xīn

The Lost Heart

When people lose their dogs and chickens, they know how to look for them, but when they lose their Hearts, then they are truly lost.[1]

Mencius

As discussed in the introduction, Hùnyuán medicine explores life through the analogy of a circle. Delving further into this concept, we elucidate the meaning of being *alive*. Forming the very foundation of medicine, this awareness will govern our attitudes and be reflected in those of our patients. Intellectual discourse moves into an appropriate Center as explained in the teachings of Liú Yuán, along with the rotation of Unification and Separation and forms a practical, tangible path for physicians. It is time to find our Heart.

Unification is our connection to nature. We absorb nature when we eat, breathe and drink. It penetrates us with colors, shapes, sounds and touch. The deepest aspect of our daily Unification happens at night when we sleep. We *plug* back into the source and recharge. If we eat healthy amounts of nutritious, fresh seasonal foods and drink clean water, breathe unpolluted air and get some sunlight on our skin, embrace the ones we love and spend our days surrounded by nature, listen to soothing music, go to bed early and rise early, it follows that we are recharging ourselves well, promoting good health and staving off illness in our later years.

全心全意

Quán Xīn Quán Yì

'Whole Heart and Soul.'

---

[1] 人有雞犬放，則知求之；有放心，而不知求. From book one of the Philosopher Gào.

> "What you hear these gentle spirits sing,
> the lovely pictures that they bring,
> are more than an empty magic-show.
> Your sense of smell will be delighted,
> your palate, too, will be excited,
> and then your sense of touch ecstatic glow..."[2]
>
> Mephistopheles

While the high tide of Unification is at night, and Separation during the day, the body also unifies during our waking hours. Our Recharging Instruments facilitate this when we eat, breathe, drink, look, listen and *feel*. A constant connection to nature through Unification *must* be maintained, regardless of the time of day. The opposite is also true. Complete Unification only occurs when we expire, so to sustain life there must always be an element of Separation present. At night during the Apex of Unification, our heart beats and our lungs breathe. Subtle movement within stillness. This is the truth of Yīn and Yáng.[3]

By missing this truth we often find that we ourselves, along with those around us, including our patients, are off Center. Frequently, we separate too far and wide, without balancing the equation. In the end though, all accounts *are* balanced, one way or another. Considering contemporary living, stumbling out of bed, dosing up on coffee, forgoing breakfast, racing to work and spending the day staring at a computer screen, listening to empty words by (*Wounded Warrior*) co-workers and supervisors, with synthetic fabrics rubbing against the skin, quickly consuming empty calories and denatured food, racing to the gym, heating up left-over take-away food, watching TV late into the night and then going to bed for a few brief hours before it all starts again...If these are the days of our lives, *life* rapidly drains away. Soon we will be a fifty year old feeling like an eighty year old. At the very end, as we lie down and reflect...what words will we say?[4]

---

[2] J. Goethe, *Goethe: The Collected Works, Faust I & II*, trans. S. Atkins, Princeton University Press, New Jersey, 1984, p. 38.

[3] In this common image of Yīn and Yáng ☯ (introduced during the Sòng dynasty), we find a description of *life in action*, as perceived by later scholars. Yáng is within Yīn and Yīn is within Yáng. To *Tonify Yáng*, a common term in modern Chinese Medicine, would mean in this instance to increase activity during the day; to *Tonify Yīn* would be to rest more. In reality, through this dialectic Chinese medicine can advance only to a limited degree. As will be seen, much deeper then this superficial dichotomy, is a far clearer picture that helps us understand our role in medicine O.

[4] This is further explored in chapter 10, *The Concealed Words*. From the example here, we see just the surface manifestations of life in disarray. All of these stem from our response to the world, which comes from our Center. So why do people respond in an often destructive way? Chapter 8, *The Wounded Warrior*, pursues this in detail.

It is the *human* Heart that takes over and whispers in our ears that we should advance more, increase Separation, be more alive. A different demand is made when we discover our *true* Heart and Xìng. A demand for balance, a yearning for a long, healthy and disease-free life. When distracted by selfish emotions of the human Heart, our physical vessel is constantly under attack from within. As more material possessions accumulate, we think our position is improving and yet the true principle of Heaven, our Xìng, diminishes at an accelerated pace. The physical material of our bodies, including our tissues and organs, are there to *assist* the process of Unification and Separation. Being off Center stresses these same structures, leading to their premature decay. The most tangible manifestation of our relationship with the external world is the Outer Water Circle.[5]

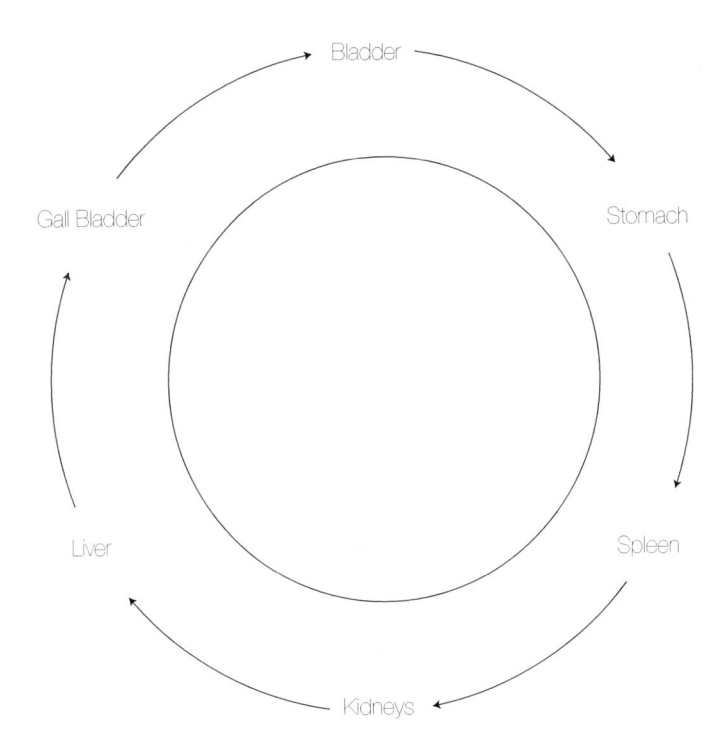

---

[5] In reference to the discussion earlier in chapter 2, we look within the kǎn ☵ trigram, viewing the core of the human being as Xìng and the physical vessel as the outer Yīn (Outer *Water* Circle). Thus, we are still dividing the One into Two.

The organs (zàngfǔ) associated with this Outer Circle, starting from the top right, are the Stomach, Spleen, Kidneys, Liver, Gallbladder and Bladder. Physically connecting us to nature and the myriad things, these *structures* assist in the ingestion and excretion of *substances*. Physiologically, nutrients and vitamins are absorbed to nourish these *structures*. In the midst of this metabolism, another far more subtle extraction takes place. The zàngfǔ are the *vehicle* by which the body receives what it requires from the environment. Our requirements are above and beyond what is contained in a vitamin pill, which is solely *material*.

An apple freshly picked from the tree contains the same vitamins and minerals as the apple rotting on the ground beneath it. Both contain *supplements*, yet only one is beneficial for human consumption. The industrial revolution has taught us how to *industrialize* our food, thereby eliminating the need for freshness. Yet the apple ripe on the tree has something the rotting one does not: or rather, the process of decay implies the *loss* of something. Often, the industrialized food we consume has lost its connection to what gave it life, and what gives us life. Chinese medicine would use the term Qì, as described in chapter 2, or *energy* to explain it.[6] Liú Yuán teaches us more eloquently, and names it *Heaven Yáng*. When consuming substances imbued with Heaven Yáng, it is this Yáng that is subtly extracted and diverted deeper into the body. It is therefore vital that everything we and patients consume, is inundated with this subtlety.[7]

天人合一

Tiān Rén Hé Yī

"Unity of Heaven and Humanity"

---

[6] Qì (氣), which can be translated as gas, vital energy, weather, air, smell, anger or annoyance, light, force. See chapter 2 for more on the complications and implications of using this *word*.

[7] In our clinics we are constantly searching for the right word that describes the living state perfectly. This word does not seem to exist. Qì, Heaven Yáng, freshness, they are all devoid of meaning until we place some upon them. In the end they all represent the principle of Heaven within the human being.

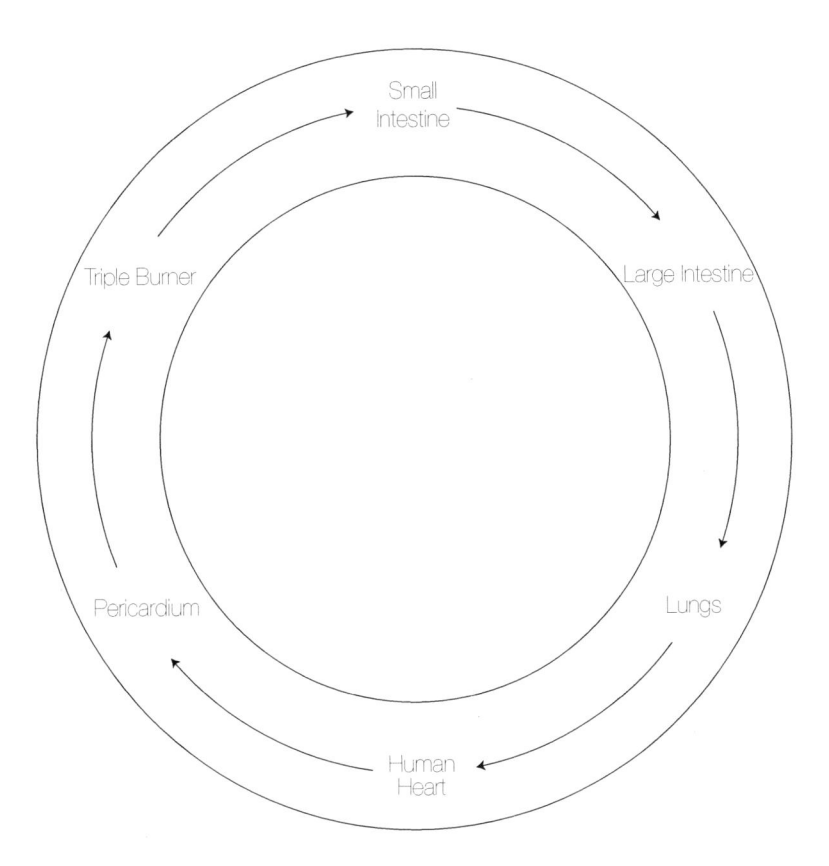

Diagram: Inner Fire Circle with organs arranged clockwise — Small Intestine (top), Large Intestine, Lungs, Human Heart (bottom), Pericardium, Triple Burner.

The Outer Water Circle is the most exterior and evident part of the picture. One step deeper resides the Inner Fire Circle, which accepts and distributes Heaven Yáng. The organs associated with this circle are the Large Intestine, Lungs, human Heart, Pericardium, Sānjiāo[8] and Small Intestine. Since the body is not a neutral realm, but must maintain a homeostasis of warmth, we call this internalized Yáng our *True Fire*.[9] Thus, the Heaven Yáng absorbed from what we ingest becomes part of our True Fire, giving the body more spark. Perishing is defined by spending more of this Fire than we save. The process of extracting and utilizing Heaven Yáng requires an expenditure of

---

[8] Sānjiāo (三膲): An interesting organ complex in Chinese Medicine encompassing the lower abdominal cavity, upper abdominal cavity and the thoracic cavity. Commonly translated as the Triple Burner or Three Heater.

[9] Chinese medicine calls True Fire, *Emperor Fire* and metabolic fire, *Minister Fire*. There have been millennia of confusion about these terms, leading to some disastrous approaches to medicine.

energy, placing further emphasis on sound dietary and medical investments. Medically, when assisting a patient with their recovery, we must ensure that what they eat and drink (including our medicines) does not denature them further.

> "My stomach pains me when I eat too much," the man said. "My throat is parched when I grow thirsty..."[10]

As Heaven Yáng arrives at the bottom of the Outer Water Circle, the Kidneys direct it inward to unite with the human Heart. This internal alchemical exchange happens at night during the peak of Unification. Shàoyīn, the relationship between the Kidneys and the human Heart, holds the key to a superior understanding of health, well-being, fertility, emotions and medicine in general. The inward movement of information from the external world becomes part of our Inner Fire Circle, helping the body recharge during sleep. A human being, though, is more than just a living vessel. We connect to nature, animals and other people through our *relationships* to them. In the diagrams above we see the placement of the human Heart in its functional relationship with the Kidneys.[11]

Foods or medicines that contain a deficit of Heaven Yáng offer the body very little, yet to metabolize them still requires energy. The amount spent on breaking down and processing this material does not equate to what is gained from them. The future fertile capacity and longevity of ourselves, our children and our patients, depends on an understanding of what it is that we *need* from what we ingest. If our food and medicines are full of Heaven Yáng, while we use an ounce of energy to process it, we gain back two ounces. This extra Yáng then becomes part of our True Fire, which can be either conserved wisely or spent frivolously.

Part of this *spending* happens when we wake up each morning. Our vessel awakes from weariness as the accumulated True Fire from the day before discharges from our Center. This gives momentum to the Inner Fire Circle, which in turn spins the Outer Water Circle into life again. These are the building blocks of our circulation, our warmth: c*ircle-ation*. Liú Yuán refers to this discharging of True Fire from the Center as *emotions*, or the seed of outwardly observable emotions. The bottom left side of the circle, the area governed by the Liver and Pericardium, is where True Fire sparks us into life. Under healthy conditions this spark simply gets the circles rotating. If excessive, however, one *displays* emotions such as rage, anger, frustration, irritability and resentment. Its purpose, though, is to be

---

[10] Feldman & Kornfield (eds), 1991, p. 230.
[11] The *human* Heart is differentiated from the *Dào* Heart in our Center, both of which are differentiated from the anatomical heart.

contained within and get the circles moving.

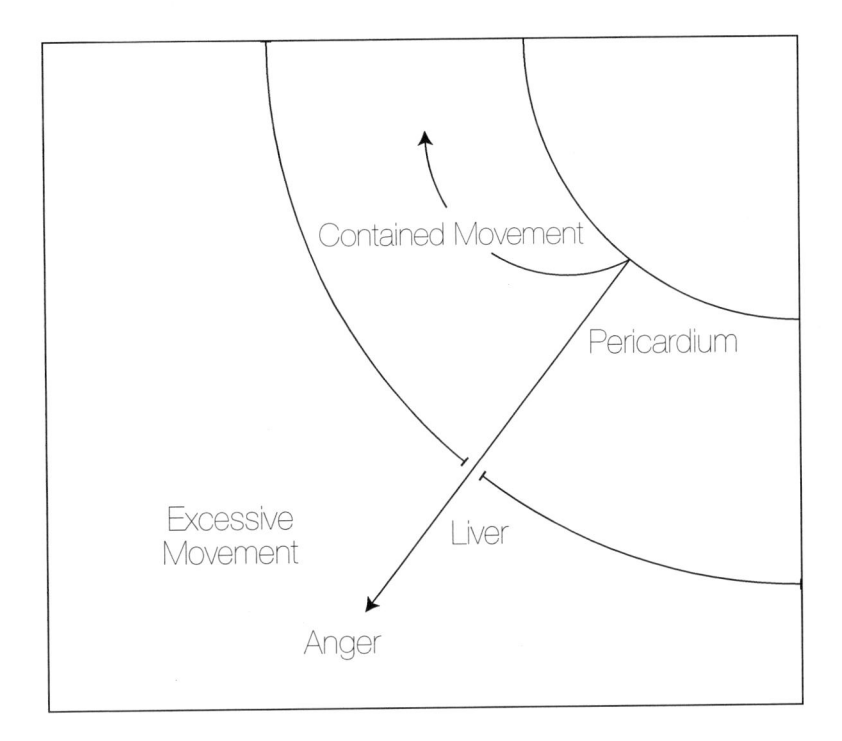

Diagram: A quadrant showing "Contained Movement" (with upward arrow) in the upper region, "Pericardium" labeled on the outer arc, "Liver" labeled on the inner arc, "Excessive Movement" in the lower left, and "Anger" with a downward-left arrow.

Emotions are needed to move the circles, and when regulated, they do so without becoming visible. When discharged recklessly, however, they separate from the Inner Fire Circle out through the Outer Water Circle, damaging the associated tissues. Otherwise, in their purest form emotions are elements of internal movement, controlled allotments awakening the vessel at dawn and settling it at dusk. The warmth from our external environment is internalized downward and inward on the right side of the circles, into Unification. It is from the bottom left side of the circles where our True Fire leaves our Center on its way into Separation. Anger, agitation and volatility are manifestations of excessive movement outward from Center, which can occur day or night. Too much True Fire is discharged and these particular emotions damage the Liver and Pericardium. In gynecological terms, for example, this relates to menstruation: a discharging movement of blood from the inside to the outside. Over time, excessive anger and frustration can damage and then obstruct this outward movement, which is often an issue found when investigating the root of menstrual disorders.

We all have *visible* emotions, expressed in the broad categories of anger, fear, sorrow and happiness. Whilst natural, these external manifestations are a reflection of our Fire leaking from our Center. Utilizing the instruments of Unification appropriately–what we take in through our mouth, nose, eyes, ears and skin, as well as good sleep–we can recharge vibrantly. Heaven Yáng obtained via the Outer Water Circle *should* give us our daily vigor, but by allowing too much leakage of Fire, our Center decays. A gradual and graceful decline becomes a rapid descent. From the dawn of birth to the eve of death is one path.[12] Our task is to alert our patients, family and friends, to the understanding that the finishing line they are sprinting towards is their own inevitable demise.

> I dream of you far, far away
> > beyond the blue sky.
> These eyes that once gave you shy glances
> > now fill with gushing tears.
> If you double my breaking heart
> > come back and look with me into this mirror.[13]

> Lǐ Bái

The Inner Fire Circle represents the deep internal circulation of True Fire that must constantly be preserved. It should be a relatively closed circuit, as when we lose warmth we lose vitality. Like the Center of the Earth, a hot core burns within us, defining our life span: once used up and extinguished, so are we. Slowing this process is the responsibility of the Outer Water Circle and through its digestion and excretion of material, we gain the immaterial. This adds one drop of Fire to our Center.

At the Center of all this transformation and change is our Xìng, anchoring life to the vessel. Xìng is *neither* the Outer Water Circle nor the Inner Fire Circle,[14] but rather it is our connection to Pre-Heaven residing within the Center. Both the Inner and Outer Circles belong to the Post-Heaven and start their rotations from our first cry outside of the womb. After we are born, we begin living and in the process lose sense of our origin as we *mature*, moving away from Center. At night as sleep overcomes us, we

---

[12] On this eve, a person may more easily experience their Center and express it with their final words. The Pre-Heaven state reveals itself and they see the unity of the myriad things. Then time stops. These last moments, and their importance, are discussed in detail in chapter 10.

[13] Lǐ Bái (李白) (701–762 CE), famous Táng dynasty poet, *Endless Longing*. Quoted in M. Cheng, *Master of Five Excellences*, trans. M. Hennessy, Frog, Ltd, Berkley, 1995, p. 45.

[14] Or, in different words, not the *human* Heart, a mistake Liú Yuán saw too often in the religions of his time. More to come on this later.

are closest to our origin. The eyes close and desires diminish, the movement within our Heart slows and becomes tranquil.

From birth our Recharging Instruments engage the new world. The discourse above articulates the importance of diet and sleep, but what of our eyes and sight, ears and sound, nose and smell, our skin and touch? If a person eats a bad banana, a few minutes later they have an upset Stomach. Twenty minutes later they may have diarrhea or vomiting. Sight, sound, smell and touch enter us much faster, however, and equally affect our health.[15] The outer world is constantly inundating us with stimuli, awaiting our reactions. People who sit in front of computer screens day after day will be exposed to a very different form of Qì than a gardener or a beachcomber.[16] What we look at and how we see things all contribute to how our emotions move within us.

> I will prescribe regimens for the good of my patients according to my ability and my judgment and *never do harm to anyone*.[17]
>
> From the Hippocratic Oath

A harsh word, or alternatively, one of kindness, pierces us and can instantly harm or heal. What penetrates through the eyes, ears and touch, streams directly into the Heart, forming a direct line of communication from the outside to our very core. From here, our emotions can be led astray as we respond to the changes around us. Our True Fire leaks and our Xìng is left unguarded. An example is when a patient sits opposite a fertility specialist, a physician in whom all trust is placed, and they are told that their eggs are old, follicles too few, or that their sperm is inferior and they will never bear offspring naturally. These words can cut straight to the core, leaving the

---

[15] Regarding the skin, for example: "[The] quality of touch...will provide the emotional comforting, the tactile information, and the integrating experience so acutely needed by the distressed individual... the human skin has a marvelous intelligence of its own, and possesses the means of carrying [healing]...to the very core of the person being touched." D. Juhan, *Job's Body: A Handbook for Bodywork*, Barrytown, Station Hill, New York, 2003, p. 56.

[16] This is our entry point into this topic and as so, it is not complete. For instance, the computer user could be planting seeds of compassion in their work, while the gardener may be poisoning trees. The outer appearance of our lives is not the critique here; rather, if our patients are unwell, our job is to assist them back to wellness. Being unwell equates to lacking or loosing True Fire, so the more that can be done to address this the better.

[17] The Hippocratic Oath is for physicians, swearing to practice medicine ethically and honestly. Interestingly, another translation reads: "I will apply *dietetic* measures for the benefit of the sick according to my ability and judgment; I will keep them from harm and injustice."

Center devastated. Whilst no pharmaceutical pill or surgical scalpel has yet been used, the patient walks out of that office wounded.[18]

> "O my God!...if I was to flourish in this world and distinguish myself in those tricks of speech which would gain honor for me among men, and deceitful riches!"[19]
>
> St Augustine

Through a well-intentioned desire to be *realistic* and prevent the promise of *false hope*, the physician has ripped a hole in the patient's sense of self-worth. Unintentionally, they cause strong movements within the patient's Heart through such statements, which leads to a self-fulfilling prophecy. It is unlikely that the desperate couple will be as vigorous in their attempts to fall pregnant naturally, as their doubts and fears about their bodies have been reinforced: they are rendered *infertile*. Similarly, some terminally ill patients upon hearing a bad prognosis, soon begin a rapid spiral of decline.

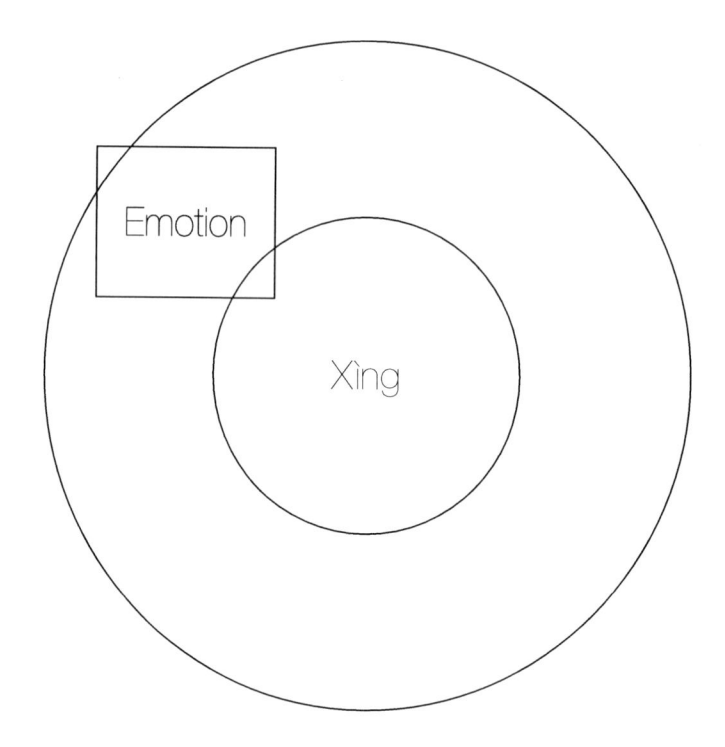

---

[18] "Dr. Xia defined medicine as "the practice of humaneness"...Humaneness, or human spirit, is the bond that links humans to nature." (Schmieg, 2005, p. 31 & 41).
[19] St Augustine *The Confessions*, Hendrickson Publishers, Massachusetts, 2004, p. 13.

The Inner Fire Circle discharges the seven emotions and the Xìng falters. Taught first by Confucius, then Mencius, Liú Yuán and now through Hùnyuán medicine, our Xìng is pure goodness. It is the *seed* of our capacity to reproduce and create, which, unless we have a great sense of self-protection, is decimated when we *believe* our eggs are *old*, our sperm *deficient*. Despite good intentions, physicians often feed this fear in their patients. When afraid, patients tend to make poor decisions regarding their health. At times, despite the most positive words, patients are defined by their circumstances to only hear negativity. Hence, our work with Xīnfǎ becomes all the more vital.

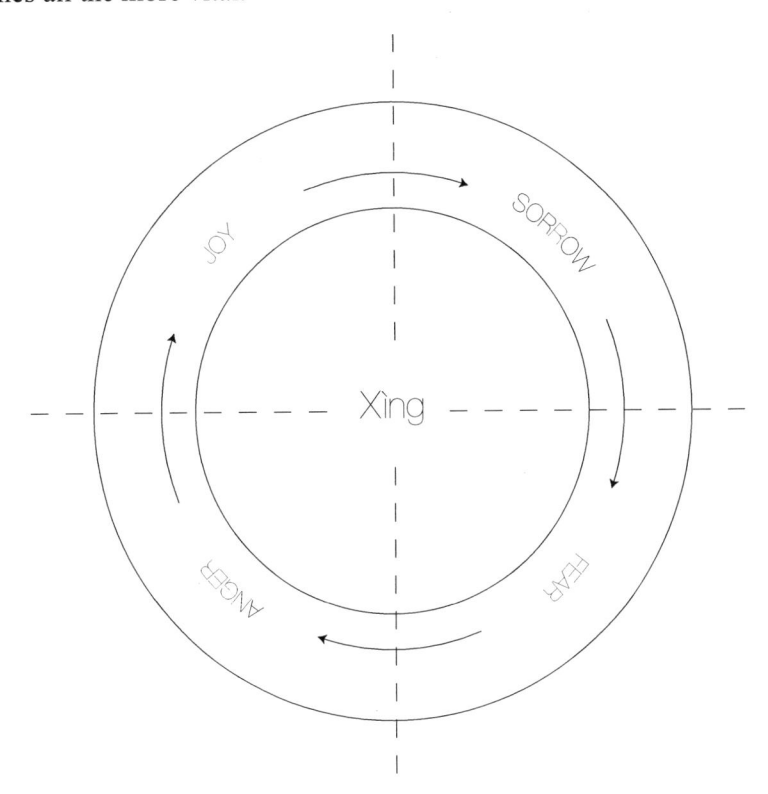

Emotions represent the rotation of Fire within our Inner Fire Circle, our *circle-ation*. Ideally, the Xìng should not be disturbed by this movement. When a physician observes a patient in physical or psychological distress, they are watching discharged emotions taking their toll on the Center, leaving the Xìng.[20] Illness reveals itself when the Xìng is neglected.

---

[20] *Are you saying that its all in my head!?* one may ask. In Hùnyuán medicine there is no division between soma and psyche, and it would be more appropriate to say that it is all in your *Center*.

Physicians actualize these philosophical constructs into practical terms, starting each and every case from the true principle of Center. Yet being Centered is not just applicable to the clinical setting. Finding this true principle is not just within the realm of doctors, monks or philosophers, but for each and every one of us. When greeted rudely by someone, how do we respond? As their emotions discharge visibly, impacting those around them, we commonly meet this with our own outburst.

Person A leaks Fire ↔ Person B leaks Fire.

Kindness and compassion come from a strong anchoring point. If we can approach such situations with kindness, which is the true reflection of our Heart, we conserve our Fire and reduce overt reactions in those around us. Being ignoble, irritated and grumpy tends to rub off on others. Unwittingly, our negativity washes out like a wave, and everyone gets wet. Instead, if we can be kind, friendly and understanding, our enthusiasm becomes infectious.

    Kindness is difficult. From childhood we have been conditioned in how to react. These lessons can stay with us for life unless they are examined and changed. Although it may be *common* for us to respond with a set of emotional reactions, it is not *natural*. Often we smile outwardly while crying inside. We have been taught to do this since we were little. Screaming on the inside while laughing on the outside are strategies for survival in the outer world.

> Indeed, inside every failed individual there is a potentially warm, loving creature struggling to get out. The trick is so to interact with the individual who has been tactually failed as to release that potentiality for something resembling the kind of humanizing experiences he should have enjoyed in infancy and childhood.[21]

Aside from writing prescriptions for drugs, herbs or acupuncture treatments, physicians must listen to their patient's words, discern them and then talk to their patient's Heart. It is a job of planting seeds of goodness, always reminding them of their inner goodness. Once all distractions have cleared, at the Heart of it our patients want to be good, kind people, both to themselves and others. In his commentary on the Analects by Confucius,[22] Liú Yuán reminds us of ourselves, of our Xìng.

---

[21] Juhan, 2003, quotes Montagu, p. 56.
[22] Lúnyǔ (論語): The Analects.

Xìng and Heaven's command are the glory of Heaven and Earth. The endless transformation of Yīn and Yáng manifests itself in the Xìng and the emotions. In Pre-Heaven the Xìng and life occupy a grand harmony: they embrace each other harmoniously. This is Yīn and Yáng at their most pure and invisible. When translated into the Post-Heaven the Xìng and the emotions become separated, and we no longer obtain this pure oneness.

The Xìng and emotions mix together. So despite the true principle, desires easily flourish. Then the joint residence of Yīn and Yáng has great difficulty in returning to oneness. We fail to see that the human Heart and the Dào Heart are in reality one Heart, with only the finest detail that can be separated from them: the propagating of Yīn and the pureness of Yáng. One must differentiate the Yīn from the Yáng to reach the essence; the one thing that must be preserved is Yáng within the midst of Yīn.[23]

The transformations and changes of Yīn and Yáng are manifestations of the exchange between Heaven and Earth. Not one aspect of these transformations are contradictory to the true principle. They are the uprightness of Heaven and Earth. One Yīn and one Yáng is the Dào. Continuing this principle is goodness, completing it is Xìng; this is the one decree of Heaven. Yīn and Yáng transform endlessly, ultimate Yīn and Yáng are the roots of Heaven. Xìng is Tàijí, the melding of Yīn and Yáng.

This instrument of creation is glorious and majestic; its appearance magnificent, as it reveals the essence of all things. True principle finds its root in the origin of Heaven and Earth, which gives birth to the human Heart. They are all complete within the Center; nimbly Heaven and man unite into one.[24]

We can express this notion of Heaven, Earth and mankind with the following diagram:

---

[23] Here we see Liú discussing what we have discussed as the Outer Water Circle (Yīn) and the Inner Fire Circle (Yáng).

[24] Analects Commentary, p. 160-2 to 161-1.

```
        ☷             ☵    ☲      ☰
      Earth         Water  Fire  Heaven
```

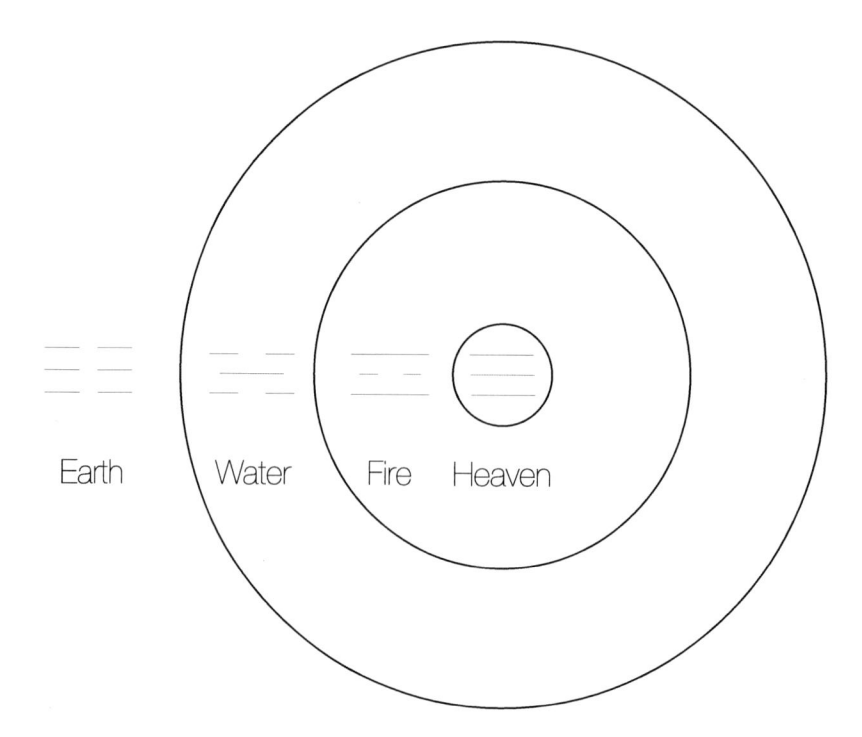

With just Yīn material (☷ kūn) there is no life; with only Yáng movement (☰ qián) there is no life. Only with the interaction of these two are Water (☵ kǎn) and Fire (☲ lí) created, giving the human being form and movement. All of these *aspects* are contained within the one Tàijí. This topic will be explored further in the following pages.

> *Principle has roots and branches; it has fine essence and crude material. Scattering, it endlessly transforms into the myriad things and affairs. In the end, it returns to one. To get to the root of it is to fix the Heart. The grand root of everything under Heaven is Center. Center is the practical aspect of oneness, meaning that Xìng and Heaven's command are in the Center of the Heart.*
>
> *In Heaven it is called Tàijí. In humankind it is called principle. Together this is the Dào. Reaching to absolute truth without Separation, principle is oneness and absolute sincerity. Within the endless creation of Heaven and Earth, this is known as benevolence.[25] Human beings receive the divinity of Heaven and Earth inside the Center, Xìng being the total pureness of Pre-Heaven.*

---

[25] Rén (仁): Benevolence, to be humane.

> *In the Post-Heaven this Xìng is mixed with the emotions. Confucius says that Xìng is how we get close to the source, close to Heaven. To Mencius, Xìng is complete goodness. Different words by different sages, but in the end it is all one principle. This principle must be put into practice, we must practice this gōngfu, otherwise how are we to teach future generations? By failing to actualize the principle, your studies and teachings exhaust your spirit in search of transformation, but the spirit within will never be understood.[26]*

Through the constant practice of sincerity, compassion and kindness, we truly reflect the endless transformations of Heaven and Earth. Eloquent and fancy words can disguise the root and, unless based on true principle, they are but branches. Shí Yīn Fū walked with three bags attached to his body, translating philosophy into practice. Each action was interpreted and understood from the perspective of principle, until this principle became his reality. Words are just floating in thin air unless grounded to Center. Through this practice we can find true meaning in our lives.

> *We attain the Heart of Heaven and Earth and are born. This is Xìng; this is benevolence, reflected in what Mencius calls the benevolent human Heart. This purity of the Heart is in the seed of Pre-Heaven in mankind. When you travel from before birth to after birth, the physical body and Qì accumulate, and through the seduction of physical matter, the ears, eyes and mouth are formed. In the Post-Heaven the body's movement is agile and nimble, being led by things outside of ourselves. Heaven's principle follows this lead, making it harder for us to be pure.*
>
> *The Pre-Heaven is purely principle, and when we make the body still and without inappropriate action, this is the place where Xìng permeates everything. In the Post-Heaven, the Xìng is too easily entangled with physical material, failing to return to the root of Heaven and Earth. Life follows along and we have the Post-Heaven Heart. The divine within the human Heart is mixed with the seductions from outside the body; therefore it cannot preserve the goodness of Heaven. Hence, the sages taught us to recover Xìng.[27]*
>
> *When we talk of the five aspects of Xìng: benevolence, righteousness, propriety, knowledge and trustworthiness;[28] these*

---

[26] Analects Commentary, p. 185-2 to 186-1.
[27] Analects Commentary, p. 203-1.
[28] Rén yì lǐ zhì xìn (仁義禮智信).

are actually just elements of our one innate moral character. In the Pre-Heaven it is all-inclusive, all within the Center, within the Heart. If you can achieve these five qualities in the Post-Heaven, you will preserve the fullness of the one Xìng. Naturally, when our Heart forms it continues its embrace of the Yīn and one cannot restrain the moving of desires.[29] However, through diligently concentrating on the vast energy of the universe with extreme gōngfu, only then the Heart truly recovers a reflection of Pre-Heaven.[30]

Our Center then becomes full with pureness, no Separation: not two things, but just one. Stillness and the ten thousand virtues are all contained within. Movement, and not even one selfish thought mixes with the Heart. Controlling our resentment and desires makes us peaceful and then we take no action discordant with benevolence. When you nurture this skill you gradually follow the principle of Heaven and selfishness lessens. Day after day in this training, the Heart becomes empty of desires and full of spirituality. No external desires can disturb the Heart. The Heart is repeatedly empty.[31]

The origin of Heaven and Earth is delivered into the human Heart. It is through nature's creation that we obtain the ultimate virtue within. So sublime, it is as if you cannot find a name for it. By itself it opens and closes; the Qì that enters recovers itself. All human affairs follow this principle. In addition, the grand harmony of Heaven's Heart is forever in the clear void of the spirit. It has no desires, no stagnation or obstructions. The human being is the Heart of Heaven and Earth, receiving energy from the interplay of Yīn and Yáng.[32]

Thus, the permeation of Heaven and Earth within the human being is reflected in our propriety. These words teach us to be *proper* in every aspect of our lives, in every relationship, in each thought and action. Liú explains further:

---

[29] Yīn here refers to the broken line in the middle of the Fire trigram ☲. This trigram represents the human Heart.

[30] Relating to the Water trigram ☵. The Center solid line represents the principle of Heaven concealed within the body.

[31] Analects Commentary, p. 204-1-2.

[32] Analects Commentary, p. 221-1.

The principle of Heaven and Earth is one and the same as the principle in the human body. In order to reach Xìng and Heaven's decree this principle must be used to the fullest. In the Post-Heaven this principle is used in the myriad affairs, and there is nothing within it that is inappropriate. Truly, it is one Yīn and one Yáng: this is the Dào. So Tàijí is the embodiment of Yīn and Yáng. When it moves, it is still, when it is still, it moves: this is Tàijí. It is movement and stillness that shapes our body and within us Yīn and Yáng separate naturally. Gradually growing and declining, Yīn and Yáng alternate, transforming into the Five Phases, becoming clear and obvious.

The Five Phases have Earth as their main element, the seed of the material making up the myriad things within the four seasons. Each phase has its own phenomena and the original Qì flows through these in a circular motion. When still, the Earth serves as a pivot. Within the Pre-Heaven the Earth is dispersed without name. In the Post-Heaven it congeals and gives Wood and Fire a place to reside and is a friend to Water and Metal.[33]

The principle of Heaven and Earth is mixed together without difference, forming endless creation and transformation. The human body is one small Heaven and Earth. Tàijí in the human body is Xìng, the master of the Heart. In the Center of Earth is Xìng; this is the Dào that makes a person come to life. The Heart is the human application of Xìng, which in Pre-Heaven is pure as if hidden in a walled garden. In the Post-Heaven, however, we must preserve the Heart of cognition and nurture the non-action of Xìng.[34] How can we tame our desires? When Heaven and the human unite into one, then there is no place where the Heart is not one with Xìng and the myriad things can no longer distract or confuse us.

Heaven, man and the myriad things are all contained within the Yìjīng, so for a thousand years the principle has been established. However, the people lost the root and sought only the branches and so Confucius' words and meaning were misunderstood. The lofty and the ordinary are all aligned in the principle of keeping Center, the origin of Heaven.[35]

---

[33] Please review the original Chinese, available from the Hùnyuán Research Institute, for information on the numerology and the *Hétú* (河圖) descriptions not translated here. The Hétú is a ancient Chinese divination system used to explain relationships between the bāguà in the Yìjīng, discussed further in chapter 8.

[34] Meaning Wúwéi (無為): Non-action, or rather non-inappropriate action.

[35] Analects Commentary, p. 223-2 to 224-1.

As physicians and patients, when we express nothing but pure goodness in our outer actions and inner thoughts, we reflect the true principle within us. Xìng is our link to life and its core is pure goodness. A lifetime, from conception to expiration, Pre-Heaven to Post-Heaven and back again, is continuous within the Heart. Even though we live our lives in the Post-Heaven, absorbing Yáng from the outer world, our connection to the Pre-Heaven comes from within. Through Xīnfǎ we naturally develop proper responses, no longer needing to excuse our emotions and ourselves.

Immense bravery is needed to overcome our desires, yet by accepting this challenge we cease inadvertently harming others. As in Shí Yīn Fū's example, once on the path of goodness he did not needlessly crush the grass beneath his feet, nor knock fruit from the tree with his hat. Beforehand, he was oblivious to his actions and inactions, his words and thoughts. We ourselves, along with everyone around us, need to learn that our absentminded intentions, which haphazardly sabotage others as well as ourselves, are equally as detrimental to us as other lifestyle choices. This same recognition is needed to shine a light on harboring harmful thoughts and feelings. We watch for them, transform them and bring them back to Center. Guilt, disappointment and despair are all far more harmful than preservatives and additives in our food. What we choose to consume, along with our state of emotional well-being, reflects the strength of our connection to Center.

> *The sole principle in Heaven is Tàijí: in man it is Xìng. When it scatters we see it in the myriad things and affairs, but it is only one principle that rules it all. The sage knows that being alive means knowledge must come through cultivating one's morals. Peaceful human relations are used in daily life, involving the principle of knowing right from wrong. These come naturally. One may ask, is the principle of Heaven and Earth within my own Xìng? Why is it so and how am I connected to the myriad things of existence? This knowledge must come from studying the descriptions of existence from the past examined today in current circumstances, in order to reach complete appropriateness.[36]*

The physician observes the patient in the present as a reflection of the past, hoping to offer a signpost to possible future destinations in health. By taking note of words and actions, we constantly direct them back to Center.

---

[36] Analects Commentary, p. 225-2.

Mencius said that through exhausting one's Heart, one knows their Xìng. These are not empty words. One must deeply contemplate them to attain his wisdom. The origin of Heart and Xìng is one and the same. It is only the human mind that makes it two. The foolish separates it. Truth is something that cannot be sought outside of the Heart, therefore the sage desires that we will only correct our Heart, become upright and recover our Xìng, our Center."[37]

Our emotions discharge from the Inner Fire Circle when the physical body comes into contact with external things. This is an interplay of Yīn and Yáng between Heaven and Earth, with us in the throes of it all. The Fire trigram ☲ has a Yīn broken line in the middle. This central position of Yīn, *the Earth within the Fire*, represents our connection to the exterior realm. The Earth ☷ and the myriad material things distract Xìng from its origin in Heaven ☰. We look out instead of in. Water ☵ has Heaven Yáng in its Center, stirring us alive in the midst of Yīn: Separation within Unification. The interplay between Fire and Water creates our ability to have emotions, desires and to reach out towards the world. Medicine walks a fine line, seeking to delay our ultimate reunion with the *origin*, the final finishing line. Yet, simultaneously it must remind us of our *connection* to this origin. Otherwise, when seeing inflamed skin we prescribe *anti-inflammatory* Heat clearing herbs. With the origin of the human being firmly in sight, the observed manifestation is seen from Center. Heat is what defines the living body from its alternative, and to *clear Heat* means to *clear life*.[38] Everything, always, must constantly be brought back to Center.

"The human being is the Heart of Heaven and Earth,
receiving energy from the interplay of Yīn and Yáng."

Liú Yuán

The totality of the myriad symptoms ☷ a patient presents with are jostling representatives of Yīn ☷ and Yáng ☰. Tàijí ☰ is the cause of life. The movement of Fire (emotions) spreading outwards (the desire for Yīn material) equates to a deficit within. Xìng is immaterial ☰ with no direct

---

[37] Analects Commentary, p. 259-2.
[38] In modern Chinese medicine the idea of *Clearing Heat* is prevalent. The physician focuses on the external symptoms that appear hot or red. By failing to observe the deeper layers, they only apply medicine to alleviate symptoms. Hùnyuán medicine teaches that for every patient, regardless of the symptoms, the one and only focus for the physician is to maintain and nourish the patient's life.

connection to *space* ☷. By looking at a patient's Heart today we may encounter issues from the long distant *past*. Despite this, the Inner Fire Circle discharges emotions in the *present*, not in the past, even if the causative factor was many years ago, many miles away. Space ☷ is irrelevant. Whilst Yīn material is often the cause of distress within the Heart, hastening the demise of Xìng, it is irrelevant in matters of *curing* the Heart. Time ☰ is constant. A Heart broken during adolescence may remain so decades later, as if the injury happened yesterday.

Excessive emotions quietly and quickly run us through, stealing the precious from our Center, mixing it with our flesh. Our Xìng is then obscured and we forget the vital importance of Unification, the connection to our origin ☰. This trigram has no Yīn lines, it has no connection to the material world; it is the pure Yáng within our Center, relating to time. Moving out one step we have the Fire trigram ☲, the bridge for Xìng to irrigate the vessel from birth to death.

On exiting the womb we desire milk, sleep and love. As a toddler we see the sun and we play. Surrounded by our circumstances, our siblings, school and parents, our emotions start to exercise themselves, eventuating in set patterns (of the Inner Fire Circle) that determines how we react to stimulus when we are older. Our formative years mold us and also our responses to the external world.[39] Being upset over someone or something is not an issue connected to space ☷. Being upset is our own response, a mirror of our Inner Fire Circle. The reflection looks back at you, not out. Reactive responses come from within and are related to the constancy of time ☰, the thread that stretches between birth and death.

The human Heart is stiffened not by physical issues or material things: it is hardened by time and memory. Time and our experiences during it, form our habits and traits of temperament. Habits learned through life distort our Xìng, resulting in distorted actions and thoughts, void of goodness. We begin to believe in our excuses, as we are eternally dependent on the flux of change to guide our emotions. Our most precious achievement is to find peace in our Center despite external changes and despite being conditioned in earlier years to react from the emotional human Heart. Achieving this results in an unshakable sense of self-worth.

The Inner Fire Circle connects the past fixations to the present. Events from the past arise and obstruct our circle-ation in the present, causing Xìng to drip, leak and perish. Through cultivating Xīnfǎ our internal

---

[39] "From infancy we concentrate happily on ourselves...We learn to distinguish life from the inanimate and move toward it like moths to a porch light...to explore and affiliate with life is a deep and complicated process...our existence depends on this propensity, our spirit is woven from it, hope rises on its currents." E. O. Wilson, *Biophilia: The human bond with other species*, Harvard University Press, Cambridge, 1929, Prologue.

and external reactions come from a point of Center, the constant goodness within our Heart.

> When anger arrives, observe it!
> When fear arrives, observe it!
> When sorrow arrives, observe it!
>
> Hùnyuán

The cycles of Separation and Unification are the rise and fall of the relationship between Fire ☲ and Water ☵. At the Center of this daily rotation is the Heaven principle of constancy ☰, our origin. The pure Yīn of Earth ☷ is the external world that attracts our desires and appetites. The material world and Heaven's principle merge together and we have life. Liú teaches us that while we are prone to consume exaggerated amounts of the external material world with our lust and desires, draining our inner Fire, the solution is not to isolate ourselves away from the world. Through training we can relate and interact with the material world with pure goodness. And that is it.

> "If you can accomplish propriety of the Five Cardinal Relationships, you have already reached a sagely level. This accomplishment is achieved through one word: selfishness. Or rather, one must remove all selfishness in order to truly accomplish these relationships. To remove selfishness means to only think of the other person, never think of oneself."
>
> Liú Bǎigǔ

Liú Yuán, along with his great grandson after him, revealed how to achieve this practically with the Five Cardinal Relationships. Our relationships highlight the amount of Heaven principle within our Heart. This is the Dào of Confucius and Mencius, where the Heart naturally expresses itself in its surroundings. Traits, habits and mannerisms dissolve and true individuality emerges, rather than a figment of society, customs, culture and circumstance ☷. Acting with kindness and compassion is timeless ☰, not relegated to a certain dynasty or era. The kinship we have with other people is our way of reflecting the quality of our Xìng.

    Presenting with palpitations, a patient wants a prescription to prevent her physical problem. However, in this case the cause is not physical as the onset of symptoms coincided with a relationship breakdown and a *broken* Heart. Xìng becomes mixed with the emotional reactions of the Inner Fire Circle programmed from earlier in life, creating a current chaos. Herbs and drugs cannot reach inside this space and instill resilience, but seeds of goodness can still be planted there.[40] Facing down sadness and fear, we must do so with kindness.

> *It is only Heaven's principle that commands mankind: this is Xìng. What is in Heaven is this command, this destiny. What is in mankind is Xìng. Earlier scholars separated this principle, calling it two. Seemingly this is an obvious conclusion–mankind is separate from Heaven–yet this is not the case. The one origin of Heaven's principle dominates the origin of all living things, a domination growing and Separating forever, never exhausted. Heaven's true principle enters mankind and we attain the true Qì, becoming alive.*
>
> *The complete Tàijí of Heaven is contained totally within our Center. Due to the transformation of the physical body, we cannot keep it completely concealed, like inside a walled garden. Whenever we lose our upright Heart, we lose the essence of being human. Once evil perverts the Heart, the transformation of Qì spoils and declines, failing to support life. Living means to be connected to the principle, otherwise you are not really living and here we see two separate extremes.[41]*

"To live is the rarest thing in the world. Most people exist, that is all."

Oscar Wilde

---

[40] "Take what you like. Plant them in your garden and let them grow." H. Jūnshēng, *Chen Style Taijiquan Practical Method/Volume One: Theory*, eds. H. & Z. Chen, Hunyuan Taiji Press, Edmonton, 2006, p. xi.

[41] Analects Commentary, p. 462-2.

Two extremes, like day and night. As we cycle through these extremes we must always have a connection to Center, otherwise we are boats bobbing in a stormy sea. With a sturdy anchor we prevent our spontaneous and impetuous *common* reactions to stimuli. During the day we connect to the exterior world. During the night we connect to the origin. Without this link, our Qì transformation perishes; life decreases and disease escalates. In all of this, though, we must remember that the Heart, *our Heart*, is not the enemy. It is our companion and when harmonious and proper, life springs from us like a fountain.

> *One's Heart cannot be restrained or forced into submission. It must be empty and still with no movement of emotions or desires. Only then does one nurture oneself and the Heaven principle replenishes. The Heart completely controls Yīn selfishness, and so without any desires one can clearly hear life's command and perceive the one pureness. Controlling and then overcoming the Heart, this is not the art of warfare between Heaven and man.*[42]

> *Heaven's principle is just one, and that is it. When this principle is invested in mankind it becomes benevolence, residing in the Heart and is the Yáng principle of pure Xìng expressed in the Post-Heaven. The Heart is not the enemy. Rather, it is the mixing of Yīn selfishness within us that separates the Heart into two: the human Heart and the Dào Heart. The human Heart must recognize the divine. One cannot do without it and must use propriety in order to dominate it.*[43]

Mastery of the Heart means we do not meander from goodness. This is a true reflection of who we can be. From Liú's perspective, denying this is a lazy excuse, an easily routed hypothesis based on habits, traits and customs. It is true indeed that it takes all kinds to make a world and true individuality is only expressed when we are honest about who we are. Underneath the layers of circumstance that we take to be the gospel of our lives, we all have Center. Practically, in medicine this should be our one and only concern. Does our treatment help the patient come back to Center, to live a longer, healthier and more peaceful life? Or is it just a panacea, natural or otherwise?

---

[42] Commentary on the Analects, p. 286-2.
[43] Analects Commentary, p. 287-1.

A patient presents with swollen lips from an unknown cause. Initially this looks like an Outer Water Circle situation, yet upon investigation we find that he only likes to consume very strong flavored foods and fluids. Spicy food, strong coffee, lots of salt and pepper. From one point of view, we could say that these substances have deteriorated the Spleen and Stomach zàngfǔ. However, from a perspective of Center, we must ask ourselves why he only wants to eat these extreme flavors. He tells us that they make him feel alive. When we suggest that he should eat bland foods for a few days, he insists on a prescription of herbs so that he can continue eating as he habitually does.

In reality, this is a Xīnfǎ case. His desires have made his diet a habit, an excuse, which has resulted in a digestive tract malfunction, revealed in his swollen lips. The body is taken to the edge, hovers, then falls. Once we recognize this as a Heart problem, our urgency is to remedy the Center, not the swollen lips. Without healing the Heart, he will not transform his habits and his digestive tract will become even more compromised, leading to further disease in the future. Therefore, treatment involves mild and bland herbs that will not aggravate the swollen lips, along with strong Xīnfǎ coming from a passionate doctor.

Here we must highlight an important exception to the attitude towards *excessive* emotions described above. Being passionate when teaching or helping others, and using one's emotions does cause a leakage of Fire from our Center. However, engaging in the propagation of goodness aids our own physiological and emotional systems. It lubricates the Inner Fire Circle, which drives more life force into Shàoyīn via the right side of the Outer Water Circle. At night we sleep soundly as our Heart is at peace with itself. Goodness also ripples outward, affecting those around us and creating a useful impulse in society. When negative emotions ooze from us, we leak from our Center, finding it difficult to get energy from our food and fluids via our Recharging Instruments and we are awash with woes. This is useless and worse, it is destructive.[44]

風口浪尖
Fēng Kǒu Làng Jiān

At the Heart of the Struggle
'Where the wind and the waves are the fiercest.'

---

[44] "Our life is shaped by our mind; we become what we think.
Suffering follows an evil thought as the wheels of a cart follow the oxen that draws it.
Our life is shaped by our mind; we become what we think.
Joy follows a pure thought like a shadow that never leaves." Siddhārtha Gautama

"Let me give an example: A physician sees the patient and endeavors to discover what is wrong, what is incorrect within their Hearts. No matter the circumstances that the physician finds themselves in, they only think of the patient. If they can only treat the body, this is fine. If they can go deeper and treat the Heart, even better, but the intent is always what is best for the patient. There cannot be even the slightest thought of selfishness in this process. Then I will say this is a good physician.

There is another kind of doctor, however, whom I hope you will not follow. They see the patient, perform the four diagnostics, then write a prescription. As the brush moves a thought creeps into their Heart; 'if I add some more expensive herbs into the mix, I will profit more...' While there are these kinds of doctors, this is not the way of your path. You will perform your diagnostics of the body and if you find that the disease is in the Heart, you help them heal at this deep level. Then I will say you are a Great physician."[45]

Liú Bǎigǔ

Physicians and teachers must use their passion like a surgeon wielding a scalpel, excising the tumors of turmoil with their goodness. The answer is not detachment, being *emotionless*, living in a walled garden sitting in our selfishness. If we can learn and *then* help our patients learn to build a walled garden around goodness, thereby protecting it from distortion. Emotions reflect Xìng and we live in Center. Using emotions to create harmony is Xìng in practice.

> It begins from deep within, burning
> it tears through me,
> shining brightly, it cannot be missed,
> glowing in my reflection
> there is no escaping.
> How light I feel, how free.
> Like the rain and clouds
> it comes and it goes,
> but briefly
> between the mists and fog,
> I see the sun.

Anon.

---

[45] 良医 (liángyī): Means a good doctor, but also implies someone who radiates ripples of goodness.

心曠神怡

Xīn Kuàng Shén Yí

'The Heart untroubled. The Spirit pleased.'

CHAPTER 4

能伸能屈
Néng Shēn Néng Qū

A Time for Giving and a Time for Taking

Heaven gives birth to the hundred grains in order to nurture the people. Upon these grains all living beings, the animals, beasts, fish and dragons are nourished. At times we use animals for our own purposes, but when we take of them we must do so for virtuous reasons, and not out of selfishness. The virtuous slaughter animals scarcely. They use a hook to catch a fish, not a net to gather many. They use an arrow to shoot a bird, not hunting chicks and eggs in their nest.

The sage's benevolence and righteousness was upright and correct and he did not abuse the living world. Future generations, however, have no regulation regarding food, doing as they wish. Daily acquiring new tastes, they poison the divine in life with their search for new delicacies. The prince and ruler can also be injured by this indulgence. Prohibition of killing and releasing caged animals nurtures the benevolence of our Heart, promoting filial piety.[1]

Here, Liú Yuán articulates the difference between *using* life and *ab-using* it. Modernity reveals this in the extreme when considering animal testing for beauty products and pharmaceuticals along with factory farming, a business paradigm dominating the supply of animal protein in the majority of the First World.[2] In a sense, this could apply to anything that we consume.[3] As humans, we are often conflicted by the thought of taking life to sustain our

---

[1] Commentary on the Analects, p. 228-1. For most people, filial piety means respect for the parents, but actually it has a broader reference, indicating the proper relationship between the human being and nature.

[2] For a detailed debate on this, see J. S. Foer, *Eating Animals*, Little, Brown & Company, New York, 2009.

[3] As, for example, is expressed in the Indian religion of Jaina Dharma, or Jainism and the practitioner's relationship with food and non-violence. For more on this, see J. E. Cort, "The Jain Knowledge Warehouses: Traditional Libraries in India", *Journal of the American Oriental Society*, 1995.

own. Modern society perpetuates this by separating consumers from the production and harvesting of their food, resulting in prepared, cleanly packaged end products housed in the walls of the sterile, local grocery. In reality, everything we consume, plant or animal, is *killed* to maintain our life, though we may prefer other, less harsh language for our comfort: harvesting, butchering, processing, preparing, reaping, and so on. We *kill* the apple when we eat it, as for us to survive we must ingest living material. It is this element of *living* that is absorbed and recharges our Center; engaging the life force contained within other *things* so we can function and achieve our purpose. Within the Post-Heaven realm there is a natural give and take to life and death, thus we can leave behind guilt and suffering and through cultivating our choices, we follow the correct path through the Center of Yīn and Yáng.

A natural giving is made by the living world for our survival and this gift must be honored. By constantly seeking the path of self-cultivation we act using empathy and kindness when dealing with other people, animals, plants and ourselves. The price paid by the life we consume is then re-paid with our virtue, helping life in return. Sustaining life necessitates a movement of giving and taking, a two-way street: an exchange. The tree absorbs nutrients and water, sunlight and carbon dioxide and gives oxygen, shade and stability. When we ingest a plant we are ingesting a physical material, one that has been formed by the process of sunlight (Heaven Yáng) being transformed into a leaf. As this leaf passes through us, our Recharging Instruments convert this material and extract out the same Heaven principle that went into its creation. From Heaven Yáng to our True Fire, we use this precious extract to engage in our life and relationships.

The capacity of the physician to be *proper* in their relationships is not defined by the continually transforming circumstances that abound and surround us (as discussed in chapter 10). There is one constant for our lifetime: the principle of our Center, which is total goodness. And that is it! For as long as we are breathing, this is constant. Everything else will change, including the Inner Fire Circle and Outer Water Circle, or rather, our anatomy and physiology along with the myriad things inundating the world around us. If dependent on sunshine for happiness, clouds bring sorrow. However, if we are only dependent upon the constancy of our Center we are anchored to peacefulness and tranquility, even in times of turmoil. This is the goal of Xīnfǎ.

"We'll see," said the Zen Master.[4]

As described above, our life is a time for taking from the environment–the Yīn material world–in order to sustain ourselves. Consequently, it is also a time for giving and if we depend only upon our Center, the niceties of others does *not* determine our benevolence. We *give* to all, not just the kind and honest. A time for giving is a time for forgiving, even those who are unkind, vain, or conceited.[5]

Self-forgiveness is perhaps most difficult and takes the most time. By taking responsibility for the mistakes they have made, the physician takes the first step to overcoming this obstacle, understanding that they are not defined by historical circumstances. Otherwise, those who have been bullied will have to remain a victim, the Inner Fire Circle continually *wounded* by the ghost of that abuse. With kindness, the physician takes time to forgive themselves and others and through their own cultivation, they give of their time to reach out their hand, assisting their patients out of their own Inner Fire Circle turmoil.

Herbs and acupuncture, pharmaceuticals and manual therapies all access and act on the Outer Water Circle. When used effectively, they reduce the demands the patient's physical body places on their Xing, smoothing the material interactions between their organs and the environment. These treatments are not only beneficial, but also necessary as they can curtail wastefulness. Endeavoring to go beneath the layers of this entry level of medicine the physician utilizes Xīnfǎ, the Heart Method, to reach deeper levels of healing that clinical practice often demands of them.

---

[4] This famous Zen story was referenced in an article in the New York Times in 2008. We give our abridged version here...
This tale tells of a Zen master who observed the villagers celebrating a young boy's new horse.
'Is this not a wonderful gift?' they asked him.
'We'll see,' said the Zen master.
The following week, the boy falls off his horse and breaks his leg.
'Is this not a terrible accident?' they asked him.
'We'll see,' said the Zen master.
The following month war breaks out, yet the boy cannot be conscripted due to his injury.
'Is this not a wonderful blessing?' they asked him.
'We'll see," said the Zen master.

[5] "Love of one's enemies? I think that has been well learned: it happens a thousand fold today, on a large and small scale...we learn to despise when we love and precisely when we love best – but all this unconsciously, without noise, without ostentation, with that modest and concealment of goodness which forbids the mouth solemn words and the formulas of virtue." F. Nietzsche, *Beyond Good and Evil: Prelude to a Philosophy of the Future*, trans. R. J. Hollingdale, Penguin Books, London, 1973, p. 148.

Along with a prescription, they plant a seed of goodness in their patient's Heart, reminding them of their true nature.

> "When a patient catches a cold, for example, the physician should administer herbs for the outer problem. Yet at the same time, through careful investigation, they must find out what else may impact the situation in the patient's Heart. Then they adjust the movement of the Heart to influence the ailment in a positive way."
>
> Liú Bǎigǔ

Intractable diseases require medicine to penetrate as deeply as possible. Physicians must evaluate and engage the Heaven principle within their patients, as this is the source of life. Focusing on Center, patients are strengthened by thoughts, intentions and most importantly, actions. Herein lies the practicability of Xīnfǎ. Clinical manifestations are endless and may guide the physician in formulating treatment, yet it is the patient's *Heart* that is *always* the Center of medicine.

Despite past events, present day attitudes can be transformed, including *how* historical influences impact the person now. Xīnfǎ can be accomplished through listening, speaking, touching, writing, living according to principle and *looking*. Eye contact is a powerful tool. Too often the physician has their head down, lost in their thoughts...*which clever herbs or points to use for which clever patterns or symptoms?* Instead, when acknowledging that human beings absorb information from the outer world via *all* of their senses, specifically the eyes and ears in this context, then these *must* be utilized *as* treatment.

This does not mean to look *at* the eyes, like getting an iris-scope to look closer and closer under a microscope. This *physical* observation would simply reveal more about the *physical* body, the Outer Water Circle. Acupuncture and herbal prescriptions along with other modalities could be formulated with this information, all the while forgetting to ask *why* the vessel would be in distress. We want to look *into* the eyes. This takes no skill or method derived from a university or college; rather, it takes empathy and kindness, observing the patient from a point of Center. The physician listens with their Heart, hearing what comes from the patient's Center. This is only possible when the doctor's Xing is not obscured. We become better at our work when we clear away obstructions of negativity from within ourselves and then apply this Centered perspective to medicine.

> If I had no love,
> then were my words as sounding brass or as a clanging symbol...
> it would all be for nothing.[6]

To honestly approach a patient from Center, the physician must have *time for giving*. Xìng is concealed within and relates to the Heaven ☰ principle. A case example revealing this in the most rudimentary of terms shows how *effective* medicine requires *time*. A patient in her fifties presents in clinic, suffering daily frontal headaches (an Outer *Water* Circle symptom). After visiting her local doctor some weeks before, she was informed of promising research suggesting the use of Botulinum toxin (an acutely noxious substance) for headaches.[7] Unfortunately, this treatment failed to relieve her symptom and so she sought an alternative approach. Our investigation into the problem, which took *time*, revealed that the only fluids she would consume was a single cup of tea in the morning. Just from these few words, clarity emerged.[8]

In this case, by allowing and giving time, the physician did not need their prescription pad: they needed to be a teacher. Two weeks later, after being *prescribed* water, she returned and had not experienced any headaches. Effective and defective medicine is largely dependent on *giving time*.[9] For all patients, even when not a Xīnfǎ case, giving extra time for a *proper* investigation changes the face of medicine entirely. For true Xīnfǎ cases, this determines the physician's ability to reach the patient's Center. R*us*hing a consultation is never about the patient. When the physician does not have *time* ☰ to see their patients, has become too b*us*y, they change into a b*us*inessperson, a technician and factory of p*harm*aceuticals ☷.

---

[6] Rudolf Steiner's translation of Paul's letter to the Corinthians (1 Corinthians 13, Holy Bible).

[7] See, for example: S. Silberstein, N. Mathew, J. Saper, S. Jenkins, *Botulinum toxin type A as a migraine preventive treatment*. For the BOTOX Migraine Clinical Research Group, Headache: The Journal of Head and Face Pain, Volume 40, Issue 6, pp. 445–450, June 2000.

[8] See: S. M. Shirreffs, S. J. Merson, S. M. Fraser & D. T. Archer, *The effects of fluid restriction on hydration status and subjective feelings in man*, British Journal of Nutrition, Volume 91, Issue 6, June 2004, pp. 951-958.

[9] "It's a question of feedback, really, of people getting the information essential to keep their efforts on track. In its original sense in systems theory, *feedback* meant the exchange of data about how one part of a system is working, with the understanding that one part affects all others in the system, so that any part heading off course could be changed for the better." D. Goleman, *Emotional Intelligence: Why It Can Matter More Than IQ*, Bantam Books, New York, 1995, p. 172.

They have lost their Heart of Medicine *even* if what they prescribe contains Heaven Yáng. To engage the unwell is to give of oneself without any trace of selfishness. True medicine, when not foc*us*ed on us, truly does no harm. Physicians remain clear about the virtue of their work ☴ and are not distracted by the material manifestations which wish to creep into their Inner Fire Circle ☲.

Effectively, our Heart is always exposed to observations of the external world. When observing confronting situations the human Heart discharges emotions and extreme movement of the One Thread of Life can occur. Unchecked, internal sickness will follow. External sights can discharge the human Heart, an outward movement often detrimental to the healing process. However, research has shown that the reverse is true when looking at the harmonious state of nature. Patients in hospital beds that overlook a grove of trees recover faster than those facing brick walls.[10] The to and fro of swaying branches in the natural world inspire us to look inward, observing our own Hearts. With this, internal movement settles, assisting our recovery.

Sensory information connects directly to the Inner Fire Circle. What we experience on the outside often triggers our internal habits of behavior and reaction. However, then observation turns inward, external stimuli cease pulling at the ache in our Hearts. The relationship between physician and patient is thereby defined; only by observing from a point of Center can the doctor successfully *know* the patient's *words*. By seeing and hearing clearly, we can instruct the patient how to search for this same internal stability. Then the real healing begins.

> "Whenever a person cannot endure humiliation or tolerate rejection,
> it is because their blood and Qì are stiff and unyielding,
> their emotions are agitated and explosive."
>
> Liú Bèiwén

---

[10] "If you were a patient in a hospital bed, just waking up from surgery, what would you prefer to see when you opened your eyes–a brick wall or a grove of trees?" E. M. Sternberg, *Healing Spaces: The Science of Place and Well-Being*, Harvard University Press, Cambridge, 2009, p. 25. The results for this research point to our interconnection to nature and how when we or our patients are close to their own nature, the Xìng, recovery is imminent. "...you suddenly notice the dappled sunlight on the blinds and no longer turn your head and shield your eyes. You become aware of the birdsong outside the window....You no longer dread the effort needed to get up..." (ibid. p. 1).

Xìng is the Heaven principle within us that determines our Center's ability to rotate the circles of physiology. Adjacent to the Center is the Inner Fire Circle that manifests in our emotions and desires. A step further out is the Outer Water Circle, the aspects of the vessel that interact materially with the outer world. The Xìng is the momentum force in our Center that allows our emotions to come out, *giving* life to the physical vessel: the molten core in the middle of the Earth. Our Xìng is guarded in the Center and innervates the body but must never be imbued with the Yīn material of the physical world.[11]

When we are conceived, the genetic strength of our Outer Water and Inner Fire Circles is received from our parents and our lineage. But we are also *given* Heaven principle, which is not a *material*, not genes (or their expression) or chromosomes. It is the life principle within our Center, the eternal principle of goodness Liú refers to as Xìng. Xìng is our life-definition, our nature:

> A scorpion asks a frog to carry him across the river. The frog is afraid of being stung during the trip, but the scorpion points out that if he were to sting the frog, they would both sink and drown. Appeased, the frog agrees and they begin their journey. In the middle of the river, the scorpion stings the frog and they both sink. On the riverbed the frog asks the scorpion why he doomed them both and the scorpion explains that it is simply in his *nature*.[12]

---

[11] Yīn material, *Yīnwù* (阴物), is the term used to differentiate exterior substances from the pure True Yáng in our Center.

[12] This fable is used to illustrate that behavior in people and animals alike will fall back onto their true nature, regardless of circumstance. The nature of humankind is of pure goodness and we will return back to it but instead of waiting to the last moments of our lives when true goodness is always apparent, we can return to it now. Regardless of this understanding, "Cautious ones would note that people are not rats..." F. Leavitt, *Evaluating Scientific Research: Separating Fact from Fiction*, Prentice-Hall Inc, New Jersey, 2001, p. 29, Contemporary scientific medicine persists in extrapolating research data from animal studies to human *beings*.

The seeds of human inception are *parents*. Hence, the utmost importance of proper care for couples seeking help with fertility concerns: future *mothers* and *fathers*. Medicine demands from us this understanding and puts into perspective our role in reproductive health or assisting in-vitro fertilization and other modern fertility techniques. To excel in reproductive medicine, doctors must contemplate the *purpose* of medicine and the facilitation of our future generation's capacity to maintain their Xìng. The physician does not stand by the banks of the River Styx.[13] One coin may be needed to cross at the end but in the *beginning* the body must be imbued with Xìng.

All Yīn material entering the body impacts the Outer Water Circle. Vitamins, minerals, medications and fertility drugs work by altering the function of the physical body. For example, if you have loose stools, you can ingest a lifeless drug and the diarrhea turns into constipation. Chinese herbs are likewise capable of altering the Outer Water Circle to ameliorate symptoms. However, altering the physical body (the Outer Water Circle) is the entry level of medicine: the barefoot doctor.[14]

Going yet a step beyond the entrance, we can alter the Outer Water Circle to become *symptom-less* and *also* guide the patient back to their Center. At the very least the medicines we dispense must resolve symptoms *and* guard the True Fire, and the latter cannot be accomplished with *dead* substances. Rather, when there is no Heaven principle to extract we can waste our Fire trying to deal with the *stale* materials we bring into our *living* body. Artificially structured lifeless chemical compounds (drugs and vitamins) belong to the social and economic trends of the 20th century. In the 21st century we should remember what is constant and embrace medicine of the Heart.

Thus, we cradle the fundamentals of sustenance. For the Outer Water Circle to accomplish its relationship with Yīn material, the Inner Fire Circle must rotate. In the morning, the Inner Fire Circle impulse starts its movement outward, our eyes open and the Heart desires the apple on the tree. Our living vessel then walks to the tree and picks the fruit. Reaching for the apple had its seed in the movement of the Inner Fire Circle. In this

---

[13] In ancient Greek mythology, the *River Styx* is the boundary between Earth and Hades. During times of sorrow, people rationalize existence, which informs ritual and culture. The ferryman, Charon, would transport souls across if they had a coin to pay him. Relatives would therefore place a coin in the mouth of the deceased. Physicians, on the contrary, and particularly those in the field of fertility, receive their fee in order to conduct life from the parent across to the child. The doctor is the kindly ferryman at the beginning of life.

[14] Barefoot doctors were invented in the 1960s in China during the *Great* Proletarian Cultural Revolution (Wénhuà Dàgémìng 文化大革命) to meet the demands of healthcare in poor rural areas. These doctors had minimal training and yet were expected to achieve great results.

example we can see two things happening simultaneously. There is the physical ability of the body to grab the apple, ingest, digest and excrete it, and there is the desire to rise, go outside and walk into the orchard. This is the *desire for life*, for survival, which comes from the Inner Fire Circle. When our eyes open and images come into the body from the material world, along with the smells and sounds, our Heart starts to discharge, and this is the awakening of Separation.

> "Aside from a few pains and aches
> that the physical body endures from external factors,
> most of physical diseases are born from the seven emotions going astray."
>
> Liú Bǎigǔ

When the eyes transmit an image of the Yīn material inward, it is just a picture. The picture in and of itself has no real power. How our Inner Fire Circle processes this image is what gives it dominance. Desire does not come from the outside, not the apple or any physical substance or place. Thus, we are often confused when seeking the origin of emotions and desires in the material realm. Rather than a physical organ or tissue, which are all contained in a lifeless body,[15] desire comes out of Center.

    The Center contains Xìng, or the Heaven *movement* principle we are endowed with at conception. In medicine, we should not be in a morgue performing autopsies. When we find ourselves there then we know we are off-track. Attachment to physical material that is not essential to our survival weakens our capacity to contain our Xìng. The more we bond with images, sounds or smells from the external material world, the more dependent we become upon them for our happiness, and the more Xìng we lose as a result. Information moves into us and we expend our energy in our reactions and actions accordingly.

    This all revolves around our Center and the Xìng guarded therein. The fact that we can go about our business and be active in the world is predetermined by the fact that we have Xìng. Therefore, this principle of Heaven movement is our focus as it defines *living*. Desires and emotions move outward from our Center using the movement potential of Xìng. As children, our circumstances mold our Inner Fire Circle, defining how we react and attach to stimuli as adults.

---

[15] Once a person passes, the body has no Xìng. It is the only thing that separates us from the deceased, hence its vital role in the application of medicine.

Often we are attached to the emotions of fear and worry,[16] naturally falling back onto them when there is sudden change around us.

> We struggle, we grow weary, we grow tired. We are exhausted, we are distressed, we despair. We give up, we fall down, we let go. We cry. We are empty, we grow calm, we are ready. We wait quietly. A small, shy truth arrives. Arrives from without and within...Arrives and is born. Simple, steady, clear. Like a mirror, like a bell, like a flame. Like rain in summer. A precious truth arrives and is born with us. Within our emptiness. We accept it, we observe it, we absorb it. We surrender to our bare truth. We are nourished, we are changed. We are blessed. We rise up. For this we give thanks.[17]
>
> Leunig

Our emotions come from nowhere. No *place*. This *no-where* is our connection to the principle of Heaven in the *now-here*. Put simply, if we are looking at a lifeless body, what we see is what we get: a decomposing physical structure ☷. So what makes the observer alive? The works of Liú Yuán describe the source of life with varying terms, yet they all point in the same direction.[18] The answer is in our Center, in quiet stillness: the residence of Xìng ☰. This is undetectable materially, regardless of the sophistication of our technology and machinery.

---

[16] "...there is the potential for a peculiar conflict in this partnership between our fears and our intellect, particularly because we have trained our intellect to consider only objectively verifiable, consistently measurable facts in its deliberations and conclusions. The problem is this: the sources of anxiety are ever-present and powerfully compelling, while the establishing of certainties which rely upon the assemblage of incontestable facts tends to be slow, methodical and subject to distressing surprises and reversals...Anxiety is neither an argument nor a piece of objective data, but a feeling state, an especially pervasive feeling state which can affect the operations of the mind in a way that mere arguments and data never can..." (Juhan, 2003, p. 6).

[17] M. Leunig, *When I Talk to You*, HarperCollins, Sydney, 1990.

[18] One could use the words life, energy, metabolism, spark, spirit, force, freshness, Dào, Qì or God...
"At the back of the classroom sat a little girl who normally didn't pay much attention in school. In the drawing class she did. For more than twenty minutes, the girl sat with her arms curled around her paper, totally absorbed in what she was doing. The teacher...asked the girl what she was drawing. Without looking up, the girl said, 'I'm drawing a picture of God.' Surprised, the teacher said, 'But nobody knows what God looks like.' The girl said, 'They will in a minute.'" K. Robinson, & L. Aronica, *The Element: How Finding Your Passion Changes Everything*, Allen Lane, Camberwell, 2009, Introduction.

Yet this is what we contemplate with Xīnfǎ, beyond an understanding of material found within a lifeless body. In reality, we are alive as long as our physical vessel has but one drop of Heaven Yáng ☰.

One's Heart cannot recharge whilst uniting with physical material as this is an outward moving process. However, during this outward movement we can still invest in ourselves. Reaching for the apple is an outward movement but then by ingesting the life from it, a drop of potential is added to our own. Anything that we can collect in this way during our waking hours is then filtered, condensed, and unified, guarding our Center while we sleep. We take a little life everyday from the material we consume, consolidating it through our recharging at night. The flower opens its petals with the rising sun, attracting the bees and butterflies, but at night they close and the Center is protected. The flower is complying with its *nature*.

If we eat and drink well but allow our Heart to be constantly anxious, we waste our collected resources and our health declines as a result. Even living in a forest and eating organically is not enough. It is beneficial of course, yet if our internal world is obstructed or discharges too rapidly, we deteriorate nonetheless. While material issues like preservatives and chemicals in our food are important to address, these are just part of the story of our health. The path material substances take as they move through us is *relatively* lengthy, first traveling around the Outer Water Circle, going through the systems of distillation and elimination and then entering the Inner Fire Circle. On the contrary, when desires and emotions are abnormal, diseases can arise rapidly. This sensory path to our Center is exceptionally short. Disharmony of the Inner Fire Circle exhausts the Xìng far more readily than poor dietary choices do. Indeed, the very Heart of those poor culinary decisions is often a result of a weak relationship to Xìng. Life and health have different layers, the superficial and the deep. Understanding the importance of diet is one, cultivating the Heart is another.

As an example, a patient sits opposite us, and we find that she eats well, drinks enough water, sleeps well and *meditates* every day. During the consultation, however, she mentions an argument she had with a friend over a differing opinion. Both parties in this disagreement were issuing excessive emotions. We advised the patient that rather than falling back on her common tendency to respond to confrontation, she could reflect inward on herself, calm herself and find Center.

The next day we received a call from her reporting that she had met her friend again, endeavored to be *friendly* and they had scheduled a dinner together as a result. After this interaction she felt very light and relieved and her friend seemed happy too. This is the ripple effect of goodness. There was no real need for conflict other than satisfying the Wounded Warrior's dichotomy of emotions.[19]

Meditation is an important tool in cultivation, helping us approach quiet stillness to gain perspective. For the patient above, however, her meditation was not being used effectively. Liú Yuán urges us to focus the insights garnered through meditation on bringing us back to propriety. Through appropriate intention, thought and action, the human Heart becomes quiet and upright. For example, when fishing one should use a rod and reel rather than a trawling net. Rather than *dwelling in void*, one must work in accord with the *nature* of things. The monk who sits in the void of meditation will still need to eat his lunch and it *is* important how his food was acquired. Liú tells us that we too often mistake the *human Heart* for the *Dào Heart*.[20]

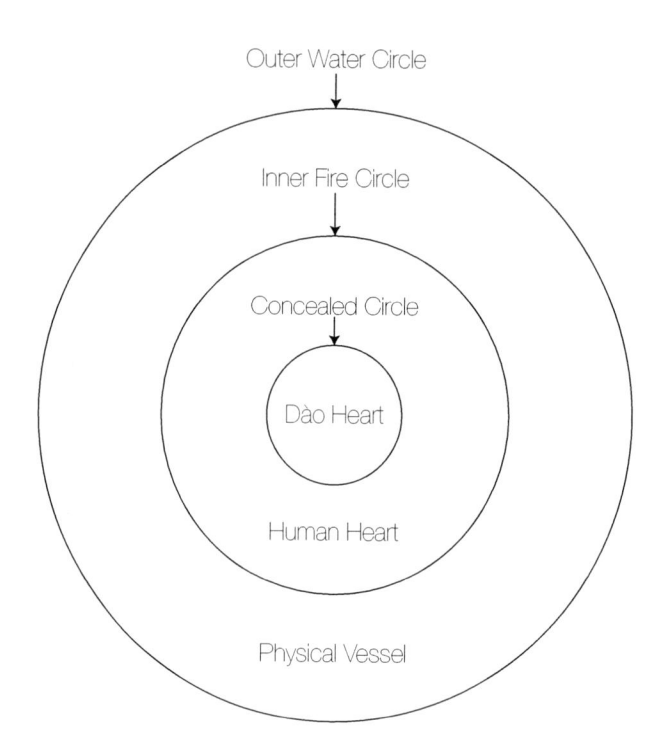

[Diagram: concentric circles labeled from outside in — Outer Water Circle, Inner Fire Circle, Concealed Circle, Dào Heart; with Human Heart and Physical Vessel labeling the inner and outer rings respectively]

---

[19] More on the Wounded Warrior in chapter 8.
[20] In the image below we refer to the Concealed Circle, which is discussed at length in chapter 7.

The concepts of *wàibìng* and *nèibìng*[21] (external and internal causes of disease) are common in medicine and we now explore them further.[22] The Outer Water Circle is the part of us most closely related to the Yīn Material of the external world. Food, fluids and medicines, along with changes in the environment can all impact the body, leading to a disease of the Outer Water Circle: a *wàibìng*. For example, eating tainted food can result in diarrhea or sudden temperature fluctuations can undermine the immune system. These are examples of the external world taking its toll on the physical vessel.

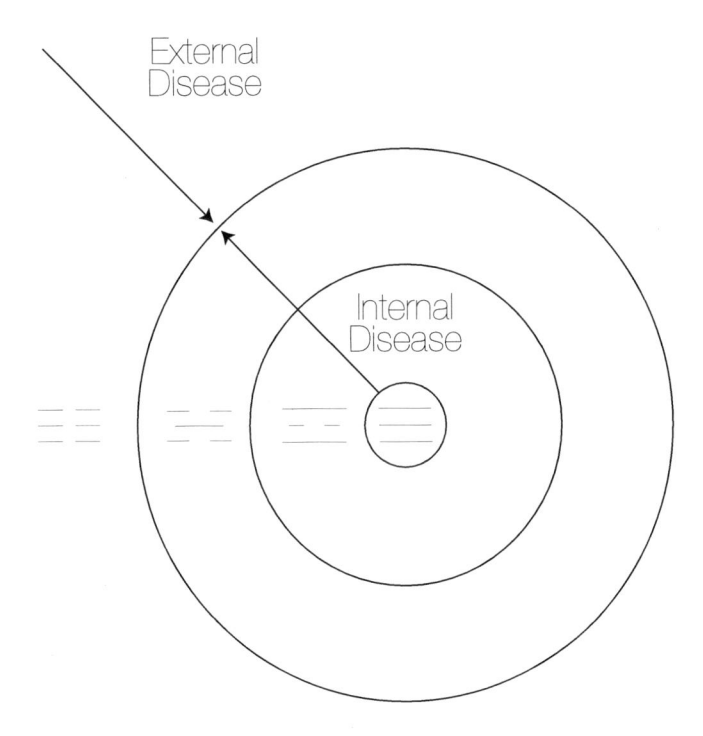

The Inner Fire Circle, on the other hand, is closely related to the Xìng and Heaven Yáng. Our emotional reactions and habits impact our Center, which can result in a *Heart* disease: a *nèibìng*.[23] Since the principle of Heaven movement is what makes us alive, derangement of this movement causes

---

[21] Wàibìng (外病): Outer disease. Nèibìng (内病): Inner disease.
[22] A western medical counterpart to these Chinese theories would be allergens or pathogens from the environment being external disease causing factors, and autoimmune or psychological disorders being internal.
[23] *Heart* disease (心病) is not referring to anatomy and physiology, but rather a disease of the Center.

major pathology. These are the diseases that modern medicine cannot cure, as everything we tend to research and treat is found in a lifeless body. Modern medicine (both Chinese and Western) looks for external and internal causative factors using pattern differentiation or a microscope, yet has great difficulty finding the *root cause* of disease. For example, a patient consumes naught but empty calories, resulting in an observable Outer Water Circle disorder. Treatment will need to address this outer disorder along with the root of the impulses guiding their choices, which are brought about by the architecture of the Inner Fire Circle, its configuration and defensiveness. Often these responses are framed by a history of abuse, trauma or neglect during the formative years.

Wàibìng and nèibìng refer to disease processes on either side of the pendulum. Despite this opposition on the external/internal spectrum, they are closely related. A body disease can become quite distressing, leading to a decline of Xìng. In contrast, diseases without a physical origin can result in a physical malfunction through the vacancy of Heaven's principle. Part of the strategy when dealing with these types of diseases is to take proactive steps toward liberating oneself from attachments and desires. The healing process for Heart diseases involve words, thoughts and positive actions, not simply medications and philosophical intellectualization. With severe disease we must rest and sleep to allow for recharging, while during waking hours, desires must be brought back to Center.

An injury when we are young, such as abuse or trauma, may have been caused by *space* and *material* (meaning that the event could have occurred in another country by someone or thing no longer present) but is related to *time*. The living body has memory and whilst the Inner Fire Circle continually attempts to mend itself, when the memory reemerges, it is as if the trauma happened yesterday or even this morning. This is regardless of how *far* away we are from it. We are *wounded*. In this state, a ton of joy will be vanquished with an ounce of sorrow. A patient can be responding well to treatment, but when a memory is provoked of some earlier trauma, this same treatment becomes ineffective. The root of their condition cannot be reached by physical medicines alone. Therefore, we need Xīnfǎ, the Heart Method.

Memories invoke the habits and routines of the Inner Fire Circle leading to the common discharging of emotions, thus the Xìng declines rapidly. We can forget that we are currently alive. In moments like these, we need to regain perspective. Standing in a forest surrounded by trees who sink their roots deep beneath the layers and continually reach towards the sun, we tell ourselves that *it is good to be alive*. Breathing comes so easily. Breathing comes so easily.

> We sat together, the forest and I,
>> Merging into silence,
>>> Until only the forest remained.[24]
>>>> Dàoist poem

This steadies the undulations of the One Thread of Life, bringing us back to Center. Emotions are recovered and we unify and begin to heal: a practical strategy creating stillness within action. It is the opposite of creating more movement, which may be induced by therapies that return to the trauma, to analyze it, relive it and dig at the wound. Once Centered, we live and relate to the external world far more efficiently and effectively. Once Centered, we are clear and yet clearer about virtue; clear about our perpetual capacity for goodness, kindness and compassion.

> "...In my current circumstances, thinking about the past can be far more exacting than contemplating the present and predicting the course of future events...I never full appreciated the capacity of memory, the endless string of information the head can carry."[25]
>
> Nelson Mandela

Habits, events, actions, words and thoughts shape our Inner Fire Circle from the moment of birth. They determine how we react to images transmitted by the eye and sounds by the ear.[26] Memories are pictures, sounds or even smells that trigger reactions in our behavior, a reflection of the traits of our Inner Fire Circle. Bad memories trigger bad reactions while good memories trigger good reactions. Without any memory, often there is no reaction, as seen in some cases of severe dementia. Bad events of the past should not be invoked and relived, especially if these processes inhibit our understanding and perception of all the good in the present. The trauma of childhood, for example, has already occurred and nothing can undo this, so the Inner Fire Circle adapts, allowing for a relatively normal life. When a traumatic memory arises, however, we are suddenly back in the maze of our historical narrative. We are no longer present.

---

[24] Feldman & Kornfield (eds), 1991, p. 33.
[25] N. Mandela, *Conversations with Myself*, Farrar, Straus & Giroux, New York, 2010, p. 112.
[26] "...we don't see the world directly. We perceive it through frameworks of ideas and beliefs, which act as filters on what we see and how we see it." (Robinson & Aronica, 2009, p. 251). Along with our other senses of taste, smell and touch.

> I met Tu Fu on a mountaintop
> in August when the sun was hot.
> Under the shade of his big straw hat
> his face was sad–
> in the years since we last parted,
> he'd grown wan, exhausted.
> Poor old Tu Fu, I thought then,
> he must be agonizing over poetry again.
>
> Lǐ Bái – *About Tu Fu*

Through Xīnfǎ cultivation these Inner Fire Circle dilemmas are more honestly observed. They are dealt with by acting upon the innate goodness within our Center. Reliving or repressing memories are strategies no longer needed as these commentaries on our past are not what define us. Rather, in spite of the past we are still and always will be capable of compassion, proper action and a happy and fulfilled life; transforming our words and holding onto absolute sincerity. This skill, which we bring out of the footnotes of history, in turn mends the wounded Inner Fire Circle, as revealed in the teachings of Liú Yuán. This is how true healing begins.

Contemplating the goodness of the present rather than the unpleasantness of the past, means breathing is treasured and being alive is great. Often we ignore this fact and adhere to internal historical archeology or unlikely hypothetical eventualities. An individual with chronic asthma understands the terrifying sensation of suffocation and the contrast between this and breathing easily. Breathing feels amazing.[27] It is not a distortion to focus on the present as long as we direct our lens towards the Heart.

Now is a time for giving and a time for *forgiving* the past. It is also a time for taking, gratefully accepting everything that is good about the present. Cultivation is the process of changing habits and mending the Inner Fire Circle. Rather than allowing the past and our ingrained habits to exhaust our Xìng, each and every person can sort good from bad; creating a new *Me*, a new *You*. With calm Hearts and abundant Xìng we live prosperous, healthy and happy lives.

---

[27] So often, however, we forget to breathe. Teaching patients how to breathe is vital. Sometimes by being caught up in the stress of their lives, they breathe shallowly into the upper thoracic cavity, increasing pressure around their heart with every inhalation. Physiologically, this respiratory pattern renders us ineffective, as our blood becomes low in oxygen, and high in carbon dioxide. It becomes very difficult to approach situations from a balanced point of Center when the body is starved of what is vital.

Two monks journeying home came to the banks of a fast-flowing river, where they met a young woman unable to cross the current alone. One of the monks picked her up in his arms and set her safely on her feet on the other side and the two monks continued on their travels.

The monk who had crossed the river alone could finally restrain himself no longer and began to rebuke his brother, "Do you not know it is against our rules to touch a young woman? You have broken the holy vows."

The other monk answered, "Brother, I left that young woman on the banks of the river. Are you still carrying her?"[28]

Zen story

---

[28] Feldman & Kornfield (eds), 1991, p. 346.

CHAPTER 5

說百病

Shuō Bǎi Bìng

Explaining the 100 Diseases

The text below was originally a chapter contained within the Dà Zàng Jīng (大藏经) Buddhist cannon, commonly known as Tripitaka. This ancient chapter, called *zhì bìng yào* (治病药), was composed in the Táng dynasty (618-907) by the monk and poet Líng Chè (灵澈法师). Recounted below are the explanations of the *one hundred diseases* with the *one hundred medicines* revealed in chapter 9.

    We received this manuscript from Master Gān Liǎo (甘了), a Heart medicine practitioner in Sìchuān. His commentary on the text is included below and we also conclude the one hundred medicines with his words. The work discusses the actions, thoughts, words and intentions that make us unwell and then those that can heal us. Illness is not solely attributable to what we ingest, inhale, or what we are born with. The one hundred diseases explain why when we act, think and say the inappropriate things, we get sick.

    The Dà Zàng Jīng has three categories: Jīng (经), Classics from the Buddha and his era, or sutras; Lü (律), laws, or rules, written by disciples of later Buddhist saints; and Lùn (论), treatises of later monks (Fǎshī 法师) such as Líng Chè, who tried to further elucidate the principle of reality. Our text translated herein belongs to this third category. The earliest version available is Korean, and the school of Dàoism also makes use of the work, referring to it as *Lǎozǐ discusses the one hundred diseases and remedies*. As will be seen, *all* the diseases arise from actions, emotions and thoughts, layered throughout the poetic style of the text. These diseases appear to be external in nature, yet they arise from within, from a compromised Center.

Preface:

Rescuing from disaster is not as easy as defending against it or preventing it from happening in the first place. Treating a disease is not as happy an event as preparing for the disease not to come. The people of today think differently; they feel that the task of the physician is to rescue, not to prevent. They do not think of being ready for it and preparing but rather just medicating it. Therefore the ruler fails to protect the grains and the Earth and the body fails to keep its life. Avoiding this, the sage looks for prosperity where there is no misfortune yet and eradicates disease by not having it at all.

Disaster is born out of very small things and diseases arise with minute details. People think that a small goodness in the Heart has no benefit and therefore will not do it. They think that a small evil does no harm; therefore they will not prevent it. When small good deeds do not accumulate, great virtue does not form. When small evils do not stop, great calamity eventually emerges. Selecting the essential is the start, these are the one hundred diseases that originate in the Heart.

治病救人

Zhì Bìng Jiù Rén

"Treat disease to save the patient"

1. Uncontrollable mood swings, suddenly happy then suddenly sad: this is one disease.

2. Forgetting one's virtue and morality, thinking only of profit: this is one disease.

3. Being lustful and ruining one's virtue: this is one disease.

4. Focusing on affairs of love whilst not functioning within society: this is one disease.

5. Wanting to kill someone you hate: this is one disease.

6. Indulging in greed and then concealing it: this is one disease.

7. Slandering others to beautify oneself: this is one disease.

8. Handling affairs without principle and going back on your word: this is one disease.

9. Indulging in outspoken, opinionated, irresponsible words and jokes: this is one disease.

10. Having good intentions but then doing wrong: this is one disease.

11. Thinking highly of oneself whilst looking down on others: this is one disease.

12. Relying on power and influence to do as you wish: this is one disease.

13. Always saying that others are wrong and that you are right: this is one disease.

14. Bullying honest people while being reliant on bad people: this is one disease.

15. Using force to make others submit: this is one disease.

16. Borrowing from others and not thinking of repaying or returning: this is one disease.

17. Using social influence for personal gain, while harming others: this is one disease.

18. Putting others down with unfriendly words:
this is one disease.

19. Belittling others and praising oneself:
this is one disease.

20. Dealing with affairs in a way that harms others:
this is one disease.

21. Criticizing others as being evil while praising oneself as being good:
this is one disease.

22. Bragging in happy times as well as times of hardship:
this is one disease.

23. Claiming that others are stupid and that you are virtuous:
this is one disease.

24. Denying common good and attributing it all to oneself:
this is one disease.

25. Reveling when famous people suffer misfortune:
this is one disease.

26. Being overworked and as a result becoming resentful:
this is one disease.

27. Falsifying truth and making it into a false reality:
this is one disease.[1]

28. Liking to discuss the faults of others:
this is one disease.

29. Accumulating wealth and then becoming arrogant:
this is one disease.

30. Having power and position, yet not helping others:
this is one disease.

31. Being jealous of the wealthy while being lazy oneself:
this is one disease.

32. Not striving to advance beyond one's rank while slandering superiors:
this is one disease.

33. Slandering one person to benefit another:
this is one disease.

---

[1] "An old aphorism explains this phenomenon: "Accumulated falsehoods become the truth." The longer—and more sincerely—such stories are repeated, the more convincing they appear." (Schmieg, 2005, p. 157).

34. Trying to promote oneself by bragging:
this is one disease.

35. Harming the accomplishments of others:
this is one disease.

36. Damaging public affairs for self gain:
this is one disease.

37. Concealing one's true intentions:
this is one disease.

38. Delegating away a crisis to maintain one's own serenity:
this is one disease.

39. Being outwardly or inwardly jealous of others:
this is one disease.

40. Inciting others to improper actions or thoughts:
this is one disease.

41. Being filled with much hate and little love:
this is one disease.

42. Judging others:
this is one disease.

43. Pushing one's own responsibility onto others:
this is one disease.

44. Appearing good and virtuous but in reality being evil:
this is one disease.

45. Manipulating others to achieve one's own objectives:
this is one disease.

46. Claiming others are frauds and that only you are trustworthy:
this is one disease.

47. Doing favors for others and expecting a reward:
this is one disease.

48. Failing to assist others and yet demanding their help:
this is one disease.

49. Helping others and then regretting it:
this is one disease.

50. Perpetually complaining and arguing:
this is one disease.

51. Cursing living things with or without reason:
    this is one disease.

52. Secretly poisoning and manipulating the minds of others:
    this is one disease.

53. Starting a rumor to slander a talented person:
    this is one disease.

54. Hating others as they have surpassed oneself:
    this is one disease.

55. Using poisonous drugs to intoxicate oneself or others:
    this is one disease.

56. Embracing favoritism and dealing subjectively with others:
    this is one disease.

57. Believing in one's own nobility and arguing with others:
    this is one disease.

58. Recalling old grievances with each and every thought:
    this is one disease.

59. Not listening to one's teachers as one feels they already know it all:
    this is one disease.

60. Distancing oneself from family while embracing strangers:
    this is one disease.

61. Incriminating others:
    this is one disease.

62. Broadcasting absurdity in order to create confusion and chaos:
    this is one disease.

63. Being harsh, impulsive, unsteady and temperamental:
    this is one disease.

64. Circulating nonsensical theories to mislead others:
    this is one disease.

65. Being self-righteous:
    this is one disease.

66. Having much suspicion and little trust:
    this is one disease.

67. Laughing at others as if they are fools:
    this is one disease.

68. Behaving improperly and against propriety:
this is one disease.

69. Using foul and abusive language:
this is one disease.

70. Being disrespectful to the aged and not cherishing children:
this is one disease.

71. Being nasty and vulgar in one's attitude towards others:
this is one disease.

72. Being opinionated and stubborn:
this is one disease.

73. Making fun of people and joking inappropriately:
this is one disease.

74. Making indiscreet remarks and controlling the freedom of others:
this is one disease.

75. Being treacherous and sly and garnering favor through false flattery:
this is one disease.

76. Greedily seeking methods to cheat others:
this is one disease.

77. Having two tongues with no trustworthiness:
this is one disease.

78. Getting drunk and cursing others:
this is one disease.

79. Cursing the rain and wind:
this is one disease.

80. Provoking conflict with vile and obscure words:
this is one disease.

81. Untowardly inducing an abortion and harming life:
this is one disease.

82. Snooping in others' private business:
this is one disease.

83. Spying upon the secrets of others:
this is one disease.

84. Borrowing without the intention of return:
this is one disease.

85. Accruing debt and then absconding:
    this is one disease.

86. Saying one thing to their face and another behind their back:
    this is one disease.

87. Allowing one's bad temper to incite arguments and irritation:
    this is one disease.

88. Taking a joke too seriously thereby harming relationships:
    this is one disease.

89. Planning to mislead others and leading them down the wrong path:
    this is one disease.

90. Invading the nest and ruining the eggs:
    this is one disease.

91. Killing pregnant animals:
    this is one disease.

92. Using Water and Fire to harm instead of heal:
    this is one disease.

93. Making fun of the disabled:
    this is one disease.

94. Interfering with the marital affairs of others:
    this is one disease.

95. Teaching how to take advantage of the deficiencies of others:
    this is one disease.

96. Teaching people how to be evil:
    this is one disease.

97. Wishing harm upon others:
    this is one disease.

98. Using immoral words and leading others into decline:
    this is one disease.

99. Allowing a greedy Heart to surge with an opportunity for profit:
    this is one disease.

100. Forcefully and unlawfully taking the property of others:
    this is one disease.

If we can remove these one hundred diseases from our thoughts then there is no accumulation of disaster. Pains and illnesses recover. One can pull through the sufferings of misfortunes with ease and our future generations will be blessed.

Here we have another tool like that given to us in the story of Shí Yīn Fū, whereby we can take charge of what transpires within. It is a detailed description, but not exhaustive, of what can go wrong practically and where we can start our gōngfu of sorting good from bad. Ultimately, it is all based on our ability to relate to the text, to the idea of cultivation and the understanding of our internal reality. By the physician only assessing the physical body when treating disease, they would be mistaking the branches for the root.

> Heaven One produces Water,
> great rivers accumulate from tiny drops.
> From here begins the great current,
> outward to the universe.[2]

> Man Jan

Dollars are made from pennies, so when health is in a state of poverty, we seek out where the pennies have been dropped. Sometimes they are found in our own choices, sometimes in those of our forebears. Many childhood illnesses along with other debilitating diseases that are prevalent in society arise regardless of personal *good* or *bad*. The text highlights the importance of cultivation and improving our inner landscape, so that when we create families of our own they are based on virtue and compassion. Earlier, Liú Yuán described a historical example of the consequences of neglecting this:

> *...if you look at those who did evil...the affairs they themselves undertook were bad. Their children...ended up being overthrown and their dynasty came to a short and bloody end. A whole generation was massacred due to this. This issue is even more prevalent amongst the common people. How many of us continue our traits of evil through our children?*[3]

---

[2] Cheng, 1995, p. 16, *Painting Ideas with Poems*.
[3] See his conclusion to the story of Shí Yīn Fū.

Distracted by what they *see* as *their* life, influence and responsibility, people can forget that they are the culmination of Xìng transmission from their ancestors to today. Keeping this at the forefront of our Hearts, however, we take up the challenge, adding our own positive contribution to the legacy we are continuing. When the mother and father, through their own cultivation achieve appropriateness inside and out, their children and grandchildren can continue this blessing of life. This transmission occurs on different levels, yet has the same origin. A healthy body will create a new healthy body (Outer Water Circle), a healthy human Heart will create a new healthy human Heart (Inner Fire Circle) and a strong connection to Heaven principle will also transcend us and imbue the next generation (Center and Xìng).

Talking about these concepts is not the same as *living* them. Preaching humility but then thinking ill of others the next day does not a *good* person make. The process of ridding ourselves of the Wounded Warrior, described in detail in chapter 8, and stabilizing the One Thread of Life is a life-long pursuit. Through our *hard work* we see the world for what it is, that life is full of joy and we can feel truly fulfilled. Suddenly it is no longer *hard work*. Being alive is no longer *work* at all. Not sprinting to the finishing line, we stroll and complement the scenery. How amazing it is just to be alive, with the sun on our skin, breathing comes easily.

"...he plucked the strawberry... How sweet it tasted!"

We conclude this chapter and indeed the one hundred medicines later, with the words of Master Gān Liǎo. Listening to him speak his words and now translating them here: this is one medicine.

When a person, regardless of nationality, becomes sick, they often bring the disease upon themselves. How so? Through the seven emotions their Center is scattered outward. They gaze at the external world, missing what is inside, hoping to find something to fill the vacancy in their Heart. So we have the words of the one hundred diseases, explaining to us the true root of disease. For example, if someone has a headache, one may think that the pain is in the head. In reality it is all the result of an evil thought. If someone, makes out to be grand or superior to garner the admiration of others, sickness is sure to ensue: the Qì escapes and they succumb to illness. At this point the physician needs to advise the patient how to alter their Heart to become soft and harmonious. With a soft and harmonious Heart, where can there still be a disease?

The words of this text teach us how to save our own lives. Through daily practice we gradually peel back the layers of the human Heart, and perhaps one day we will see the true story of our lives: the understanding of the Dào. It is this situation that we call Hùnyuán, as this term implies a state of being beyond the dichotomy of Yīn and Yáng. How can we reach to this state of Hùnyuán? We develop in the womb without the toss and turning of Yīn and Yáng, we naturally grow within Hùnyuán, gaining our body and become a person. As soon as we enter the exterior world, however, this state of Hùnyuán disappears.

From this early moment we lose our original connection so that when we come of age we seek virtue and follow the path returning to Hùnyuán. Then we reach the Dào. Starting this process seems difficult, as we have piled upon ourselves obstacle after obstacle, creating a scenario where we lose faith in ourselves. Regaining our self-worth comes from understanding our own capacity to improve ourselves. Through the instructions in one hundred diseases paired with the one hundred medicines that come in a later chapter, our goal is not to become a saint or sage, but to practice diligently every day to reach our own accomplishment.

For those who depart from this Dào, this state of Hùnyuán, are they still people? A person, but not a human being. Each person has the Dào within them, the capacity to become human, yet we tend to lose sight of this. So the first step is to seek and locate it again. Once found, we bring it back to Center. Expressing this outward to others, you are then a teacher of the Dào. For the physician, regardless of theoretical persuasion, their role in society is to assist the patient to find their soft and harmonious Heart.[4] Teaching how to focus their intention on Center, they become enlightened to their emotions and agitation and are able to dissolve them.

So how do we practice this in medicine? If a patient is stuck in a lifelong state of confusion, how can a few words change their manner? First, we must be soft and harmonious ourselves! Only then can we talk to the patient and hear their words. By asking them where they think their disease has arisen from, you open the way for their understanding. For example, a patient suffering from a Spleen and Stomach disease complains

---

[4] See the entry by Liú Bèiwén at the end of chapter 10.

of a distended and painful abdomen. Rather than reaching for herbs or needles, the physician must immediately seek any seeds of dishonesty hiding in the patient's Heart. While the patient articulates the particulars of their symptoms, the physician listens to their words, hearing the disordered desires and emotions and where the Xìng is obscured. Then the prescription is to instruct them how to remedy their Heart. If we can master this, then that is it. First and foremost, the physician helps the patient's Heart and does not just hand out medicinals. Getting this fundamental principle of medicine backwards results in an inferior physician, as seen in Chinese culture. The level of cultivation will be revealed in their actions and words. If the physician can see into the patient's Heart then they can cure diseases at the very root of the problem. Otherwise, they treat the skin, body and hair.

In reality though, no one, doctor or not, regardless of nationality and theoretical predilection, can force another person to change their ways, knowledge or posture. The only thing each and every one of us can do is mend our own Heart. Then when talking to a patient, we simply explain how we personally experience life: 'I find that if I approach things this way, things go well.'

Unfortunately, the medicine of today has taken a separate road to that of the Heart. If we can remember the Heart, healing will be far easier. This kind of medicine should always be pursued! There is not one instance where it is not needed!

Caution is needed, as the physician who practices Heart medicine must not feel loftier than others, as this is just another trap of the human Heart and desire. When seeing a patient, we must not think of ourselves as great doctors, or if the patient is rich or poor, successful or educated. Whoever the patient is, it is our destiny to meet them here and now, and our destiny to direct them back to Center. Without using the four methods of diagnosis, the physician knows the condition of the person's Heart by hearing a few words. When giving herbs after a consultation with the Heart, the physician's own Hùnyuán Qì melds with the medicine. This is a time for giving to the patient and assisting in their recovery.

The physician walks the Center path to serve their patients. Heart full of virtue, they try their best to help. This is called Center. In reality the patients heal themselves. This is what the one hundred medicines chapter is all about. Every few days I look at this text and lament how inadequate I am. Mimicking a good person does not equate to goodness. The human being is a human 'being' good. By practicing virtue repeatedly, gradually we feel at peace, agitation settles and we find harmony. The myriad divisions of materialism merge into one unity.

Gān Liǎo, Sìchuān

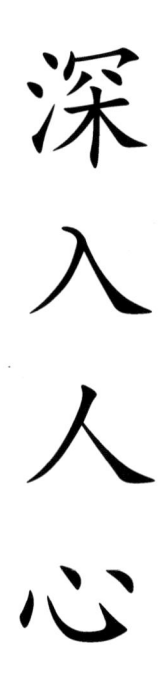

深入人心

Shēn Rù Rén Xīn

To deeply enter someone's Heart

CHAPTER 6

我知言

Wǒ Zhī Yán

I know words

'May I dare ask the Master: what is the difference between you and other philosophers?'

'I know words...' Mencius says."[1]

This chapter utilizes Liú Yuán's commentary on the Book of Mencius to further explore Xīnfǎ and finding the true Heart. Mencius, who lived around the 4th century BCE, was a follower of Confucius, and after him is considered the second greatest Confucian scholar. Regardless of the historical issues surrounding this text and who compiled it, the book has influenced Chinese philosophical thought greatly. Words are pointers to meanings: yet looking at a word can confuse us. Endeavoring to *know the words* of Liú Yuán and Mencius, we would ideally contemplate the original pictogram. Taking Xìng for example:

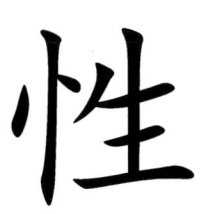

性

Suddenly this is no longer a word, but a picture painted to reveal an understanding. On the left side is a picture of the Heart 心 (xīn), in its presentation as a radical component of the character, and on the right is a

---

[1] Commentary on the Book of Mencius, p. 428-2.

picture expressing birth and life 生 (shēng), which together form Xìng: *the Heart of life*. In ancient times, 生 was an illustration of a seedling growing and pushing out of the ground and reaching for Heaven, representing the constant movement of life in nature. When combined with 心, the human Heart has a constant connection to birth and movement, giving the material vessel life.

I know words...

This statement by Mencius has great significance for our work and explorations into Xīnfǎ, as words are the expression of the Heart on the exterior. When a patient speaks, they convey their Heart to the physician, who can recognize the difference between the angst of the human Heart and the purity of the Dào Heart. In this way, the physician assesses how desires, fears, likes and dislikes, wounded words and skewed intentions present themselves in both the patient and themselves. Using this knowledge, the goal of therapy is to reflect the true nature of Xìng. Thus, to know words we must know the path that they take from within, out to our lips. Discussed below using a five-step progression outward from Center, this path not only gives the physician a clear and yet clearer understanding of their patients. With it they can also formulate strategies to help them believe in themselves again.

Liú's analysis over the next few pages highlights the words of Mencius, starting with a discussion on *hàorán zhīqì*[2] and the *conscious Heart*, which we use as one of the five steps later.

> *'Dare I ask what you mean by Hàorán zhīqì?'*
> *'This is difficult to explain with words...'* Mencius replied, *'This that we call Qì, it reaches to the vast and the all-encompassing. Between Heaven and Earth it only nurtures and never harms.'*[3]

> *Benevolence is where Xìng is heading to, and the domain of Xìng engenders it. Consciousness of Heart*[4] *is where belief is headed to, belief is where emotions are headed to, and emotions emerge from Xìng. All people have Xìng but their Hearts are not fixed in the same way.*
>
> *Only after being excited by objects do they reach for it. Only after they are pleased do they take action. Only after they have learned patterns does the Heart become fixed. Joy, anger,*

---

[2] Hàorán zhīqì (浩然之氣): The expansive vital energy of the universe.
[3] Commentary on the Book of Mencius, p. 429-1.
[4] Of Heart, not of mind...

sorrow and grief emerge from Xìng. Xìng comes from Mìng. Mìng descends from Heaven.⁵ All worldly affairs begin with emotion, whilst emotion is engendered by Xìng, which begins with Heaven.⁶

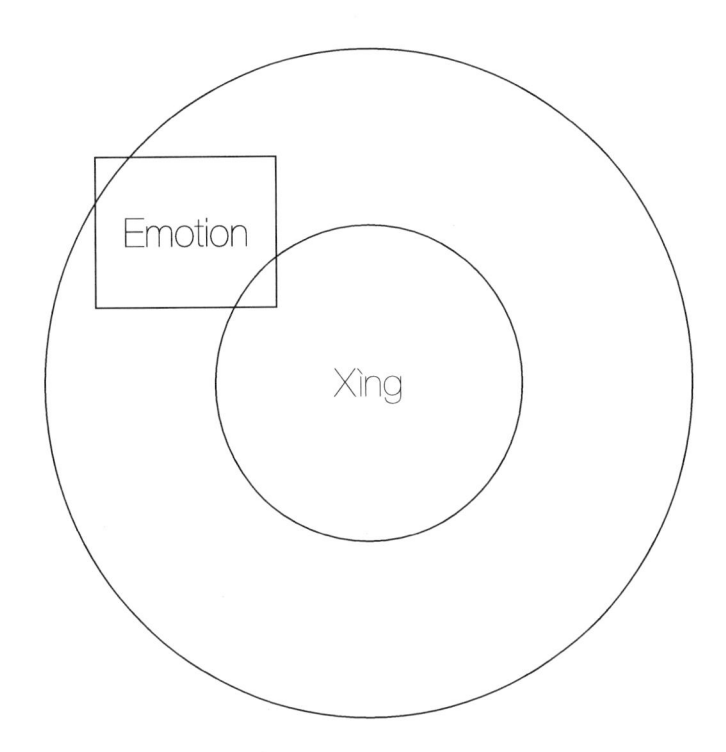

The ultimate application of the Dào Heart is benevolence, a topic dealt with by Mencius in depth. Benevolence is comprised of being kind-Hearted and mirroring the principle of Heaven by having an inextinguishable enthusiasm for life. This principle lies within our Center, a rippling of the life force of the universe–hàorán zhīqì–within us. Having negative thoughts about life goes against this principle, highlighting the relevance of Xīnfǎ to help us back to benevolence. There is a progression from Xìng outward to benevolence, which illustrates how the One Thread of Life influences our attitude, as shown below.

---

⁵ Tiānmìng (天命): Mandate of Heaven, destiny, fate, the span of one's life.
⁶ Guōdiàn Chǔjiǎn (郭店楚簡) tomb bamboo slips, from the Chǔ state (722–221 BCE), titled Xìng Zì Mìng Chū (性自命出) *Xìng comes from Heaven's Decree*. These bamboo slips were first excavated in 1993 in Jīngmén (荊門), Húběi (湖北) province, allowing for a whole new investigation into the words of Mencius as they are contemporary to his works.

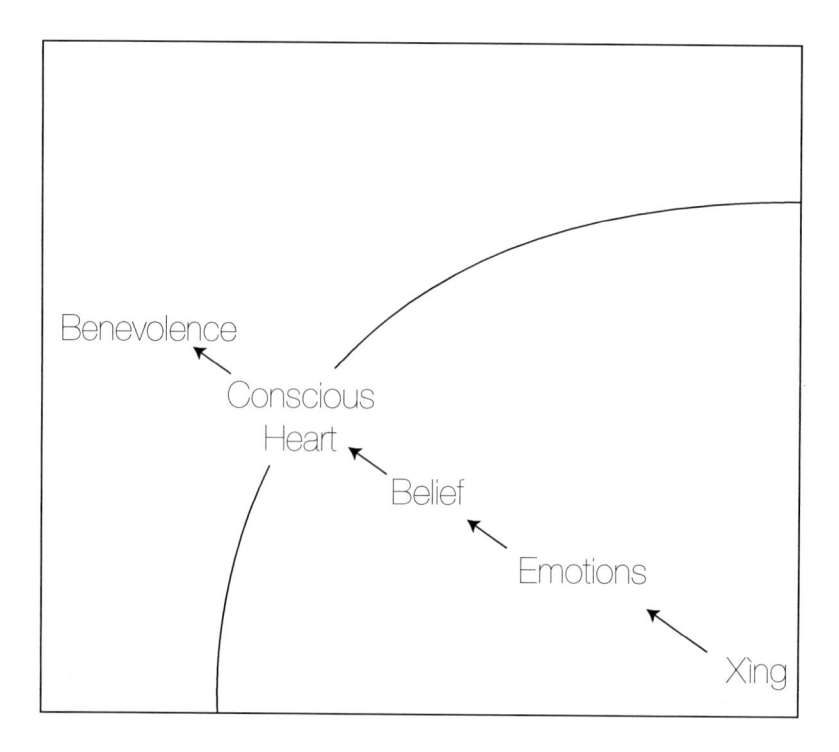

[Diagram: A square with a quarter-circle arc in the upper right. Arrows point inward from "Xìng" (outer) → "Emotions" → "Belief" → "Conscious Heart" → "Benevolence" (outward).]

From Xìng to emotions and belief to the conscious Heart, Xīnfǎ utilizes this progression from our Center outwards into benevolence. Emotions, the first stage of movement away from Xìng, permeate every cell of the vessel and make us alive. Anger wakes us, happiness opens, sadness brings us back and fear unifies, all at a level where they cannot be seen outwardly. Our Inner Fire Circle rotates according to this inner momentum, and only when unregulated and discharged do emotions cut through the Outer Water Circle and are seen as *reactions*. Any and every physical action and *word* had its seed in emotion moving out of Xìng.

> "Xìng exists with life itself.
> Emotions, however,
> are engendered with the exposure
> to external things."[7]

---

[7] Hán Yù 韩愈 (768–824 CE), Táng dynasty poet.

Emotions and desires stir through our innate longing for life. Hunger propels the body into action as we desire the apple on the tree. For this to occur, the *image* of the fruit must enter us first, until our Inner Fire Circle has formed a memory of it. Then an emotion is discharged, which feels like an attachment to the *thing* in the outer world. From this one example to the myriad attachments we form during our lives, we see how responses and desires are developed as we grow, and our Inner Fire Circle becomes our character.[8] We are all individuals with differing circumstances revealed in our *character*istics, yet despite this we all have the same Xìng inside of us and the same capacity for benevolence, regardless of our circumstances.

Xīnfǎ is especially important for cases of childhood trauma or sexual abuse, as this occurs during the formative years of the Inner Fire Circle, with ramifications throughout the entire cellular body. Sexual abuse cuts into the deepest layers of the Heart and can severely hamper the Inner Fire Circle, influencing behavior even decades later. For physicians, this makes treatment more complicated. As mentioned in the previous chapter, treatment can be progressing smoothly until a memory arrives, an internal trigger, which shoots through the physiology. Health can decline overnight, confusing both the physician and patient alike. As there is a Xīnfǎ problem created by verbal, physical or emotional abuse in childhood or from sexual abuse later on, herbs and acupuncture alone are unlikely to result in a cure. It is true, however, that by making the Outer Water Circle operate more effectively, this gives the Inner Fire circle some breathing space. It is hard to feel benevolent when in severe pain or suffering diarrhea, for example.

With a Xīnfǎ disorder, one's approach to treatment is not simply to be *nice*, as in being *a nice doctor*. To seek out the core problem and plant the seeds of healing it may even necessitate being brusque. An Inner Fire Circle obstructed by misguided beliefs and justifications requires careful confrontation in order to transform itself. Part of the therapy is this recognition, and seeking any disjunction in the natural flow from Xìng to benevolence. The human Heart can play tricks, hiding signposts to the five stepping-stones from Xìng, so the treatment principle is to bring this progression into order. Most commonly there is a rift between emotion and belief.

---

[8] Our character and Xìng are not one and the same. Xìng is the Heaven principle within the person, giving them life. Their characteristics are behavioral patterns formed through growing up, responding to their surroundings. Natural character (Xìng), on the other hand, is not molded by the dichotomy of the external world of Yīn and Yáng, rather, it is inherent in the womb and at birth. The natural goodness radiating from a newborn baby is the Xìng of a person.

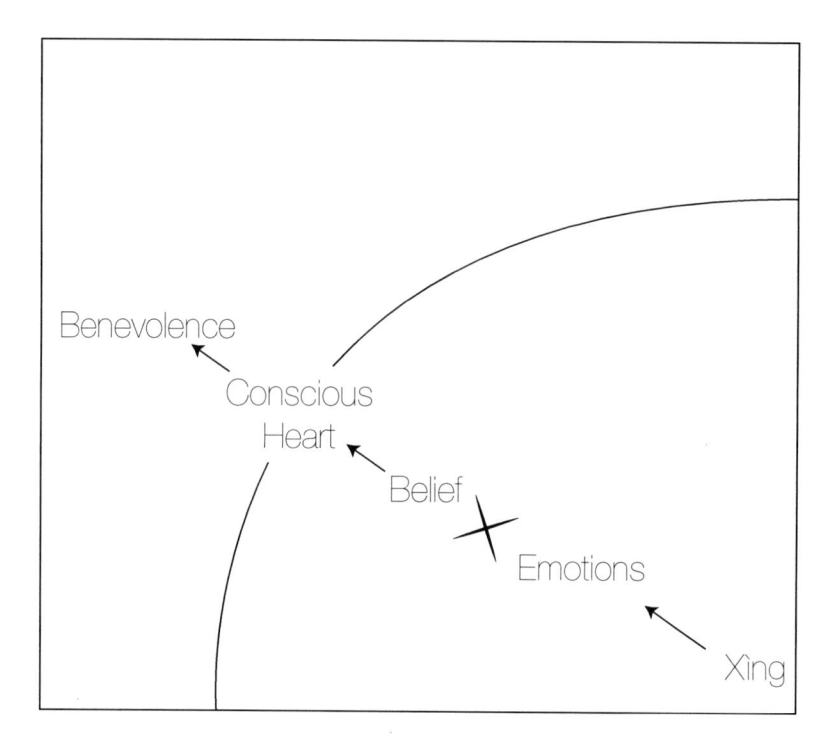

> Benevolence is where Xìng is heading to,
> and the domain of Xìng engenders it.
> Consciousness of Heart is where belief is headed to,
> belief is where emotions are headed to,
> and emotions emerge from Xìng.

> Guōdiàn tomb bamboo slips

The precursor to hesitation lies in the disconnect between our words and our Center. Xìng engenders an *emotion* (E), yet it cannot reach to *belief* (B): it cannot become a conscious Heart and materialize as benevolence in the physical world. This is often due to self-manipulation and contortion as we try and manage our experiences. Physiologically, this leads to problems, as Xìng should permeate out of Center in a controlled way to irrigate every cell of the body. Trauma breaks a link in the chain, which must be welded together again so belief can reach the *conscious Heart*. When the physician hears words they know the integrity of the path to the Heart, as when the patient speaks they are reflecting their Center.

> From hearing just this one sentence,
> Yù Kāi could tell from the sound of his voice
> that this man had sadly been walking an incorrect path.[9]

When someone has this internal rift (B✘E), rather than being *broken*, they are at a junction: a crossroads. Acknowledging this difference is important, and is the key to mending the tear between emotion and belief. By looking forwards at options rather than looking backwards, inciting memories of the cause of breakage,[10] we can close the distance between illness and recovery. Every ounce of our strength must be diverted to the *now-here* and where to from now.

> Where is sad?
> Sad is everywhere.
> It comes along and finds you.
>
> Michael Rosen

Some of the deepest pangs of sorrow come when a couple has fertility concerns. Often, cases of infertility due to Inner Fire Circle disorders are related to some earlier trauma. Negativity abounds, with a sense of failure at not being able to conceive, disappointing an expectant partner and the pessimism prescribed by their fertility *specialists*. A destructive health spiral can result, physically and mentally, furthering the rift between our Xìng and the reality we create. Cases like these need a gentle approach with lengthy consultations allowing appropriate time to speak *to* the Heart so the physician can address the root of dis-ease. The treatment principle here is to *change the length perception* (B↔E).

BENEVOLENCE ← CONSCIOUS HEART ← BELIEF – – – – EMOTION ← XÌNG

---

[9] From Shí Yīn Fū and the Ledger of Good and Evil.
[10] "In my view it is only from one's *experience* – experience always means a bad experience, does it not?" (Nietzsche, 1973, p. 129).

From the Center we have Xìng, then emotion and then the physical body. When a couple have intercourse this should be born out of this progression: Xìng moving emotion, emotion moving the body. So often with fertility concerns the *perceived* distance between emotion and belief can seem vast. Treatment, therefore, is to transform this perception, achieved by bringing emotion and belief closer: *when I believe I can achieve it, then at least I will try...*

When we see the apple tree our Xìng will exude and naturally will reach for it. Physiologically this means we will become hungry. However, when there is a rift between emotion and belief, the tree appears as if across a mighty canyon; too far to reach, too wide to jump. We fear drowning in the memory of a painful event. This illusion prevents us from even extending our hand, as we do not believe we can succeed. Accordingly, when facing this situation the physician will hear the abyss in their patient's words. By changing the length perception, emotion is brought closer to belief or belief closer to emotion and the patient realizes that there is no canyon, just a little crevice that is easy to negotiate.

Recognition of our true potential directs belief back to emotion (B→E) and our Center: we can *be* harmonious. Our passion and enthusiasm is refreshed and this translates into our attitude along with each cell in the body. By invoking strong positive emotions, reinforcing the importance of our goals and the importance of achieving them, our defensiveness along with the negativity of others fades into obscurity, allowing us to extend our hand. This is stretching emotion towards belief (B←E) and we can *be*come *be*nevolent.[11]

Depending on the level of trauma this can be a challenge, even for the strongest soul. Yet with a Centered physician this path becomes a journey to true healing. Trauma lodged deeply within the Heart may require many months of Xīnfǎ, gently bringing the patient (and ourselves) back to Xìng, along with appropriate herbs and acupuncture to facilitate from the exterior. The more positive impulses coming towards the patient from both the physician and their social setting, the better.[12]

---

[11] *Be-never-violent.*

[12] There are extreme cases of severe psychological disorder that require intensive medication to just gain some semblance of control. However, the need for treatment with kindness, understanding and time is most vital. There is no case in the world where these elements would be detrimental to healing. The only reason we are so dependent on medications is that our society does not allow for kindness, understanding and time. There are not enough resources, mental health is not prioritized and mental health workers are overworked, underpaid and not given the respect they deserve. So the solution is more drugs, stronger drugs. At the Heart of it all and where we are lost, is that when we look deeply into the causes of disease, mental or otherwise, we must start from an understanding of the living body and how life has passed through generations

Resolving trauma is a challenge, and the process of knitting our link from Xìng to benevolence through softening our Inner Fire Circle can sometimes result in anxiety. Acute episodes of anxiety are best moderated with deep relaxed breathing to calm the system. As cultivation develops, when the beginning of an anxious episode is perceived, it is dealt with appropriately, smoothing the interruptions between Xìng, emotion, belief, conscious Heart and benevolence. Eventually overt anxiety has no place to hide in the Heart. The nuts and bolts of this interval exchange are not accomplished through herbs, acupuncture or medications out of the doctor's toolbox. Rather, they are achieved through *knowing words*.[13]

What you cannot obtain from a person's words, there is no point looking for it in their Heart. What you cannot obtain from a person's Heart, there is no point looking for it in their Qì.[14]

Understanding people in general, but specifically patients, is through knowing their words and *where* these originate. A physician can become distracted by blood test results, signs and symptoms, pulse and tongue, the Outer Water Circle. First and foremost we should establish a clear and yet clearer connection between the patient's Center and the situation as they perceive it. This calls for Xīnfǎ, an inquiry into the machinations of the Inner Fire Circle and sorting body diseases from Heart diseases.

"If you do not know words, there is no way to know people."[15]

A patient in her forties had been attending clinic for three months, hoping to fall pregnant. Looking down at her basal body temperature chart we were concerned, and wondered about herbal options. Yet today something is different. It *takes time* for us to register this. Looking up, we *see* her and *hear* that her *words* have transformed from her first attendance where she related all of her internal *wounds*, to the present where she is speaking from a new point of reference. Beautiful words are resounding around the room

---

before us and will continue into generations after us.
[13] An analogy we often use in the clinic to describe the activity of herbs, acupuncture and medications is to set the scene of when we are watering our garden. If the hose has a kink in it, the water will not come out. Acupuncture releases these *kinks*. If the tap is turned off, no water will come out. Herbal medicine (if prescribed and understood correctly) turns the tap on. Me-*dictate*-ions tend to make us forget all about watering our gardens. In all of this, we had to understand in the first place that our plants were suffering and often this is something we had to be *told*.
[14] Words from Gàozǐ.
[15] The Confucian Analects, Yáoyuē (尧曰) chapter: Bù zhī yán, wú yǐ zhī rén yě (不知言 無以知人也).

about how wonderful her life is and how she feels so much stronger and self-assured. The human Heart has become a reflection of the Dào Heart.

A fortnight later she discovered that she was pregnant. Not yet aware of the good news, her fertility specialist called her with the results from some earlier biomedical tests. Looking down at the laboratory findings, her physician informed her of low Anti-Mullerian Hormone levels along with abnormal genetic markers, suggesting that she will not be able to fall pregnant naturally. The patient *knows these words* are off Center because she *is* pregnant and revealed this to her stunned doctor. Not wanting to disappoint her family if the pregnancy falters, the patient will wait until after the first trimester to announce her accomplishment. Sitting at her sister's house, her young nephew who cannot talk yet, waddled up and started to gently caress her tummy, looking up at her smiling.

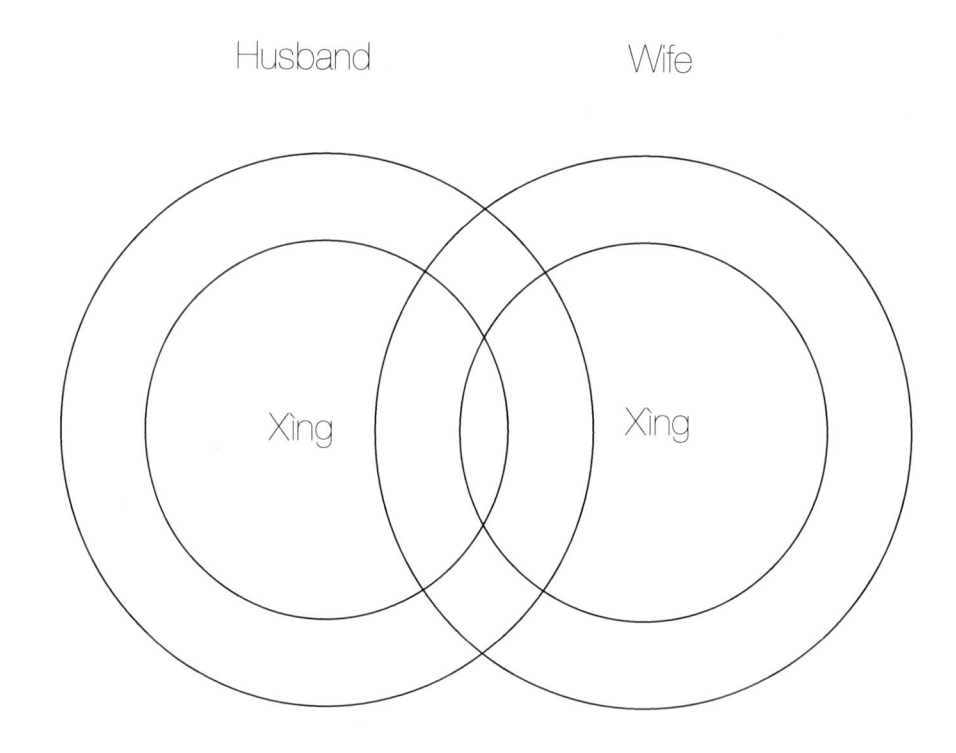

In general, the human Heart is not a solitary one, tending to develop close kinships with those around them. We join circles with family, partners, parents and children, siblings, friends, strangers and *doctors*. Of these, the strongest is that of the husband and wife, or lovers. The husband and wife are the parents of the following generation, the foundation of their children who see and learn how to interact with the rest of the world from their primary role models.

And so the Heart is not alone but rather joins with those of others. As shown in the image above, we are not independent units but are constantly linking up with those around us. Quite literally, this occurs in the intimate relationship between couples as the Xìng of each individual merge, the Two becoming One. Creating a new life naturally is the result of this mingling. Viable conception and successful implantation of an embryo are determined by the strength of this connection, allowing the union of Xìng to form a new Center. Infertility solutions based on modern fertility medicine are so often unsuccessful because they only base treatment on stimulating an admix of physical material. At the same time most couples are told *you have old eggs and deficient sperm*. These remarks tend to drive the circles apart when the very foundation of the relationship is based on this proximity. Why would the couple even bother trying if they think they have faulty gametes? It is far too common to see this situation of drug therapy and inappropriate words furthering the divide between emotion and belief.

> Look at his actions, observe where they come from.
> Examine what he rests upon, where can a man hide?
> Where can a man hide?[16]

> What is within must manifest itself outside.[17]

Recently a couple had been attending clinic for unexplained infertility.[18] After three months of treatment with herbs and acupuncture the husband underwent a detailed semen analysis, the results of which were less than favorable. *You will never be able to have a child naturally with that sperm*, they were told by their well-intentioned doctor, thinking to himself that it was best to annihilate any false hope. The very next day the couple discovered to their great surprise that they were pregnant! In medicine, with all the best intentions we are too often led astray by what we see, either in

---

[16] The Confucian Analects, Wéizhèng (為政) chapter.
[17] The Book of Gàozĭ by Mencius.
[18] In Hùnyuán medicine we disagree with the notion that medicine can treat *unexplained* problems. If a condition is unexplained and you still apply treatment, then you are throwing darts in the dark. We say instead: *If in doubt, do not treat the patient!*

signs or reported symptoms, or in our very advanced biological reports. In the example above, there was a disconnect between modern medicine and reality.[19]

When treating infertility it is helpful for the physician to observe the couple together, assessing the dynamics between them.[20] Let us compare two hypothetical case scenarios. In the first, the wife has many health problems and is here because she believes in Chinese medicine. The husband does not and yet attends regardless, supporting his wife. Not wanting herbs, the love for his wife overrides his selfishness and he accepts the prescription. He will do whatever it takes. Here, the prognosis is very good. In the second case, the wife and husband are both quite healthy and are both very eager to use Chinese medicine, but they are obviously not interested in each other. They move their chairs further apart than necessary and make no eye contact with each other during the consultation. When asked about their sexual relationship, they state that they only copulate at ovulation, when trying to conceive. This dynamic is off Center and regardless of the herbs and acupuncture we may use (and their eagerness to use them), it is their circles that must amalgamate to form a new life. In this case, the prognosis is not good. Outer Water Circle treatment alone will not get to the root of this dilemma, so the physician will use words to access their Center, speaking from the Heart, to the Heart.

Discovering *how* to *hear* what is within the patient's words is the challenge for the Xīnfǎ physician. When listening they should be aware of the circles involved in relationships that may interfere or assist the patient's health. Commonly, when one half of an elderly couple passes, after a lifetime together, the other can often quickly decline. This is due to the absence of their partner's Inner Fire Circle that they had merged with over a lifetime; the Heart remembers and longs for this extra warmth and the physical body starts to collapse. Lost love draws the Xìng out through the cellular vessel, where the physician sees the manifestations. Yet the remedy is not Outer Water Circle treatment. A lonely Heart needs appropriate words, which come to the physician instinctively when speaking from Center, unperturbed by the likes and dislikes oscillating on the periphery.

---

[19] Hùnyuán medicine is critical of *any* medicine that observes the physical body and forgets about the Heart. We hope to advance the cause of merging all one-sided medicines into something complete, an advanced system of healing, where the body *and* life are considered.

[20] For a thorough exploration of infertility and approaches and understanding of its treatment, please see: Y. Seidman & T. McLaren, *Hunyuan Fertility: Conception, Babies and Miracles*, Hunyuan Group, Inc, Connecticut, USA, 2012.

> Fondness brings about desire, whilst anger brings about dislike...
> desiring is joy, disliking is grief.[21]

> Dislikes engender with Xìng, anger engenders with dislike.
> Fondness engender with Xìng, joy engenders with fondness.[22]

Broad brush strokes of Unification and Separation can be applied in more detail to the human Heart, which reflects these energetic properties in its *liking* and *disliking*. These two broad divisions for the myriad emotions of the Inner Fire Circle are the outward expression of Xìng.

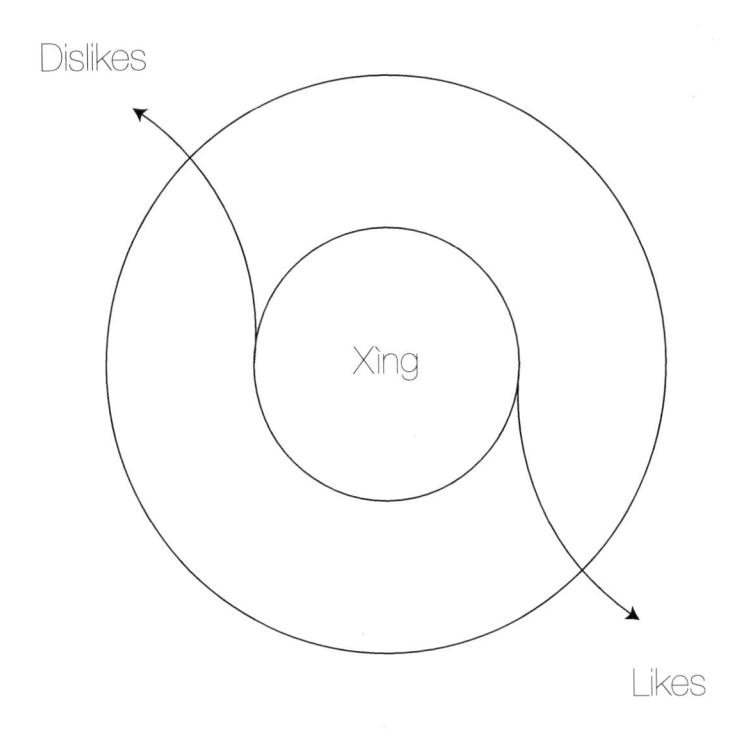

Dislikes

Xìng

Likes

> Desires and dislikes belong to Xìng,
> whilst anger, grief, sorrow, fear and joy are called emotions."[23]

---

[21] Zuǒ Zhuàn (左传): *Mr Zuǒ's Commentary on Early History* (400 BCE), attributed to the famous blind historian Zuǒ Qiūmíng (左丘明).
[22] Guōdiàn yǔcóngèr (郭店語叢二): Guōdiàn bamboo slips, *Thicket of Sayings Part 2*.
[23] Xúnzǐ (荀子), (310–237 BCE): A Confucian philosopher and author of Quànxué (劝学), *On Learning*.

Anger grows from the seeds of our dislikes, both of which are elements of a separating movement away from Center.[24] Joy and fondness on the other hand, are born out of desires and likes, which are all elements of Unification. When we desire something we bring it closer, wanting it near at hand, yet if we dislike something or someone we want to keep them at a distance. For a couple, they must desire each other to enable and empower the Unification capacity of their reproductive systems. Linking the chains that create a stable foundation for a new life requires the True Fire of desire.

Articulating this in a general sense, a hypothetical patient has cravings for sweets at night and suffers headaches during the day. On the Hùnyuán circle, night is our time of Unification where desires settle. In this case, they discharge and the patient craves sweets. During the day, in our time of Separation, she suffers the seemingly unrelated symptom of headache. Each point on the circle influences the whole and so her Separation at the time of Unification manifests as an Outer Water Circle malfunction during the day. By addressing the problem accordingly and bringing the discharging back into healthy parameters, the outer symptoms dissipate on their own.[25]

> Whether 'tis Nobler in the mind to suffer
> The Slings and Arrows of outrageous Fortune,
> Or to take Arms against a Sea of troubles,
> And by opposing end them: to die, to sleep
> No more; and by a sleep, to say we end
> The Heart-ache, and the thousand Natural shocks...
>
> William Shakespeare – Hamlet

To be (or not to be) in a state that Mencius refers to as *knowing Heaven*,[26] the movement of our likes and dislikes require strict moderation. Physicians determine the nature of disharmony within the patient through revelations from their lips. For example, a patient attends clinic who suffered a miscarriage twenty years ago followed by several surgeries to remove the fetus, multiple complications and heavy bleeding. Over two decades have passed and she lives in this memory as if it happened this morning. As

---

[24] Remembering that on a circle, at every point the movement along the perimeter seems to be moving away from you, only to return in the end. This is part of the principle that keeps our circulation circulating.

[25] We may be tempted to describe our patient's headache as being *Liver Qì Stagnation*, replacing one name for another and therefore leading us to replace one panacea for another. In this way, in our search for the *Universal Remedy* we find ourselves drifting down the Panega without a paddle.

[26] Commentary on the Book of Mencius, p. 571.

evidenced by her words, there is no distance between her current reality and the emotions of that trauma. In this case, herbs and acupuncture alone will not be of much use.[27] Rather, we would see her as a Xīnfǎ patient who has a chasm between emotion and belief, held at bay by her trauma. She needs reminding that having a baby is actually possible for her, otherwise from where will this impulse spring forth? *I know words* means understanding the patient's Center from hearing just one sentence, along with the words the physician releases, reaching into their Heart. Gently they are brought back to Center, which should be the core principle governing *all* medicine. When this becomes fixed, the myriad treatment strategies fall into line with benevolence.

Another patient walks in who six months ago had a miscarriage with twins at the end of her second trimester. This was a severely traumatic event and yet she has come through it relatively well. On examination we find that she had pre-existing menstrual issues, which were treated by various pharmaceuticals, implying a possible disorder and injury of the Outer Water Circle, which eventuated in miscarriage. Hence, the root of the problem did not begin in her Heart. Rather than gentle words, she requires strong herbs and regular acupuncture for a successful cure. Very easily we could mistake this for a Xīnfǎ scenario, assuming the history of trauma equates to a Heart disease.[28]

Our response to severe emotional trauma or shock will depend on the integrity of our Inner Fire Circle. Over the years we have developed survival mechanisms, layering themselves over one another, which can present as a web of signs and symptoms on the Outer Water Circle. Irrational emotional responses and reactions ensue. Commonly, when facing another failed month of trying to conceive, a couple can get more and more frustrated which increases their Separation. After months of this, the spirit breaks, vanquishing hope. They become forlorn when their friends or sisters conceive. Wanting to feel joy at the good news, they find themselves frustrated and resentful instead. Out of this darkness the physician opens the curtains, letting in the sun. The couple needs time to recharge and unify, to persist in getting themselves stronger and healthier.

---

[27] Meaning *appropriate* herbs and acupuncture encouraging Unification. To the contrary, giving her *sedatives* or *movers*, natural or otherwise, will just add another layer to her Inner Fire Circle obstruction and chaos, starving the root further and defeating the purpose of medicine. Incorrect treatment is not only not beneficial to the patient, it is destructive.

[28] In our modern society, however, it seems that most people could use at least some help in this department.

Bringing emotions and belief back into line by shortening the length perception allows the Xìng to effectively saturate the body with benevolence, making the couple more fertile.

'Dare I ask about your view on the concept of not moving the Heart?' Gōngsūn Chǒu (公孙丑) asked Mencius, 'Both Gàozǐ and yourself say this,[29] do you mean the same thing?'

'Gàozǐ says that if you fail to attain it with words, do not seek it in the Heart, and if you fail to attain it in the Heart, do not seek for it in the Qì. Without attaining it with words you cannot find it in the Heart. The will is the general of the Qì. Qì fills up the whole body, and so the Will arrives and Qì follows. Therefore it is said, support the role of the Will and its Qì will not burst abruptly.'

'How is this so?'

'The Will is one, and therefore when it moves the Qì, the Qì becomes as one, and therefore moves the Will. For example, if someone falls to the ground, this is Qì. If this then moves his Heart then there will be worry and anxiety.

'This Qì, the physical body, is secondary. Its role is to support the Will. How can the Qì not be abrupt?'

'It is easy to see it in the physical form...'

'May I dare ask the Master, what is the difference between you and the philosopher Gàozǐ?'

'I know words,' Mencius says, 'I nurture my own Hàorán zhīqì.'

Liú Yuán: Mencius knew words and therefore knew people. He knew evil and uprightness through the words of others, finding what lay behind them. He completed Xìng with the greatness of Heaven and Earth and explored to the extreme the appropriateness of the myriad things and affairs. Therefore, he was good at nurturing the purest aspect of his interior and then outwardly discarded all that was irrelevant.[30]

The origin of the qián ☰ and kūn ☷ trigrams are actually just one, and when people attain this, they truly become human. Talking about Qì is talking about principle. The realm of it, however, does not surpass this vastness. So we call it reaching

---

[29] Gàozǐ (告子): A Chinese philosopher during the Warring States period (420–355 BCE) and a contemporary of Mencius.

[30] Commentary on the Book of Mencius, p. 428-2.

for the big or reaching to the Heart, which directly shows movement and stillness, inside and out, and Center uprightness. Whatever we find within us that is not upright will damage us. When someone's Qì is complete between Heaven and Earth, then Heaven and Earth become the root of the person.

This is what is called 'Qì going together with righteousness and the Dào', and in this state there is no starvation or collapse. This is born out of our accumulated righteousness and cannot be appropriated through random acts of kindness. When one acts below the standard set in their Heart, any uprightness will collapse. The philosopher Gàozǐ never understood this as he only looked at the external manifestation.[31]

When you nurture the Center, the root of Heaven ☰ is retained. There is no discharging and so the Tàijí of Heaven mixes together as one Qì within you. When it moves and you attain it, then this is called the harmony of Central control. It becomes one Qì, which scatters into the myriad things. The idea of Mencius, of not moving the Heart, is reflected inside and out as they exchange and cultivate. Movement and stillness exchange and nurture each other. This is not an easily obtained skill. Its principle is difficult but its form is firm.[32]

Concerning the complete Heart, Mencius said 'to fully understand the Heart, we need to know the likes and dislikes, which means to know the Xìng. If we know Xìng then we know Heaven.[33]

For the physician, knowing Heaven means prescribing medicine that allows patients to heal themselves. Through knowing words, the Center is revealed. Words come from Center, guided outward by likes and dislikes, joining the myriad juxtapositions of Yīn and Yáng. Constantly moving away from the principle of Tàijí within us means our health is in an endless free fall. When harmonious, however, the Xìng is securely anchored to benevolence, regardless of circumstance and the constancy of change.

---

[31] Commentary on the Book of Mencius, p. 429-1.
[32] Commentary on the Book of Mencius, p. 431-2.
[33] Commentary on the Book of Mencius, p. 571-2.

CHAPTER 7

太极: 無終點

Tàijí: Wú Zhōng Diǎn

Tàijí: Without an Apex

> "No man ever steps in the same river twice,
> for it is not the same river and he is not the same man."[1]

Whilst this statement from Heraclitus is true in one sense, it is looking at the world through the panorama of change, the Yīn and Yáng. Indeed, all *things* change. In this chapter, however, we explore life through the paradigm of constancy.[2] Finding this element of timelessness we then apply it to the principle guiding our medical endeavors.

> Born of Heaven and Earth.
> Silent and void
> It stands alone and does not change...
> I know not its name
> so I style it *the way*.[3]
>
> Lǎozǐ

Whilst the individual drops of Water may not be the same, the river is constantly flowing and is constantly wet. Looking for this persistent principle within the river, the distracting details abate and the observer chooses not to descend into the theoretical and intellectual rabbit hole of

---

[1] Variation on the quote by Heraclitus (Ἡράκλειτος) of Ephesus (535–475 BCE), a Greek philosopher, who, in a similar style to the Yìjīng, was fascinated by the idea of *change*. He is also cited as saying: *The waking have one world in common; sleepers have each a private world of his own... Even sleepers are workers and collaborators in what goes on in the universe.*

[2] "The river looked at him with a thousand eyes – green, white, crystal, sky-blue...He saw that the water continually flowed and flowed and yet it was always there; it was always the same yet every moment it was new. Who could understand, conceive this?" H. Hesse, *Siddhartha*, Picador, London, 1973, pp. 81-82.

[3] Lǎozǐ, *Lao Tzu: Tao Te Ching*, trans. D. C. Lau, Penguin Books, London, 1963, p. 30.

uncertainty. Liú Yuán teaches about this certain principle as it applies to the human being, translated in his terms as Heaven, the one Origin, Xìng, Dào or Tàijí. In the previous chapter we introduced and explored the concept of likes and dislikes along with the five steps bridging the Xìng with our outwardly expressed emotions. These likes and dislikes, or desires and distastes, can either be moving too fast, too slow, or harmoniously on the Inner Fire Circle.

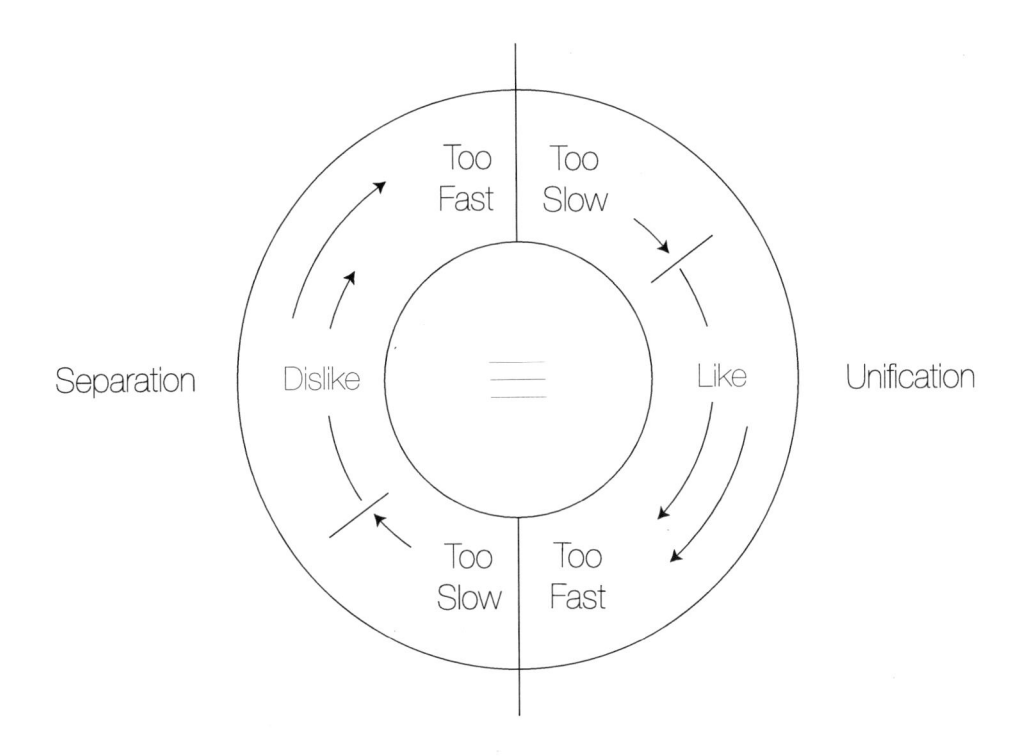

Separation — Dislike | Too Fast / Too Slow — Like — Unification
(Too Slow / Too Fast)

Here we see the structural components, the nuts and bolts of our emotional underpinning. What follows is deeper investigation beyond the mechanical manifestations and further into the Center. Our likes and dislikes (and by extension all of our emotions) surface visibly, observable on the exterior, induced by external affairs and determined by our circumstances. Where we were born, our family dynamics, exposure to conflict, warfare and suffering, laziness, greed and selfishness, along with compassion, love, kindness and peace, all formed the basis of how we will respond to stimuli as adults.

For a clinical example, consider the medications used in in-vitro fertilization procedures. One woman offered these drugs may *dislike* the idea of injecting these into her body and seek out alternatives, while a second woman *likes* the idea as she is more inclined to believe in their efficacy. Each woman's decision is based on her individual circumstance and historical perspectives. Another example is choosing to purchase either organic or genetically modified foods. People's opinions and beliefs about these issues will vary, just as the river does. The way we respond to the external world will be full of these examples as we are individually dictated to by our likes or dislikes. If the cause is the same and yet the response is different, then it cannot be the *cause*. Our likes and dislikes are not determined by the outer world but rather how our internal world has formed and how we interact with the exterior from our Center.

> "Without regulations or rules regarding our likes and dislikes, when external things present themselves we transform to become that which we desire or distaste. We want it so much it is as if it becomes us, consumes us; Heaven principle is then made extinct."
>
> Liú Yuán

Clinically, this has significance. For example, a patient comes to us who has just had surgery to remove a tumor from their kidney. They present with severe anxiety, loose bowels and exhaustion from working long hours. It is unlikely that our treatment on and for the Outer Water Circle will reach the root of their condition. This patient has a serious disease and our job is to seek tirelessly for a remedy, so we must go beneath the superficial layers of...*this surgery for the tumor, this acupuncture point for the kidney, this herb for the anxiety, this drug for the stools, this stimulant for the energy*...Whilst important in their work on the Outer Water Circle, herbs and acupuncture will only take the physician and patient to the river bank. Reaching to a deeper principle, they take another step towards the Water with the virtuous intention of *really* helping their patients. Liú Yuán is unafraid of the rapids; he hoists us up onto his shoulders and takes us to a state *without an Apex*.

> *All under Heaven are imbued with and created from the one principle: therefore it is called Dào. When scattered, this principle transforms into the myriad variations of creation and*

when it congeals it returns to the root of oneness. Amongst the myriad things, the human being is the most nimble. The Qì of mankind attains the uprightness of Yīn and Yáng and is filled with Xìng, the principle of Heaven and Earth. Through arduous study seeking the very root of this principle, people exhaust their Xìng in order to abide by Heaven's decree. And so mankind is like one Heaven and Earth. All of the myriad things exist because of it, and this one principle must be grasped. Only then can one attain a harmonious Center.[4]

The essence of Heaven and Earth is pure and complete through the principle of Qì. All of the myriad things flow from and return to this principle. This is the Apex, reaching to a place where you cannot add any more, therefore we call it Tàijí. Tàijí, however, does not name its Apex, as it has no Apex. There is nothing outside of Tàijí, there was nothing before it, there will be nothing after it. There is no Wújí outside of Tàijí.[5]

    Tàijí resides at the birth of Heaven and Earth and governs their Center. It has no name and no form, yet to visualize its complete pureness we draw a simple picture, without addition or subtraction, without deficiencies or excesses. The myriad things all join within this, so it is called the Dào.

---

[4] Commentary on the Yìjīng, p. 1057-1.

[5] Wújí (无极) is the concept of supreme emptiness, which first appeared in the Dào Dé Jīng (道德经) in reference to returning to one's origin. From the Warring States period (476–221 BCE), the meaning of this term was *ultimate, boundless, infinite* and then later it came to be understood as the *primordial universe, a limitless void*.

When you attain this within your body then it is called virtue. It is a state of no excess and no deficiency, and is thus called Center. When you reach this truth without any doubt, then this is sincerity. The principle of endless creation is contained within it, so we call it benevolence. In its root is the beginning of all life.

And so within it Heaven and Earth bring forth life and mankind's Xìng, establishing polarity and an Apex. All Earthly and Heavenly things have it, allowing them to spread forth and have meaning. This is the principle we must follow to understand life thoroughly. When we follow the sage on his journey through the Apexes and juxtapositions of Heaven and Earth in order to fulfill their Xìng and life's decree, then we are following a path of scales and claws.[6] For example, from ancient times we have the transmission from Zhōu Liánxī[7] of the Tàijí picture. Inside the circle there is black and white, the shapes of two Qì, the Yīn and Yáng. In the midst of each there is a dot of the other, showing transformation, the birth of Yīn within Yáng and Yáng within Yīn. Tàijí, however, is the summary and convergence of true principle.

Yīn and Yáng are contained within Tàijí naturally. Due to the difficulty of naming and shaping this principle, it has been called Wújí. In reality Wújí is Tàijí: there is nothing outside of Tàijí. More so when making a picture of Tàijí, we simply draw an empty circle. This is the image of complete pureness.[8]

Distracted by the ebb and flow of life, people tend to perceive polarities, differences and contrasts over similarities. When looking at the Sòng era Tàijítú image, ☯, we *tend* to only see black and white shapes, hence placing importance upon them, translating into how we operate as physicians of medicine. Looking for Yīn and Yáng means we will find Yīn and Yáng. Liú Yuán teaches us to guard against this mentality of grasping the scales and claws,[9] hoping that we see the truth: one unending circle O.

---

[6] Meaning what can be seen on the outside, the superficial level.
[7] Zhōu Liánxī (周濂溪), also known as Zhōu Dūnyí (周敦颐) (1017–1073 BCE), who is famed for formalizing the Tàijítú, or Yīn Yáng symbol with two entwined fish, one white and the other black ☯. The opening line of his book, Tàijítú shuō (太極圖說) "Explanation of the Diagram of the Supreme Ultimate" is wújí ér tàijí (無極而太極). Over the last 900 years this was taken to mean, *first there is Wújí, then there is Tàijí*, which is an assumption that Liú Yuán disagrees with entirely.
[8] Commentary on the Yìjīng, p. 1061-2 and 1063-1.
[9] Chinese idiom: Dōng Lín Xī Zhǎo (東鱗西爪). *Dragon scales from the East and Dragon claws from the West.*

Clinically, this is the one and only concern and is the path to the true root of disease. For example, if treating a headache or eczema, the physician first observes the exterior and yet resists the temptation to applying treatment based on the flux of Yīn and Yáng. Liú encourages us to avoid changing one dichotomy for another, where we would say *Yáng* instead of *headache* or *Yīn* instead of *eczema*.[10] Rather, Liú shows the physician the way to Center and the principle of no Apex. This scenario from a medical paradigm could be translated into every aspect of our perception; instead of seeing the differences and distractions ☯, we can look at the world from a whole O new perspective.

> The five colors make man's eyes blind;
> The five notes make his ears deaf:
> The five tastes injure his palate...[11]

> Lǎozǐ

Tàijí is often translated as the *supreme ultimate*, yet it does not imply the *top most point* as it has no dichotomy, no Apex. Regarding the creation of the universe, Liú addresses the error that there was *first* Wújí and then out of the emptiness Tàijí emerged.[12] In his deep contemplation, creation does not arise out of the void. Dào *is* One: it does not give birth to One.

---

[10] Meaning we observe the flux of ☯ and erroneously base our treatments upon it. From this entry level of understanding, the physician would then apply therapy, logically treating Yáng with Chái Hú (*Radix Bupleuri*) and Yīn with Shú Dì Huáng (*Radix Rehmanniae*), for example. Adding more Yīn or moving Yáng. Rather, the principle of medicine must be to bring the Heart back to Center, thereby facilitating the body's ability to cope with constant change. To exemplify our concern, modern Chinese medicine tends to see Heat in the superficial tissues and call it *Toxic Heat* or *Fire Poison*, equating it to *inflammation*. Medicine is then used to *treat* the Heat using bitter and cold substances. The living human being is defined by warmth. When the One Thread of Life is completely still, we pass on, and the vessel is *stone cold*. Fire, Heat and warmth are the experiences of circulation, a cycle that should avoid Apexes. *Seeing Heat* and then *clearing Heat* equates to wāi mén xié dào.

[11] Lǎozǐ, 1963, p. 16.

[12] Dào gives birth to One.
One gives birth to Two.
Two gives birth to Three.
Three gives birth to ten-thousand things.
The ten-thousand things carry Yīn and embrace Yáng.
They mix these energies to enact harmony.
Dào Dé Jīng (道德经) chapter 42.

Heaven utilizes the one origin in order to generate life and spread throughout existence, so the myriad things have shape, form and order according to their rank and nature. This is the origin of propriety, as mankind acquires the excellence of the five phases from Heaven, so their Xìng is the most nimble, refined and clever within the principle of Tàijí.

Encompassing Heaven and Earth, Tàijí disseminates the five phases, forming the myriad things, and thus mankind attains its Xìng. The Five Cardinal Relationships are all Separations of Tàijí, which, when coming in contact with the human Heart become the foundation of moral ethics. To sum up, its principle is one. It is this oneness that lets life take its course to the utmost reaches. Inferior people focus on external things, lose what comes first, and so find that propriety evades them. They fail to see that Xìng is naturally within, that propriety is constantly at their Center. Only after this realization can there be harmony, as without this Center there is never and will never be true peace...[13]

Under Heaven, from ancient times to the current one, social customs have changed constantly. The sages who cultivated themselves by nurturing their Qì, encouraged peace under Heaven. How would this be possible? The myriad affairs and principles all find their root in the Heart, which has a human Heart and a Dào Heart. The principle of restraining oneself and going back to propriety[14] means to expel Yīn selfishness, as the body constantly lusts over external and material things. The one principle allows the human Heart to hear the decree of Heaven, which is held within the Dào Heart. The sage puts this into practice with all human relationships and thus penetrates the laws of nature. Both the roots and branches are nurtured, and then Center harmony is achieved, embracing the entire world. It clarifies not only the average affairs of daily life, but also encompasses everything leading to peace...[15]

This principle of one origin has no beginning or end, no sound or smell. It is the instrument of opening and closing which splits and thereafter Heaven and Earth form and come into existence. Even though there is Separation, everything still has this one origin. It is this origin that makes things come to life.[16]

---

[13] Commentary on the Book of Rites, p. 1264-1.
[14] Kèjǐ fùlǐ (克己复礼).
[15] Commentary on the Book of Rites, p. 1381-2 and 1382-1.
[16] Commentary on the Book of Rites, p. 1412-2.

The one principle, Liú explains, is the constancy found within the Center, a place *without Apex*. In previous chapters, the Outer Water and Inner Fire Circles have been discussed, analyzing their structure and function, emotions, likes and dislikes. These two circles engage with the exterior material world, absorbing life and discharging it. Unlike Tàijí, they both reveal an Apex. People can swing from their likes to dislikes, a pivot where one thing leads to another. Our emotions discharge from the Center according to our circumstances, as the *social customs have changed constantly*. Inconsistencies, like not being able to step in the same river twice, show that social norms along with our emotional reactions cannot be pure principle, which is by definition unchanging. To advance into this perception is to approach complete oneness.[17]

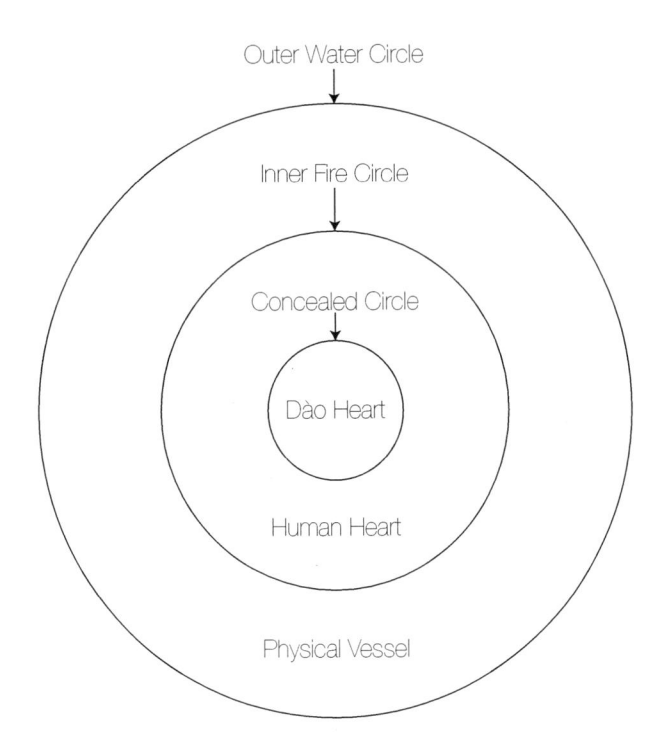

- Outer Water Circle
- Inner Fire Circle
- Concealed Circle
- Dào Heart
- Human Heart
- Physical Vessel

---

[17] "There have been philosophers...who would weaken, or destroy, the claim of science to understand reality by questioning the very existence of cause and effect." B. L. Silver, *The Ascent of Science*, Oxford University Press, New York, 1998, p. 21. Yīn and Yáng exist, just as the sorrow and happiness do, yet they are just the manifestation, not the cause. Cause and effect, the to and fro, are not the *true cause*.

The Dào Heart is in the Center of the Center, a place Liú refers to as Tàijí: the one origin, the one principle. Hùnyuán medicine calls this the Concealed Circle, and is the resting place of Xīnfǎ, away from the swell of desires and distastes, the tides of Yīn and Yáng and impervious to time and space. Within the Dào Heart (心) is the Xìng, our connection to all that is living (生). This Concealed Circle is the only true circle as it has *no Apex*, the true principle of Xìng.

> *The human is born and has life and stillness through the Xìng of Heaven within the Heart. As we come into contact with external things we move our desires out of Xìng. As external things become clear in one's knowledge, then our likes and dislikes appear. When these are without any internal regulation and one becomes acquainted with outer seductions, one cannot reflect inwards and then Heaven's principle vanishes.*
>
> *The possibilities for external things to come in contact with us are endless. Without regulations or rules regarding our likes and dislikes, when external things present themselves we transform to become that which we desire or distaste. We want it so much it is as if it becomes us, consumes us: Heaven principle is then made extinct. It is this process that exhausts our desires and we are afflicted with perversity, licentiousness, chaos, weakness and being counterfeit. A fake Heart.[18]*
>
> *Thus the strong become weak, the many become few, the knowledgeable become foolish and the courageous become fearful. When this disease is not addressed the old and the young are alone in solitude and cannot find their proper place: this is the Dào of the great chaos.[19]*

> *For a person to be classified as a human being they must live by and apply the one principle of Heaven. And that is it! This principle is all goodness, whilst the seven emotions discharge and can be seen as likes and dislikes. If these are well behaved and suitable, how could the Xìng not be content? Only when material desires and lust are slanting our Hearts do we become disturbed to the extreme.[20]*

---

[18] Therefore, the opposite of benevolence.
[19] Commentary on the Book of Rites, p. 1472-1.
[20] Commentary on the Book of Rites, p. 1572-2.

The myriad affairs and principles are all contained within the human Heart and the Dào Heart. Through becoming upright, the human Heart attains the pureness of the Dào Heart. How is it possible to reach this state in just one morning?[21]

Correcting the human Heart to reflect the pure Dào Heart requires lengthy cultivation, yet the mere process of walking this path and that we traverse its highs and lows, leads us into a peaceful state of being. The reward is here and now, *in the middle of the road*, not at the end of our journey. Every minute we walk this path with benevolence, we receive a yellow bean and our vessel fills with life.

"Step by step walk the thousand-mile road."[22]

Miyamoto Musashi

Recently a patient we had been treating for fertility concerns who had not ovulated or had a period for the last three years, reported having a vivid and highly emotional dream involving a hospital (a place of dislike), a baby (like) and issues regarding the birth (dislike), which ended up being wonderful (like). She awoke crying and was then intimate with her partner. A few weeks later she had a positive pregnancy test. Looking back at her basal body temperature recordings, the morning after her dream showed a sharp temperature spike indicating that ovulation had occurred.

Many women experience dreams of having babies and yet in this case the impulse came from somewhere deep within her, passing through her likes and dislikes, through her physiology (hormones and ovaries) and out into the external world as material tears. This is an example of an internal impression evolving into maturity in her Outer Water Circle. Quite easily, these same impulses can be exuded by a Wounded Warrior and the implications for the Heart and physical body are not positive ones.

Mencius explains that at birth the human Heart is naturally good due to its proximity to the Dào Heart. Contained within the Concealed Circle, Tàijí reflects our origin, the ever-rotating motion of the planets around us, or we around them. There is no Apex, no beginning or end. At the moment of conception when the sperm enters the egg, Two (二) elements merge to become One (一). Inside the new circle rapid division takes place transforming into the myriad cells and tissues of the physical body, yet this all takes place within the whole. While this division appears an outward and

---

[21] Commentary on the Book of Rites, p. 1558-2.
[22] M. Musashi, *A Book of Five Rings: The Classic Guide to Strategy*, trans. V. Harris, The Overland Press, New York, 1974, p. 66.

forwards movement, the momentum being generated is not an example of a straight line that moves away from the fetus. Rather, it is part of a curved line that appears to be moving away, yet eventually it returns along that curve to the original site. Similarly, the sun looks like it is moving away from us in the afternoon, only to come towards us in the morning.[23] A complete circle which we tend to observe in segments and divisions, yet the end finds itself at the start: this is Tàijí.

When standing at one point on a circle it seems that the path ahead is leading away, yet it always returns to the origin: there is no Apex. Apexes are evident in states of growth and decline, such as our lifetime from birth to decay. We are born and then we are extinguished, a process governed by the dichotomy of the human Heart. The principle of the human Heart is to desire and distaste through its interaction with the material world, whilst that of the Dào Heart is always to move away whilst always returning, cycling without end.

Shí Yīn Fū and his ledger of good and evil, taught us the skill of using black and yellow beans to monitor ourselves, a means to sort out the human Heart so it conforms to and reflects the Dào Heart. This is a tool for avoiding Apexes, as reflecting the Dào Heart equates to reflecting our origin within the Concealed Circle, which has no Apex. Disease, disharmony and ill health are planted and nurtured when we create an Apex through our connection to the exterior world. Indeed, each and every cell within us is at the whim of our human Heart, and its propensity for creating Apexes (our likes and dislikes). Discharged emotions are energy movements outward from Center that do not return. We have created an Apex. Thus, the meaning of being alive *is* to create and have an Apex, yet this same process is what leads to our decline. It is the natural way of things, as we are born into the external world of Yīn and Yáng. While *natural* for us to age and decline, this does not imply that we should expedite the process. Life is a precious gift for us to achieve our purpose in the world and through Xīnfǎ the physician and the patient can improve and promote their capacity for kindness and compassion.

仁民愛物

Rén Mín Ài Wù

'Universal Benevolence.'
Mencius

---

[23] From a geocentric perspective.

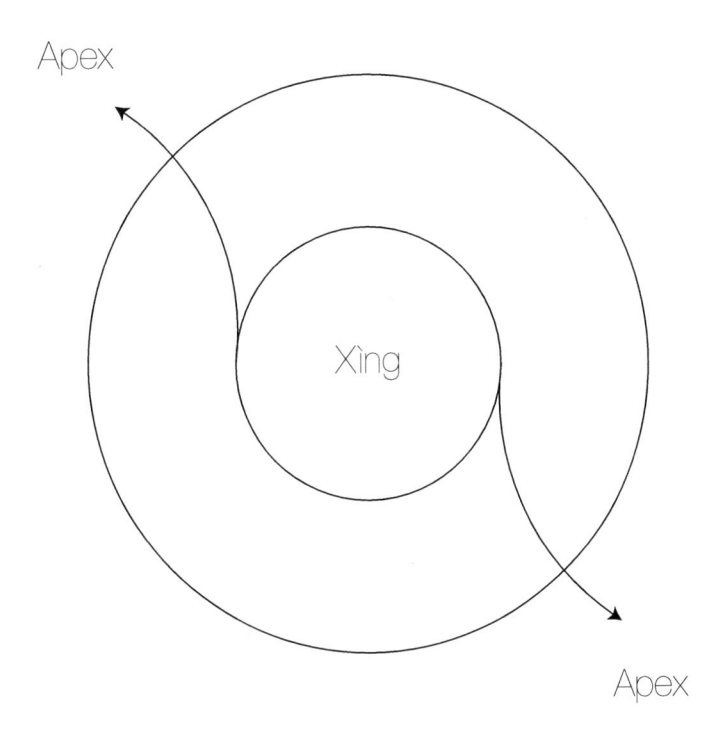

Diagram: Two concentric circles with the inner labeled "Xìng" and an arrow curving through both circles with "Apex" labeled at each end.

We need to have these desires to live, otherwise we would never desire to approach the apple tree, to reach for its fruit. Yet it is not just sustenance people reach for; through circumstances they are *taught* to extend their desires into every crevice, greedily using up every resource in order to feed their wounded human Heart. Unbeknownst to them, this *learning* is the root of their undoing, illness and suffering. Unfortunately, the more we desire, the more we need and the more we need, the more we desire. All accounts must balance in the end, and if we have spent beyond our means, we will be in a debt of our own choosing.

> Some of you say,
> "Joy is greater than sorrow,"
> and others say,
> "Nay, sorrow is the greater."
> But I say unto you,
> they are inseparable.[24]
>
> The Prophet

---

[24] Gibran, 2008, p. 59.

As the human Heart draws its impetus from the Dào Heart, separating it into a dichotomy, the physical vessel is brought under increasing strain. The human body lives, but then dies through Tàijí becoming a division between two opposites. The Concealed Circle, after a hundred years of being taxed by the momentum of the human Heart, finally succumbs and moves in a straight line that does not return: it gains an Apex and life in the vessel ceases. Every cell begins as a Concealed Circle, containing the entirety of life within it: a tiny acorn holding the potential to stand taller than any peer. The One is separated by the human Heart into Two, and then into the myriad miracle of cell division. We grow and then perish as we pull at the seams; weakening the integrity of the vessel's capacity to contain the Xìng. The Apex of living is dying. And herein lies the magic. Once we were all merely gametes and then through a miraculous union our bodies grew. Later, we unite with another Xìng and a child is born; a true circle, a cycle of creation, a continuous life. This is the life cycle from one generation to the next where the One Thread stretches out eternally, and we see just segments of the curve as ourselves. It is this miracle that drives Hùnyuán medicine, particularly in the field of infertility, as this should be shared by everyone, turning immaculate sorrow into joy.

> "Oh yes, we've reached the very stars!
> My friend, for us the ages that are past
> must be a book with seven seals.
> What's called the spirit of an age
> is in the end the spirit of you persons
> in whom past ages are reflected."[25]
>
> Faust

Unification and Separation are the means by which the physician enters the conversation with the physical vessel, encouraging appropriate relationships to food, water, sleep and season. Then the Inner Fire Circle will be sufficiently supported and able to accomplish the gōngfu of cultivation through Xīnfǎ. Medicine moves closer to Center and harmony. All emotions, whether they are likes or dislikes, move outward and do not return, taking with them a drop of life. True health can only be accomplished through regulating this, and when the Center emanates nothing but benevolence, infertility will just be a distant memory, a dream.

---

[25] Goethe, 1984, p. 18.

> I do my utmost to attain emptiness;
> I hold firmly to stillness.
> The myriad creatures all rise together
> And I watch their return.
> The teeming creatures
> All return to their separate roots.
> Returning to one's roots is known as stillness
> This is what is meant by returning to one's destiny.[26]
>
> Lǎozǐ

As described in the case above involving the patient's dream, her outcome was not achieved through the Outer Water Circle but rather it started from the Center, and then manifested in the cellular body as the potential of the Xìng was unlocked. It started as an impression in Xìng, resonating with the One Thread of Life ready to be woven into another vessel, then evolved and matured into physical reality. The work of the physician in improving the patient's Outer Water Circle is relevant and contributes to the process, but the final result is always due to the internal workings of the patient, *not* the doctor.

> *As Mencius said, 'The difference between humans and animals is very slight, so what is the distinction? It is the Heaven principle and that is it!' The human being attains the principle of Heaven and is therefore part of mankind, endowed with the good Heart of Heaven. The sages knew they just had to fulfill these words. We, the average people, due to this slight difference between ourselves and the beasts, are also human beings endowed with the kind Heart of Heaven's principle.*

> *This is Xìng.*
> *This is Benevolence.*
> *This is Dào.*
> *This is virtue.*
> *This is sincerity.*[27]

---

[26] Lǎozǐ, 1963, p. 20.
[27] Commentary on the Spring and Autumn Annals, p. 1662-1.

Our Heart reaches to the invisible and is completely concealed, becoming complete with virtue. Only Heaven knows it. Preserving our Heart and Xìng is what is defined as serving Heaven. The Heart and Xìng may reside within me but have their origin in Heaven. As Heaven and mankind have but one principle, how could it be anything but one Qì?[28]

Heaven's Dào has no words to describe it. Despite this, the myriad things come endlessly into being from its spreading forth: how is this so? The one origin has no end and no beginning; it flows with the myriad materials and finds itself within human ethics.[29] Each has its place, each has its path and appropriateness.[30]

Heaven is vast and hazy and one cannot know it. Its principle, however, comes into every human being. Whatever the circumstances, the human Dào is reliant totally upon the Heavenly principle. When following this principle, you move forward and every thought is included in the Heaven principle of oneness. And so Heaven's Dào comes upon us, as Confucius says, 'Knowing the Heaven in me, then there is nothing that can rile against it.'

Later generations have not been excited by propriety. They lost discipline and restraint of their body and Heart. They thought that Heaven's Dào was too high for them to reach and began offending the divine. Absentmindedly they followed their emotions instead of the true principle. How can you be ignorant of this principle and be without error?[31]

Life is constant and continuous. Regardless of our opinions and desires, we are given our time and that is it. Yet the days and nights leave their mark and the rift between emotion and belief result in a lifetime of blindly arguing: *they thought that Heaven's Dào was too high for them to reach, and began offending the divine...*Hence, our time is short with life being drawn outward to the myriad things, an osmosis of Center. So the physician knows their place and is without offense, following the true principle, seeking the Tàijí within the patient and that is it! The physician looks, eyes shining with

---

[28] Commentary on the Spring and Autumn Annals, p. 1908-2.
[29] Human ethics here means proper kinship relationships between people. See chapter 10 for more on this.
[30] Commentary on the Officers of the Zhōu Dynasty, p. 1924-2.
[31] Commentary on the Officers of the Zhōu Dynasty, p. 2020-2 and 2021-1.

benevolence. The physician hears, knowing words and then knowing the patient. By investigating beneath the layers they acknowledge the immense potential within the patient's body. Locking this potency down, the Inner Fire Circle has become habituated, making the key harder to turn. Remembering that the physical body is the last stepping-stone out from Xìng, the physician gently guides the patient back to Center. Knowing through their own experience, the physician understands that the patient tends to be out of balance with Unification and Separation. It is easy to get lost but difficult to find the way back. A lighthouse in the storm of desires and despair, the physician helps the patient breathe; respiration, the most fundamental of cycles, acts as an anchor. The Heart calms, the mind clears and we take hold of sincerity and uprightness.

Center means *the Center of each cell* and yet more broadly it refers to an area of the body where we commonly experience emotion. A broken Heart is not felt in the head, but in the Center. It is the place we experience when seeing another living being suffer. Although strong emotions drain us, they can guide us to this place of sensation, fixing our point of reference for our cultivation. From here we are reminded of our innate longing to be benevolent, to be compassionate.

Compassion, unlike our desires and distastes, does not perish into an Apex. It circulates within the Dào Heart, following a curved line without end. People are brought into this sphere of kindness, feeling safe and at home. Exuding sympathy and sorrow must translate into compassion; otherwise this good intentioned discharging creates an Apex. When our bag is full of yellow beans, compassion has become our natural constancy. Being filial towards one's parents, loving a spouse, caring for a child, respecting a sibling, being a trustworthy friend, these are all acts of compassion derived from our Center and what make the person a human being. Keeping these relationships constantly in our Heart is to be in concert with Tàijí. The Yīn and Yáng can clash and clang around us, but no matter how loud the cacophony, we are only defined by the principle of Heaven within us.

When off Center, the physician takes time to appreciate the gift of the present, bringing the patient with them. Walking to the riverbank, they feel the breeze on their skin, the sun on their face. Taking in the natural world around them, they see its colors and forms, listen to its sounds, and breathe it all into their Center. There is neither happiness nor sadness: there is simply *living*. They are *being* alive, one with the principle of Heaven. Not coming or going, always leaving and always returning. The physician and patient have returned, compassion reverberating out from their Center into the world. Reaching a sagely level, they manifest this state of being in each step and breath, regardless of setting, as they are constantly with Tàijí.

Carry the Sun to the Earth
O, Man, you are placed
between Light and Darkness
Be a warrior of Light...
transform yourself.[32]

Zarathustra

---

[32] From the *Zend Avesta*, a classical text from ancient Persia.

CHAPTER 8

扭兵

Niǔ Bīng

The Wounded Warrior

Alone must it seek the ether...
...alone and without his nest shall the eagle fly across the sun.[1]

From an understanding of Center and Tàijí we now look in detail at the Inner Fire Circle, our molten river that spans the distance between the Dào Heart and the external world. This chapter explores Xīnfǎ by discussing the works included in book nine of Liú Yuán's Huái Xuān compendium where he mentions an historical figure named Shào Yōng (邵雍), (1011–1077 CE). A northern Sòng dynasty poet and rationalist scholar, Shào was the originator of Pre-Heaven theory–*Xiāntiān Xué* (先天学)–and explained Tàijí as being the source of the myriad things. Liú utilizes one of Shào's works entitled *Huáng Jí Jīng Shì* (皇极经世), *The Rules of Imperial Statecraft Passed to the World,* to articulate errors and correct corruptions therein. Along with Shào's work, Liú uses several famous texts by first quoting them and then offering his elaborations.

> *Shào Yōng told us that 'the science of investigating Pre-Heaven is called Xīnfǎ. Originating in the Hétú (河图) river picture,[2] all life starts from the Center and the number five. From this place all the myriad things and affairs come into existence. This is the Heart.'*

---

[1] Gibran, 2008, p. 28.
[2] The Hétú (河图) is an ancient Chinese divination picture and system used to explain relationships between the bāguà within the Yìjīng.

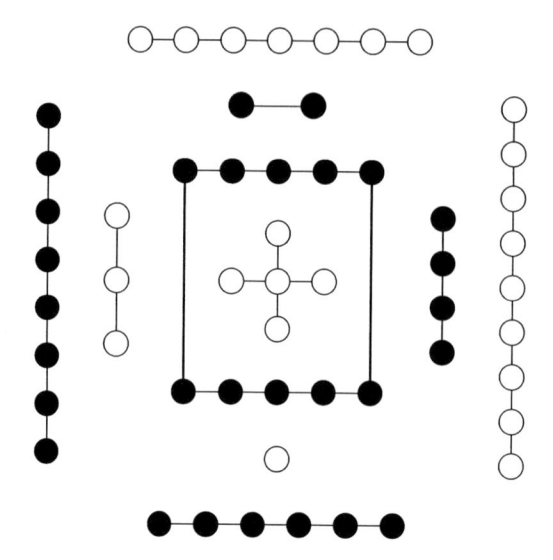

The term Xīnfǎ started with Master Shào and the Confucians that followed him have repeated his words. When one studies, one does so in order to understand the true principle–the principle of Heaven–and through this endeavor we can become truly human. So how could the sage simply infer a technique for this? Rather than a technique, we are given a method: Xīnfǎ, the 'Heart Method'. Here, the superficial student may grasp at words that go astray. When Master Shào says that in the Hétú the originating number is five, which resides in the Center, in this context the picture resembles Tàijí in Pre-Heaven. In contrast, the human Heart exists in the Post-Heaven and therefore finds itself distant from a state of pure oneness. The Pre- and Post-Heaven are not the same and we who dwell in the Post-Heaven realm do not attain our Center through analyzing the Hétú.[3]

Great Masters teach the world, leaving their words for us to follow, yet sometimes words are misunderstood and misinterpreted. What is written on the page can confuse as easily as clarify. Words are important, yet without the spaces between them itisalljustabigjumbledbefuddlingmess.[4]

---

[3] On Correcting Errors, p. 3584-2 to 3585-1. Liú clarifies the idea that the five in the Center of the Hétú, representing the Tàijí principle, is being equated to the human Heart of Post-Heaven. These are two different things, he explains, which are closely connected, but different nonetheless.

[4] For more on this inference, please see P. Coelho, *The Witch of Portobello*, HarperCollins, Sydney, 2007.

Seeking the Lost Heart of Medicine, the breathing spaces between the rules, regulations, definitions, prescriptions and formulations let us see the *foundation* of all these manifestations. It is the true principle behind the words *not marred by ink* that is constant. Our strategies and treatments may morph and adapt with the rolling of time, but when words are understood from the principle behind them, the myriad applications of medicine are imbued with virtue.[5] The physician finds the Heaven principle within themselves and their patients, within their Hearts. And that is it!

> "One must *always* help a good person, no matter the circumstances.
> One must *never* help a bad person, no matter the circumstances."
>
> Féng Zhìqiáng (馮志強)[6]

Embracing the difficulty of *good* and *bad* as studied in the tale of Shí Yīn Fū, the physician and patient choose their daily quota of black and yellow beans. *Not helping* someone would seem to gain a black bean, yet not helping *a bad person*, as advised by Féng Zhìqiáng, means not helping them to accomplish their foul play. Yīn Fū helped Xīn Dé not by aiding and abetting his trickery but by helping him become good. The physician is not a bu*sin*essman and must not gain profit from the negative affairs of others, nor support them in these affairs, no matter the circumstances. Yet the physician must help a good person, regardless of material gain. Constantly, without an Apex, we reflect inwards and apply our medicine from the Heart as if the patient was our own child or parent. Intentions tilt the scales to either good or bad words and actions, and it is often our inner *Wounded Warrior* who settles the score of this pendulum.

> "There is a saying,
> when with good people,
> you study good things,
> while when with bad people,
> you study bad things."
>
> Liú Bǎigǔ

---

[5] We can only see the meaning of words when they are surrounded by nothing: *the empty void*. For example: the secret to success is ▮▮▮▮!

[6] Féng Zhìqiáng (馮志強), (1928–2012) was one of China's great Tàijíquán and Qìgōng masters.

As soon as a person is born, they begin the study of life, and through this the Heaven principle within begins its decline; they mature, age and then pass. In one sense, life is constantly being lost or stolen through the process of living. The Wounded Warrior within us is a product of the human or Post-Heaven Heart, which naturally rails against losing its territory, finding itself in a perpetual state of defense. This part of us that attaches and relates to the outside material world uses the sword of the Inner Fire Circle to constantly and erroneously defend life, as if trying to hold onto it and plug the hour glass. Yet life, regardless of this effort, *will* run out. Wounded Warriors desperately try to defend that which they cannot, resorting to desperate measures that do not succeed. In the end they just wave their arms in despair: the worrying Warrior.

As discussed in previous chapters, our human Heart discharges emotions, making us hungry, seeking *things*, craving safety and security. Through this we can have balanced cycles of Unification and Separation, drawing in and pushing out appropriately to achieve our purpose in our allotted years. Yet when attempting to defend against life from disappearing, paradoxically, the more we try to defend the more we lose. This effort of defending and controlling takes enormous amounts of energy, weakening us. The Warrior is Wounded and can no longer defend their kingdom, more holes appear in the sieve, more vitality leaks. When life is dominated by this mindset, or Heart-set, people's good intentions are often based on shaky foundations; thinking their actions are on the right track, instead they find themselves lost.

> Cogito ergo sum.
> *I think, therefore I am.*
>
> René Descartes

I think, therefore I am...lost.[7] As we discovered in the previous chapter, in spite of the inconsistency of our years we take Heart that within us resides the true principle of Heaven, our constant reference point. The river is *always* wet and we are *always* imbued with the Dào Heart. Human Xìng is all goodness with utter compassion for life and living, and by returning here with Xīnfǎ we find our Center and quieten the One Thread of Life. Our mental, emotional and physical health improves and life leaks less. Thinking and acting from a balanced Center, we respond and react positively and appropriately in our relationships.

---

[7] Mencius tells us that *we feel*, therefore we are, while his compatriot Xún Zǐ (310–220 BCE) agrees with Descartes. For more, see P. K. Bol & W. C. Kirby, *China: Traditions and Transformations*, Harvard lecture series.

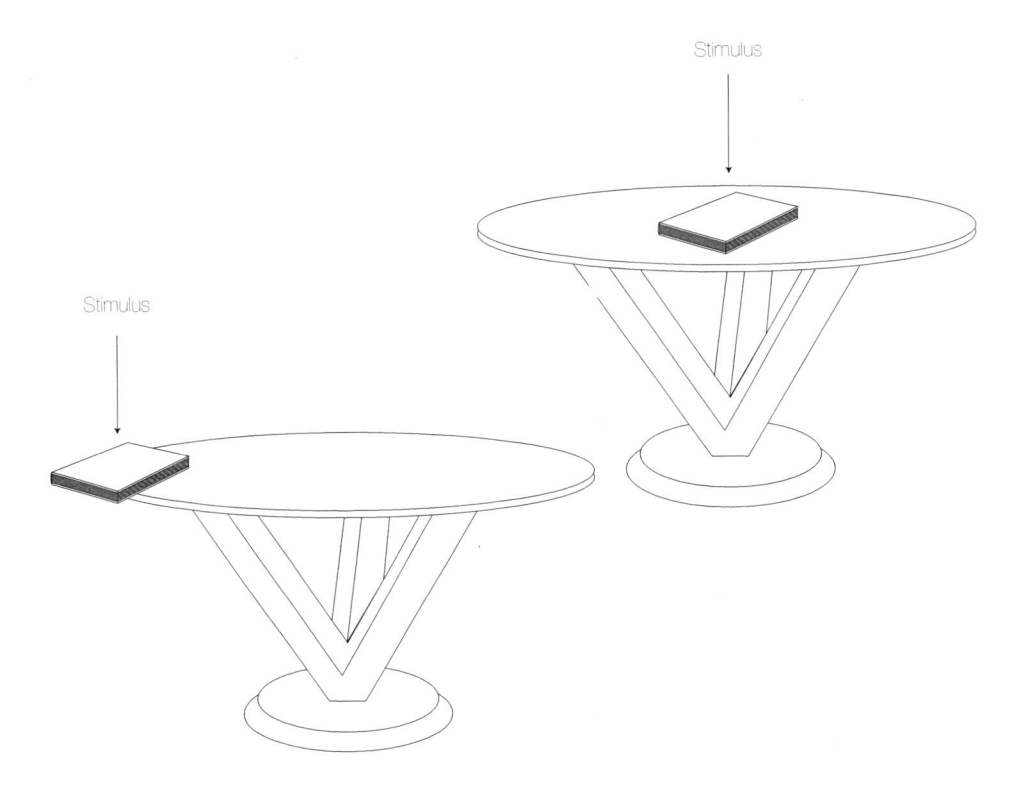

This image was first described by Tàijíquán Master, Chén Zhōnghuá (陳中華), in the context of finding one's Center or that of one's opponent.[8] When the book is flat on the table it is balanced and does not fall. Yet when positioned on the edge, with just the slightest of movements the book will topple. For us, the same principle applies; when Centered we act and think harmoniously, yet when we feel on-edge it becomes difficult to radiate benevolence. For the physician, opening the book of the patient and exploring the inner workings must be done from a fixed point of Center. When safely in the middle of the table we can peruse the pages without predicament. Opening it while quivering on the precipice, we are bound to fall. First the physician comes into the Center and only then can they help the patient back to their lost Heart.

Giving the human being the present of housing the Heaven principle, the vessel is brought to life *by* Xìng. Being defensive or afraid of life *or* death will obscure our clarity of purpose, health and the broader consequences of our actions and abstention. Protecting Xìng from defensiveness, we work with géwù and through self-examination we remove selfishness. Life is not ours to grasp firm and *own*, rather, it is ours to

---

[8] Chén Zhōnghuá (陳中華) is one of the prominent Tàijíquán masters of the 21st century. The only disciple of the two legendary masters, Hóng Jūnshēng (洪均生), (1907–1996) and Féng Zhìqiáng.

complement, sustain and then graciously hand on to the next generation. Excuses and justifications formed over years or decades of circumstance are not rudely confronted, but gently left at the riverbank.

> A society grows great when old men plant trees
> whose shade they know they shall never sit in.
>
> Greek proverb.

Being defensive equates to a perception of being under attack. Feeling threatened, fearing the loss of something that is *ours*, the Warrior waves their arms, wounding their surroundings. On edge, they become deflated and lean towards being a *bad* person. What Fēng defines as *bad* we explain as a Wounded Warrior who adversely effects those around them: *I need to defend against something being taken away from me = what I claim as my own will deprive someone else.* Intellectual intentions may be positive, yet fail to materialize into benevolence.

> Having good intentions, but then doing wrong: this is one disease.

Medicine protects and nurtures that which is most important: life. Thus, the physician must rid themselves of the Wounded Warrior before engaging the patient. When the body is in a defensive internal posture, emotions easily discharge beyond appropriateness with likes and dislikes forcing more gaps in true understanding.[9] Each relationship and interaction is thus defined. Despite good intentions, the person finds themselves asking, *why is my health in such a poor state and why are my relationships in such turmoil?* Enter the physician, who should have the answer and yet if this comes in the form of a pill, or point, or herb, without Xīnfǎ they play darts in the dark. No one wants to feel the sharp end of the projectile.

    The practice of medicine is full of merit as long as it is based on principle and comes from a point of Center. *So how could the sage simply infer a technique?* Medicinal techniques are as varied as the myriad things so *rather than a technique, we are given a method, the 'Heart method'*. For the physician this means starting each consultation by asking themselves, *the human being has an innate love of life and an innate ability to <u>heal itself</u>, so how is it possible that my patient's body is in disarray?* The answer could be as simple as dehydration or as complex as abuse, which will be

---

[9] "...how would you guard *your* back?"
"Ah," he smiled. "An excellent question. The way to guard your back is to act in such a manner that the people about you love you so much that they would never allow you to be attacked from behind." (Schmieg, 2005, p. 1).

clearly differentiated by the Centered physician. Their responsibility is then to teach and guide the patient with compassion and kindness until they both see the true root of the dis-ease. Recovery may indeed involve the application of physical medicine either applied or ingested, which will be based on an understanding of Xìng and delivered with strength, speed and confidence. Both physician and patient can sleep well that night, completing the fullness of Unification as their Hearts are at ease.

> What a wonderful sleep it had been!
> Never had a sleep so refreshed him, so renewed him, so rejuvenated him!...
> He had slept wonderfully. He was remarkably awake, happy and curious.[10]
>
> Siddhartha

Oh, for such a sleep! Being awake, happy and curious has a positive ripple effect within ourselves and also within our patients and in turn, their relationships and interactions outside of the clinic transform. The kind Heart of Heaven[11] is tarnished in mankind through the reactions of the Wounded Warrior, which likewise ripples out into our relationships. Oblivious to Xìng, people protect their own territories and fear for their *cubs*. This natural animalistic response has us constantly on guard, but not guarding the Dào Heart, rather it guards the human Heart and the perception that we are constantly losing something. In the end we live and die as if we have not lived at all.[12]

A *bad* person bases their choices in life from a defensive stance, which is a posture of selfishness. Observing this in ourselves or others, we are provided an opportunity to flex the muscles of géwù. The cultivation of the Wounded Warrior requires a determined approach.

---

[10] Hesse, 1973, p. 72.

[11] This kind Heart of Heaven is referred to by Liú and the ancient Classics as *tiānlǐ liángxīn* (天理良心).

[12] "Ah never cried as a baby. That is to say, throughout mah babyhood never once did ah cry – no, not a peep. Nor did ah brawl away mah childhood either and during mah youthhood ah resolved to contain all mah emotions within and never to allow one sob without – for to do otherwise surely laid one open to all manner of abuse. And now, as ah count away the final seconds of mah manhood – as ah don the death-hood – ah will not crack. No. In all mah lifehood ah have never once cried. Not out loud. No, not out loud." N. Cave, *And the Ass Saw the Angel*, Penguin Books, London, 1989, p. 18. Literature, along with other arts, as discussed below, is the perfect medium for the Wounded Warrior to express itself. The reader takes what they want, leaving what does not impress. The patient, however, takes the medicine their physician prescribes. And that is it.

When we feel attacked and go on the defensive, we bring ourselves back to Center; we turn to the next chapter and read and re-read *Revering the 100 Medicines*. Reading the 100 medicines: this is one medicine.

> *The Great Learning states that to be clear about virtue, one must get close to the people. However, getting close to them does not mean just physically, but also means we must actually love them. This requires gōngfu. The Doctrine of the Mean states, '...the king said, every person in the kingdom, all are better than me.' We dare not slowly inspect these words or be lax with their meaning. We dare not be indolent with observing our lust and greed. Instead, we must always think of how to place ourselves below others. This is defined as reaching for goodness.*[13]

This strategy of not raising ourselves by lowering others is part of the skill of virtue, of how to minimize our Wounded Warrior and increase our relationship with Xìng. The physician is the perpetual student relinquishing the Wounded Warrior. This brings us to meditation, a practical way of reaching a profound place.[14]

> *The root of all action must be in the Heart. Nonetheless, the human Heart has many selfish desires that lead us astray; how can it not deceive us with laziness and recklessness? It is by knowing to stop only at ultimate goodness, and in this way one can collect the emotions back to Center. The Heart that is already discharged can be stilled and then enter into divine emptiness: the divine void.*

---

[13] Commentary on the ancient Great Learning, p. 3298-2.

[14] Just by looking at the word *meditation*, we may have already written a story in our minds about what the word means. Liú Yuán asks us what good we achieve by sitting in void in our temple? In this context, meditation means self-reflection, which is not defined by time or setting. Meditation may indeed take the form of sitting quietly, or walking through a forest, lying next to a stream, or doing Tàijíquán, Qìgōng or yoga, or painting, singing, dancing, writing, gardening, breathing. It is a tool used to iron out our internal wrinkles and bring us back to Center. This is not to isolate ourselves within a bubble, but rather give us insight and perspective and respond more favorably to our Cardinal Relationships.

"...the old man said: I live alone not because of my virtue, but rather because of my weakness. You see, those who live among people are the strong ones." (From the Desert Fathers, Feldman & Kornfield (eds), 1991 p. 151).

> *By supporting one's Will in order to contain one's Qì, one reaches to void and stillness: the place where one thought does not arise.*[15] *When residing in this place, one knows the stopping point. The Heart then finds itself naturally flowing and moving with the Dào.*
>
> *Forcefully restraining the Heart in order to heal internal disorder is not the answer. On the contrary, to know the stopping point we must not use force to restrain the Heart. Rather, we nourish the concept of preserving Xìng, nurturing the Qì and guarding the Center. By guarding the movement of the Heart and Xìng our illusions are purified; surrounded by the empty void, our Heart becomes firm and complete.*[16]
>
> *With this we have yǒudìng,*[17] *a point of reference, so that when the Heart moves away from goodness, we have a compass needle pointing North and South. This is our precise guide, immediately allowing us passage back into stillness. A sage can fix their Xìng and still their Heart through constantly referring to this point of reference when their intention strayed from Center.*
>
> *For the beginner, even if we simply know about the stopping point and only acquire it for one brief moment, this distils our spirit. If we meditate for hours and experience this stopping point in just one mere inhalation, we have found in this one breath a profound place."*[18]

When a patient who has been in utter despair for what seems an eternity– *whose Heart wants to abandon Center*–experiences just *one* moment of joy, one brief flash of light in their bleak sorrow, that is enough; it is proof that no*thing* is constant. Sorrow and joy are *things* we experience because of *things*. They do not define us, they are not us: they are transient and we observe them.[19] For both physician and patient, one flash of light proves that light exists.

---

[15] Xū (虚): Empty, void, humble, guiding principle. Jìng (静): Still, calm, quiet, without apparent movement.

[16] *Above all else, Guard your Heart, for from it flows the springs of life.* Proverbs 4.23.

[17] Yǒudìng (有定): To have a fixed point of reference, a stabilizing anchor on a stormy night at sea.

[18] Commentary on the ancient Great Learning, p. 3298-2.

[19] "I have lost them, or they have lost me – I am not sure. The wheel of appearances revolves quickly, Govinda... The transitory soon changes, Govinda..." (Hesse, 1973, p. 74.).

The gulf between emotion and belief is bridged by that flash of light, for that one breath, and *this* is the fixing point, the Center of the compass, the North Star. Then, despite a lifetime of forming a foundation of emotional reactions to their surroundings, the physician and patient have this anchor. They can stand up to challenges and see life differently.

> He saw beauty everywhere, and once said,
> "Even the lines in a dog turd on the pavement can be beautiful!"
> He taught me to see beyond the immediate substance.
> Like I said, some of his words made no sense at the time!
>
> Mr Kunio Kobayashi quoting his teacher, Mr. Sasaki

A colleague mentioned that when she sits with one of her exquisite Pénjǐng (Chinese for bonsai), and is focusing all her attention on that little tree, gently moving a branch that took her years to grow, nothing else exists. Hours can pass as if minutes. The only things present are her and that branch. In this profound place she feels utter peace. She understands her little tree; it needs sunlight, water, fresh air, some nutrients, a little love and that is it. Should a human being be so different, she asks, with all our likes and dislikes shaping our disposition?[20]

This example shows us that we can create a sacred space for our meditation like she has with her trees, and in that space we easily melt away into Center. It may be a temple, a church, a martial arts studio, a yoga mat, a shrine. Yet this sense of being is something that comes from *within*, not from *without*. It is *always* within us, regardless of our surroundings and so is available to us at all times.

> Before enlightenment, chop wood, fetch water.
> After enlightenment, chop wood, fetch water.
>
> Zen proverb

Step by step the physician walks this path of Xīnfǎ; it is not via grand leaps that they catch up to the sages. Little by little, drop by drop, comforted that we are walking in the right direction, we are guided by Liú Yuán who offers feedback to mediate our meditations:

---

[20] Ergo, when we become unwell, we can approach ourselves as she does her trees. Are we getting enough light, enough rest, enough water and food, enough love? If these fundamentals of existence are all in place and yet still there is a problem, only then is it time for medicine.

Surround your intention with a wall of goodness; thick and condensed it congeals and stills the thoughts. When it goes astray you eradicate it. The earlier sages said that they were not afraid of thoughts; rather, what they feared was negligence in their recognition of them. Whenever it rises, I gather it; I bring it back. This is the method of seeking the discharged Heart. The Great Learning teaches us this with géwù.

As soon as the Heart instigates a movement, recognize it. As soon as we have the sprouting of material desires, our aspiration becomes lucid and the true Heart immediately removes it. We must know the stopping point in order to nurture the origin. By being cautious with ourselves and our internal machinations we can make our intentions sincere. One cannot allow the situation to arise where one thing leads to the neglecting of others.

Without knowing this gōngfu of the ultimate stopping point, the Heart perpetually floats and meanders ceaselessly, then at times it wants to abandon Center. When desires for things reveal themselves, remove them, heal them. And then when yet other desires come, remove them, heal them. It may ensue that our intentions are sincere, yet they cannot be fixed and we find ourselves exhausted, wondering how we are to reach the Xìng. In this case, we have attempted to make our intentions sincere and we have failed. We need géwù, reaching toward knowledge of self-investigation. Then the inside and outside will be spoken for.

Outside, this is our external work, our investigations, studies, inquiries and careful pondering, all leading to a clear differentiation of the principle. For our internal géwù, Confucius guides us, 'if it is not in accord with propriety, I do not look at it, I do not listen to it'. It is not through an empty struggle with restraining of the Heart or flippantly seeking phenomena everywhere in the material world, that we find Center. Without a bright teacher this is very difficult to obtain. Without eternally pursuing this with your Heart, how can the myriad layers of experience be pieced together? With even the smallest missing piece, how can your mind be complete?[21]

---

[21] Commentary on the ancient Great Learning, p. 3307-1-2.

Intentions without a basis in Center and a proper fixing point result in unintended outcomes. As a true reflection of Xìng, sincere intentions are no longer assumptions. Taking our pottery tools, our hammer and chisel, we use Xīnfǎ and the removal of selfishness to clear a path to the Dào; the path to extracting beautiful jade from crude stone.[22]

> "In every block of marble I see a statue as plain as though it stood before me,
> shaped and perfect in attitude and action.
> I have only to hew away the rough walls that imprison the lovely apparition
> to reveal it to the other eyes as mine see it."
>
> Michelangelo

The human Heart discharges easily but finds it difficult to come back. It is easy to move but hard to keep still. Thus people with self-deceit are many. Attempting to collect the Heart and to bring it back to Center, but then to tremble in fear of a deity in Heaven, this brings a great hardship to people.[23]

The Great Learning tells us that getting to self-cultivation is grinding and polishing. This is géwù. It is the Heart of yes and no, of knowing right from wrong. All people have this Heart, yet how is it that so many are clouded and so few are clear? The culprits of this phenomenon are our selfish desires. The ears, the eyes, the mouth and nose, along with the four limbs, they all have these desires and they then separate in disorder with the seven emotions.

If we fail to inspect the Heaven principle to guide our intentions, and then we take action, the physical form exhausts the Xìng and material desires are born. These then shackle and chain us down, keeping us from reaching true knowledge. Without nurturing on the inside and studying on the outside, selfishness will never melt away. The brightness within will never expand.

By stopping our self-cultivation only at ultimate goodness, this path leads constantly to peacefulness and stillness. With being careful with movements of the Heart, every day our aspiration becomes clear and purified. We dare not be

---

[22] "...when in the midst of quiet, the energy of the physical body becomes like silk or jade..." T. Cleary, (trans) *The Secret of the Golden Flower: The Classic Chinese Book of Life*, HarperCollins, New York, 1991, p. 35.

[23] Commentary on the ancient Great Learning, p. 3316-2 to 3317-1.

lazy or reckless for even one moment. Thereafter, day after day, inner knowledge arrives. It is like curing jade rock; we grind away at the stone until we attain the jade.[24]

The crude rock around the jade within the human being is largely shaped by unawareness. Liú writes beautifully about how one can escape ignorance like flowing Water. He uses the fourth hexagram in the Yìjīng, méng (蒙), which means childhood ignorance, youthful folly, the young shoot and discovering. The lower portion of this hexagram is made up of the kǎn trigram ☵, representing Water and the upper portion of the hexagram is composed of the gèn trigram ☶, representing a mountain. Therefore, the hexagram depicts Water being obstructed or held down by a mountain.

The Xìng of Water is to flow and move and yet here the mountain obstructs it. It is like the human Xìng; at their core they are naturally good, yet desires cover them, obscuring and hiding it. This is what is revealed in the méng hexagram of the Yìjīng, the darkness of ignorance.

Yet Water, when it flows out of the mountain is clean and pure like a spring. The sages saw our ignorance as a youthful folly and even though temporarily obstructed, in the end we can all still reach our destination like flowing Water. We then no longer dwell in ignorance. When our Heart finds Center, the obstruction is resolved and immediately we can go through it. Water is good when it is flowing.[25] *One must not rest in ignorance, but rather seek the exit point of ignorance.*[26]

By dwelling in unawareness, people do not realize how much they invest of themselves in material things. This childish mindset is appropriate for a child but a physician must understand that the nature of Water is to flow and that Water is always wet.

All of the myriad things are born from Heaven and Earth. Within the myriad things mankind is the most divine as they alone attain Heaven's principle. This principle resides in the Heart, which is divided into the Pre-Heaven Heart and the Post-Heaven Heart. The Heart of Pre-Heaven is Xìng. The Heart of Post-Heaven is

---

[24] Commentary on the ancient Great Learning, p. 3318-1.
[25] "Think of mosquitoes. They seek stagnant water, but do not cause the pool to become stagnant." Microbiologist Antoine Béchamp, who believed bacteria were not the cause of disease, but the consequence of it.
[26] On Correcting Errors, p. 3528-2.

emotion. And so our Heart starts moving into Separation and disorder as one material thing interacts with the other. The emotions we attach to these interactions with external materials eradicate the Xìng.[27]

Benevolently, the physician stands on the shore with hand outstretched to the Wounded Warriors, who flounder against the fleeting nature of their lives, thrashing in the currents trying to hold back the river. By washing away the obstacles of their own creation, the physician and patient choose to awaken from ignorance and the Wounded Warrior finds Center.

O Fortuna,	O Fortune
velut Luna	changeable
statu variabilis,	as the moon,
semper crescis	you are always either waxing
aut decrescis...	or waning...
Sors immanis	Vain,
et inanis,	monstrous Fate,
rota tu volubilis,	you turning wheel,
status malus,	you can, when you will,
vana salus	destroy bad circumstances
semper dissolubilis...	and delusive success alike...

Carl Orff – Carmina Burana

Creative arts such as music and painting are the perfect place for wounds to clean and heal. Some of the world's greatest works of art are expressions of the Wounded Warrior. The observer then takes what they will from the piece. Sergei Rachmaninoff practiced his 3rd piano concerto on a silent keyboard while traveling from Russia to America by sea, a clear expression of angst experienced by the Wounded Warrior, translated out of himself into quavers and crescendos.

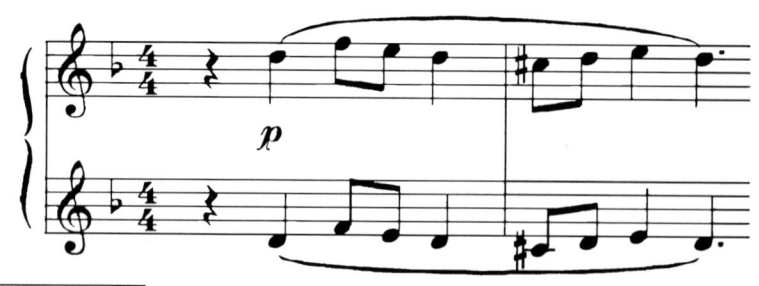

---

[27] Commentary on the ancient Great Learning, p. 3322-2.

Wielding neither a music score nor paint brush, the physician's instrument is Xīnfǎ and benevolence. Unlike notes from black and white keys, when the physician prescribes material substances that the patient consumes, the ramifications for propriety are far greater than for the musician. Thus, the art of medicine is not in the rampant application of medicinals (Yīn and Yáng) at the whims of a Wounded Warrior. Instead, the physician enthusiastically lives, works and breathes from a point of Center, taking their patients with them...*not even one of us has been forgotten.* Liú furthers our contemplation by discussing the merging of emotion with Center and reaching apparent stillness.

> *Because the human Heart is so easily discharged, the purity of the Dào Heart is tarnished. If we are not reaching toward void and stillness, we cannot nurture the Xìng. When seeking the discharged Heart and reaching for Center, even one thought cannot be born or entertained. Submerged and still, fixed, void and tranquil; all can be seen when we reach this Center.*
>
> *That which is already discharged is harmonized with what remains in the Center. Not even one selfish thought presents itself when preserving the spirit within this void. Impartial and one-minded, immediately this is reality. Without reaching this void, this nothingness, we cannot reach the Center, regardless of how we try to preserve the Heart and nurture the Xìng. Without clarifying ignorance and becoming purified of desires, our emotions intermingle with the Xìng. And so the issue of void and nothingness, purification and tranquility, absence of desires, they are the formation of reaching stillness.*[28]

Stillness is actually a constant rotation, the Tàijí state, without movement *away* from Center. Discharging emotions all have Apexes and move outward, taking our warmth with them. The skill is to recognize any emotion springing forth that is not in line with sincerity and compassion and then gently bring it back to guard the Xìng. We remember the five stepping-stones over the Inner Fire Circle leading from Xìng to benevolence. Liú Yuán teaches the gōngfu of *Gazing at the Subtle*, described further below, as a means to stand guard over our Wounded Warrior.

---

[28] Huái Xuān Assorted Compilations, p. 3367-2.

The human being is the Heart of Heaven and Earth: not even one of us has been forgotten. There is only goodness and no evil, as our root is in Heaven. So the human Xìng is goodness, and connects with the good that surrounds it. When aligned with this, good affairs respond to us. And likewise with evil: when we are detached from Xìng, evil affairs are attracted to us.

Within the myriad things it is only mankind who have self-selected actions. The Doctrine of the Mean says, 'when you plant a tree, Heaven will cultivate it, but if it is planted askew, Heaven will topple it.' This mutual impact is immediate. The great Yìjīng is from cover to cover a narration of good and bad fortune, leading people towards goodness. Later generations did not understand that Heaven and man have but one origin, are but one Qì. And so they instruct people to cultivate the body, but fail to speak of fortune and misfortune.

The wise kings of old understood that fortune and misfortune were the natural Dào of Heaven. So to seek fortune and to avoid misfortune is within everyone. When our mind is clouded with misfortune we know that these moving thoughts must be brought back to the Heaven principle in our Center. The true principle is pure; Heaven and man naturally contain it and inspire each other. Without reaching exhaustion you can already reach the highest level of knowledge. With a middle or lower level of ability, we have a Heart that wishes for good fortune, yet we do not know the root of goodness. We are afraid of misfortune, yet not afraid to do evil.[29]

Acting from our fixed point of Center, good thoughts and actions bring good fortune, while for actions based on desires and defensiveness, the alternative is true. Wounded Warriors, by default, grasp, hold and struggle with life, using energy and effort in vain. More holes are punctured in the chalice and soon all that is left is a sieve that leaks Xìng and yellow beans. Physiologically, this relates to tension in the vessel; the muscles seize up and ache from reduced circle-ation. A case example elucidates the point. A woman suffering from long-term anorexia nervosa presents with icy cold extremities and fingers and toes in the throes of decay. Her biomedical doctor has advised her to take a blood thinner for her woes, as the observation of her hands and feet reveal that there is very little blood circulating to them. Thinning her blood is therefore the answer as more blood will be able to irrigate her fine distal capillaries.

---

[29] Huái Xuān Assorted Compilations, p. 3370-2.

"Physician, heal thyself."

Luke 4:23-30

Returning to Center, we ask ourselves, *how is it even possible for her to be in this state of disrepair?* The human being has a profound ability to sustain itself, yet after years of starvation it must decline. Medicine's role is to facilitate the body's self-healing capacity and to never get in the way of it. Our patient has a scarcity of blood in her fingers and toes because these areas are less vital for her survival and under duress, the body diverts warmth to more vital areas. There is very little blood in her extremities because her circumstances and Wounded Warrior have dominated her relationship with food. Thinning blood with synthetic or natural products would divert what little blood that is remaining away from what is vital. Rather, our treatment involved herbs to guide Heaven Yáng down and into the Center via the Unification side of the Outer Water Circle, and Xīnfǎ. Xìng is in our Center, *not even one of us has been forgotten. There is only goodness and no evil, as our root is in Heaven.* Encountering some *good fortune*, she has made a full recovery and her improved health has been reflected in an improved relationship with her husband.

> *The Heart naturally floats and then you need to sink it. When it reveals itself, then you submerge it. Our Center is the root of everything under Heaven. When we reach our Center we reach harmony. We must nurture the goodness of each thought and restrain the evil within each thought.*[30]

A patient once said of her young niece, *'...but she does not know that I am nobody...'*. Emotions emerge from Xìng and through moving to belief and the conscious Heart they should manifest in our thoughts, words and deeds as pure benevolence. Recognizing words, the physician helps the patient become aware of inappropriate thought patterns that weaken the connection to Xìng. In each and every moment, the patient gains an unshakable sense of self-worth and in turn they are no longer a Wounded Warrior. They become themselves again.[31]

---

[30] Huái Xuān Assorted Compilations, p. 3431-2.
[31] "If we therefore isolate our 'nature' from everything that encumbers, conceals, or hobbles it; if we liberate ourselves from ideological perspectives and constructs, then we can restore our nature to what it truly and uniquely is: the vital potential that we are." F. Jullien, *Vital Nourishment: Departing from Happiness*, trans. A. Goldhammer, Zone Books, New York, 2007, p. 33.

> "...and if you can't see anything beautiful about yourself
> get a better mirror
> look a little closer
> stare a little longer..."[32]

Shane Koyczan

Xīnfǎ cultivation is for both the physician and patient as they inspect every movement of the Heart, which transmits out from Center into and through the cellular vessel. Taking responsibility for themselves and their health, they metastasize goodness. Thus, the physician's practical skills and techniques are married with Xìng and the patient's intentions, actions and relationships resonate with purpose and harmony.

學生:	'Shīfu, how do I get out of this headlock?'
師傅:	'Student, how did you get into it?'

People tend to see a problem only when they are stuck in it; finding it hard to see the wood for the trees, the creative solution eludes them.[33] The process of transforming the Wounded Warrior, however, gives us Heart, as the mere act of trying is an impulse coming from Center. You are reading these words and turning these pages, actions coming from within you. Once on this same path, Shí Yīn Fū became aware of the subtle. He did not unknowingly, haphazardly knock fruit from the trees in the orchard with his hat, or squash flowers with his feet, as he started noticing the consequences his actions had on his surroundings. Once on this path, step by step he never meandered, walking it until his last day.

    Géwù teaches that a Wounded Warrior wallows in a reality shaped by the circumstances of a life history. From start to finish, underlying all drama and mayhem, the human being is only defined by the Heaven principle within the Dào Heart. We are only our true individual selves when we are true to Center. The vitality of this understanding comes from viewing the continuum of the One Thread of Life, not just our segment on the curve. Thus the ramifications of our choices echo throughout the ages.

---

[32] S. Koyczan, 2013, *To This Day*.
[33] Yī yè zhàng mù (一葉障目): *Vision obscured by a single leaf*.

> Treat the Earth well:
> it was not given to you by your parents,
> it was loaned to you by your children.
> We do not inherit the Earth from our Ancestors,
> we borrow it from our Children.
>
> American Indian proverb.

When considering our children and grandchildren, perhaps Liú's summation of Shí Yīn Fū and his ledger clarifies the situation:

> *Look for example at the Zhōu family, who founded the dynasty of the same name. For many generations, their virtue was great, with many sages coming forth in those eight hundred years. When the Qín took over violently, the Zhōu family were not massacred but lived into their eighties and nineties without disease, dying in peace. However, if you look at those who did evil, like Cáocāo at the end of the Hàn dynasty, or Sī Mǎyì whose grandson founded the Jìn dynasty, their forebears had virtue, so thereby they arrived at power, but the affairs they themselves undertook were bad. Their children, although born into this same position of power, ended up being overthrown and their dynasty came to a short and bloody end. A whole generation was massacred due to this. This issue is even more prevalent amongst the common people. How many of us continue our traits of evil through our children?*[34]

There is no Apex to life and the continuum of the true circle is a transference, both materially and energetically, through the linking of Xìng. Regardless of inheritance, the physician and patient follow the principle and the words of Liú Yuán. We are all capable of reaching the Heaven principle; eventually we do not need the ferryman as we have taught ourselves to swim.

"Have you, my good man, by any chance studied swimology?"

---

[34] Please refer to chapter 1 for the full citation.

There is the true principle of Heaven and that is it! The human being is the divine among the myriad things as when it receives the beauty of Heaven, then we are alive. We live through attaining the upright principle, which is Xìng. If we want to experience the fullness of Heaven our Xìng must be at its fullest. So with each thought, with each affair, we must join them all together with the true principle. This is our constant connection to Heaven. All who are human can reach this.[35]

The student who studies the Dào must see the Dào in their human relationships. Our relationships must have their root in our Heart. When the Heart is upright, the body can cultivate. When the Heart is not upright, the apprentice may use fancy words about filial piety, yet these are all floating, void of meaning and virtue; the kind Heart of Heaven principle is not reflected. Heaven principle is Xìng. When this is fulfilled, we know Heaven and the human relationships, both the grand and minor, the refined and coarse, are all coordinated appropriately in our daily life.[36]

In each and every breath, our human relationships must be engaged with an upright Heart, making them prosper. By putting themselves below others, the physician and patient no longer look down with judgment. They keep close to principle and look only from the Heart. Our compass needle points the way until all our relationships, be they between student and teacher, parent and child, between brothers and sisters and with our friends, are in alignment with propriety and free from suffering.[37]

When the Wounded Warrior looks out at the world and their relationships, they are losing life with every breath that they breathe. Days and years are forever vanishing and they battle against this in vain. Reaching out, the physician reminds them that at this precise moment they *have* life, a life that must be lived! The licking flames of the Inner Fire Circle hear these words and settle, fear and angst calm, and warmth is kept in the Center...*In this we must not err, not even slightly*...The perfection of our circle is determined by the stability of the Center of a compass that defines its outline.

---

[35] On Correcting Errors, p. 3437-2.
[36] On Correcting Errors, p. 3483-1.
[37] "The ultimate power of the boxer is not his advanced skill, but his righteousness." (Schmieg, 2005, p. 83).

Love and hate are two outcomes of the seven emotions, which are born in the temperament and disposition of a person. The ministers who govern this disposition are the human Heart and Xìng. Xìng has no action, whilst the human Heart has perception. This perceptive Heart wanders astray many times, making the emotions disorderly, distorted and polluted with desires. One must use the true principle to regulate these emotions and bring them back to Xìng.

The Great Learning gives us these four methods: self-examination and scrutiny, reaching for knowledge, making our intentions sincere and making the Heart upright. So when we return and regulate our emotions, this is the gōngfu taught by the Great Learning. In this we must not err, not even slightly. On track and the Heart will be upright, the body will cultivate and the Xìng and emotions join in Center harmony. Then the emotions of love and hate simultaneously come out of the grand void.

This is the Tàijí with its root in Wújí, with no Apex. Then you come to the root of the seven emotions. Furthermore, till death they will attempt to return to materialistic desires. One step it is born, one step it is formed and completed and so it becomes the spirit. Those who do not know that the spirit of Heaven and Earth is pure do not know that Heaven and Earth are without desires or emotions.[38]

The human Heart is so often led astray as it so often is filled with selfishness; the Post-Heaven does not return to the Pre-Heaven. The student works this gōngfu, collecting the discharged Heart, and so they enter into Center. They nurture the empty void and no thought comes. All of the ten thousand causes of disturbance are brushed aside, reaching the extreme accomplishment of attaining stillness. Then the true Xìng of Pre-Heaven is spontaneously born and comes to life. When Mencius speaks of 'knowing myself', if we fail to attain this ultimate goodness and cannot collect the Heart back in order to nurture the Qì, then everything becomes very difficult. Until the end of our lives we struggle to reach any clarity.[39]

---

[38] On Correcting Errors, p. 3545-2.
[39] On Correcting Errors, p. 3616-2.

To clarify the whole issue, Liú gives us some simplified guidelines. This is a summary of what we need in order to achieve an *Harmonious Center*. It is called *cúnxīn yǎngxìng* (存心養性), *preserve the Heart in order to nurture Xìng,* meaning deliberate internal cultivation. When we doubt ourselves, his words guide us back:

> *Our tolerance has to be big, while our defensive Heart and desires must be small. All of our affairs must be respectful, the Qì has to be harmonious and our desires few. True principle must be clear. When engaging with people we must be kind. Propriety and appropriateness must be seriously observed. Everything must be sincere and guarding the Center must be long lasting.*[40]

When the physician and patient peer into the bags on their chest and see very few yellow beans, they take time to return from wandering amongst their wounds. Liú shares his method of achieving this homeward journey of cultivation, calling it *Gazing at the aperture and Gazing at the subtle*.

> *Generation after generation, without exhaustion, transformation without end: this is the Center of Heaven and Earth. You cannot name it. This is the origin of the myriad things, the extreme of which we call Tàijí. The Tàijí of Heaven and Earth reaches toward emptiness. When at its fullest, it is the principle of one origin.*
>
> *The Qì mixes with the one aperture*[41] *and so before birth the human being receives Center within the womb, and then in the dāntián, which is also like Heaven and Earth, immediately after they are born. Then the spirit and Qì scatters to all the bones and joints of the body, and so this aperture becomes empty, while life enters through the mouth and nose, eyes and ears.*
>
> *To preserve the Heart and nurture the Xìng, the physician knows the principle of the Tàijí within the human body. When it moves, they gather the discharged Heart, direct it to this aperture, fix it here and then peace is produced. This is defined as observing the aperture when diseases arise. This is the gōngfu of preserving the Heart. Even when we are without*

---

[40] On Correcting Errors, p. 3655-1.
[41] What Liú is referring to here is the umbilical cord where the baby is connected to life (Heaven) via the mother (Earth). After we are born and this link is cut, this same area is referred to as our dāntián (丹田), the place where our Qì resides. This is the *aperture*.

desires, we still quietly guard the Center aperture.

We reach emptiness and stillness, the Qì is quiet and tranquil and the true principle starts to manifest itself spontaneously. This is the skill of nurturing Xìng: observe the subtle to be without desire. Gazing at the aperture and gazing at the subtle means that respect starts at home. This is the study of the generous and peaceful Heart.

Like the Yellow Emperor who would always look inward and question, we too must stop only at ultimate goodness. The aperture and the subtle are in one place, the origin is remote and quiet. By observing the aperture and the subtle, we reach emptiness and stillness. When the Heart is still, Xìng arrives. It recovers Center and collects the discharged emotions. It makes pure our outer harmony and eases the opening and closing within the human body. The body connects back to nature and creation.

Observing the aperture and the subtle is only possible if you do not allow a single thought to be present.[42] *The grand void becomes the same as your body and so attaining this subtlety is very difficult to describe with words. This is the origin. More so, through this method the inside and outside are simultaneously cultivated with benevolence and righteousness. This is the root of all under Heaven.*[43]

Before each treatment the physician draws an unadorned circle. This is their starting point, observing the ultimate aperture and finding an understanding of completeness. From here they can add in their segments, herbs and acupuncture, all from a point of Center. When the patient lies on the treatment table, they are safe and included in the stability within the physician. *Given time* to breathe, the patient *takes time* to contemplate the leaves that move smoothly with the wind, yet are firmly rooted to the Earth. For the physician, the treatment principle is simple; assist the patient to get back to Center, and that is it! Wounded Warriors then rest their heavy boots, letting their weary feet cool in the shallows as they repose on the riverbank.

---

[42] "In order to be in a state of no thought, you must be very balanced and peaceful within yourself. A sense of unity is felt inside that comes from being honest...with yourself and others...If honest, I have nothing to hide. If I have nothing to hide, then I am free. I do not have to keep up so much effort maintaining a false appearance." S. F. S. Chin, *Nei Jia Quan: Internal Martial Arts Teachers of Tai Ji Quan, Xing Yi Quan and Ba Gua Zhang*, ed. J. O'Brien, Blue Snake Books, Berkeley, 2004, p. 101.

[43] On Correcting Errors, p. 3488-1.

And the river flowed with the sky.[44]

To be secure on the shore, the constant movement of Water over our skin does not shift our Center. Our book is placed firmly on the middle of the table and we observe the subtle. This nurtures our Xìng and makes us more effective in our work and in our relationships. If we can touch on this experience for even the briefest of moments, this is a great achievement.

Once, there was a man traveling across a field...

...when he encountered a tiger. He fled, the tiger after him. Coming to a precipice, he caught hold of the root of a wild vine and swung himself down over the edge. The tiger sniffed at him from above. Trembling, the man looked down to where, far below, another tiger was waiting to eat him. Only the vine sustained him. Two mice, one white and one black, little by little, started to gnaw away at the vine.

The man saw a luscious strawberry near him. Grasping the vine with one hand, he plucked the strawberry with the other. How sweet it tasted![45]

Zen story

---

[44] T. A. Jaensch, *Yì Shén (意神): Remember the Spirit*, Self-printed, self-bound, Sydney, 1997, p. 50.
[45] Feldman & Kornfield (eds), 1991, p. 23.

CHAPTER 9

崇百药

Chóng Bǎi Yào

Revering the 100 Medicines

Preface:

When it came to goodness, the sages of ancient times attained even the smallest aspects of goodness. When it came to evil, there was not the smallest aspect of it that they did not remove. If you can also do this, it is like taking a prescription of the purest medicine.

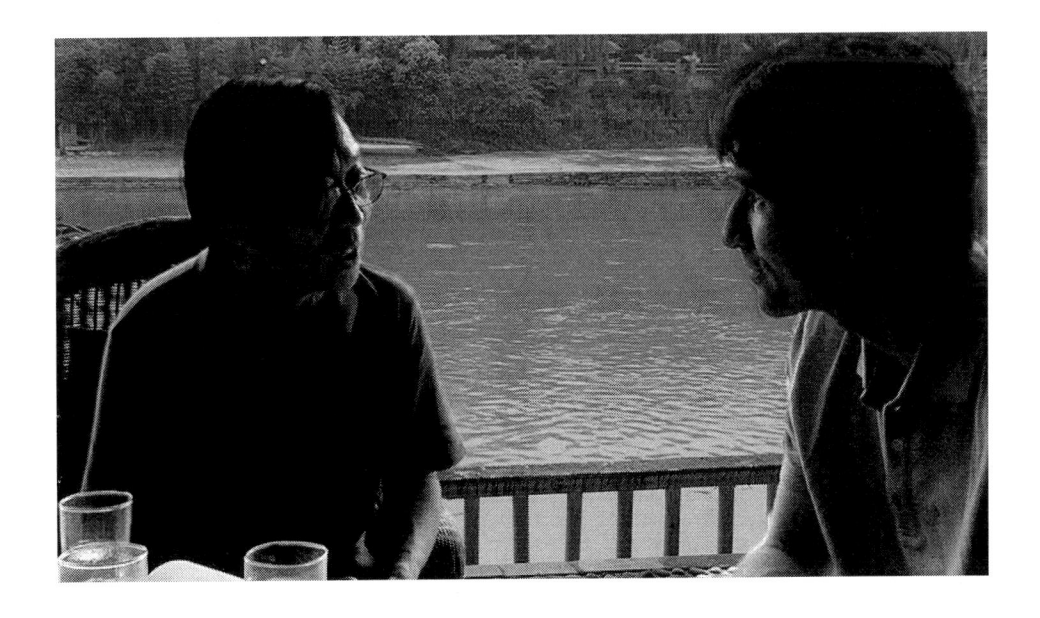

Master Gān Liǎo and Yaron Seidman discussing matters of the Heart.

1. Making oneself humble and not seeking conflict and struggle:
   this is one medicine.

2. Making all actions kind, with a tolerant and conciliatory Heart:
   this is one medicine.

3. Maintaining proper behavior when sitting, standing, talking and eating:
   this is one medicine.

4. When one's sleeping, eating and exercise are appropriate:
   this is one medicine.

5. Constantly investigating virtue and distancing oneself from lust:
   this is one medicine.

6. Eradicating greed from the Heart:
   this is one medicine.

7. Examining one's duty, morality and justice:
   this is one medicine.

8. Not taking that which does not belong to you:
   this is one medicine.

9. Meeting the hateful with a pleased look and loving Heart:
   this is one medicine.

10. Spending time seeking talent and then supporting it:
    this is one medicine.

11. Looking to help others prosper:
    this is one medicine.

12. Helping save others from calamity:
    this is one medicine.

13. Educating the ignorant and guiding them towards enlightenment:
    this is one medicine.

14. Advising the crooked and rebellious on how to become upright:
    this is one medicine.

15. Teaching children how to do the right thing:
    this is one medicine.

16. Straightening out the unintended mistakes of superstitious people:
    this is one medicine.

17. Assisting the sick and aged:
    this is one medicine.

18. Using your physical strength, money or power to help others:
    this is one medicine.

19. Providing for the poor and the widowers:
    this is one medicine.

20. Having compassion and bringing salvation to the poverty stricken:
    this is one medicine.

21. Respecting subordinates and giving them a courteous reception:
    this is one medicine.

22. Speaking with humility:
    this is one medicine.

23. Politely addressing everyone, even those who have no social stature:
    this is one medicine.

24. Repaying debts promptly:
    this is one medicine.

25. Being honest and sincere with others:
    this is one medicine.

26. Embracing truthfulness in deeds and words:
    this is one medicine.

27. Inquiring into the correct principles to guide the crooked:
    this is one medicine.

28. Not engaging in arguments about who is right or who is wrong:
    this is one medicine.

29. Meeting the vulgar and yet not disdaining them:
    this is one medicine.

30. Being humiliated, yet not resenting those who humiliate you:
    this is one medicine.

31. Electing decent officials and removing the indecent:
    this is one medicine.

32. Politely declining goods so that they can go to others:
    this is one medicine.

33. Giving the large portion to others, only taking the smallest for oneself:
    this is one medicine.

34. Admiring and praising the able and the virtuous:
    this is one medicine.

35. Observing those of virtue and then critically examining oneself:
    this is one medicine.

36. Not standing out or showing off:
    this is one medicine.

37. Modestly declining credit and giving to others:
    this is one medicine.

38. Not bragging about oneself being good, wise or kind:
    this is one medicine.

39. Not hiding the good achievements of others:
    this is one medicine.

40. Not resenting hard work and toil:
    this is one medicine.

41. Cherishing the sincere Heart, being faithful and generous:
    this is one medicine.

42. Not propagating the ill doings of others:
    this is one medicine.

43. Working diligently, not wasting time or being miserly with wealth:
    this is one medicine.

44. Holding in esteem those that surpass you and not obstructing them:
    this is one medicine.

45. If poor and living a hard life, to still feel fulfilled:
    this is one medicine.

46. Not being pretentious and feeling that you have reached greatness:
    this is one medicine.

47. Helping others to achieve grand accomplishments:
    this is one medicine.

48. Not prying into other people's private matters:
    this is one medicine.

49. Not being happy with gain and sad with loss, but taking it as it comes:
    this is one medicine.

50. Performing good deeds and giving favors in secret:
    this is one medicine.

51. Never cursing others:
    this is one medicine.

52. Never criticizing anyone:
    this is one medicine.

53. Only saying words of kindness:
    this is one medicine.

54. When suffering disaster or disease, first reflecting upon oneself:
    this is one medicine.

55. Not blaming others during times of hardship:
    this is one medicine.

56. Thanking those who give you favors:
    this is one medicine.

57. Not cursing animals:
    this is one medicine.

58. Harboring only good wishes for the success and health of others:
    this is one medicine.

59. Maintaining a calm Heart and harmonious mind:
    this is one medicine.

60. Fixing the mind so that desires and thoughts cannot roam free:
    this is one medicine.

61. Forgiving and forgetting all past disputes and wrongs:
    this is one medicine.

62. Rectifying and correcting the thoughts and deeds of the wicked:
    this is one medicine.

63. Listening to advice and receiving instruction from the enlightened:
    this is one medicine.

64. Not interfering in the lives of others:
    this is one medicine.

65. Controlling one's anger:
    this is one medicine.

66. Dismissing negative stray thoughts:
    this is one medicine.

67. Respecting one's elders:
    this is one medicine.

68. Being respectful at home:
    this is one medicine.

69. Respecting one's parents and older siblings in the family:
    this is one medicine.

70. Highlighting the good in people rather than their shortcomings:
    this is one medicine.

71. Being honest, upright and content with what one has:
    this is one medicine.

72. Happily offering food and drink to others:
    this is one medicine.

73. Earnestly and devotedly assisting others to carry out their deeds:
    this is one medicine.

74. When disaster strikes, only desiring to save others:
    this is one medicine.

75. Distancing oneself from suspicious affairs and people:
    this is one medicine.

76. Being indifferent to fame and gain and being free from worry:
    this is one medicine.

77. Being respectful to the ancient texts:
    this is one medicine.

78. Focusing on the Dào and virtue to preserve the spirit:
    this is one medicine.

79. Propagating teachings of sages to transform the Hearts of the people:
    this is one medicine.

80. Giving beneficial service tirelessly to help the Hearts of the people:
    this is one medicine.

81. Respecting Heaven and Earth:
    this is one medicine.

82. Paying homage to the Sun, Moon and stars:
    this is one medicine.

83. Quieting one's mind to be without desires:
    this is one medicine.

84. Modestly allowing others their needs with a loving and kind Heart:
    this is one medicine.

85. Loving life and hating killing:
    this is one medicine.

86. Not accumulating riches with greed:
this is one medicine.

87. Not violating taboos:
this is one medicine.

88. Not becoming corrupted, but rather staying loyal:
this is one medicine.

89. Whilst wealth may be necessary for life, not becoming greedy:
this is one medicine.

90. Not burning the mountain forests:
this is one medicine.

91. Helping others to carry their loads on the path:
this is one medicine.

92. Remonstrating to one's face with an honest and trustworthy Heart:
this is one medicine.

93. Feeling happiness and joy when others find luck and virtue:
this is one medicine.

94. Throwing oneself into difficultly and hardship for a noble cause:
this is one medicine.

95. Supporting the elderly and helping them bear their burdens:
this is one medicine.

96. Removing emotion and desire, expelling corruptions:
this is one medicine.

97. With a kind Heart, looking at others with sympathy and empathy:
this is one medicine.

98. Liking to announce the good deeds of others:
this is one medicine.

99. Utilizing one's riches to assist those in need:
this is one medicine.

100. Helping the commoners with your power and position:
this is one medicine.

Conclusion:

These one hundred medicines reveal that when mankind suffers disease, it is all due to evil mistakes. The Yīn evil is hidden within and cannot be seen or understood, yet it manifests outwardly as disease. For some, it is through destiny, diet, or external influences (heat and cold) that disease comes. Some offend the spirit to such a degree that the Hún (魂) separates and the Pò (魄) sinks; the vessel is abandoned.[1] The body becomes hollow and fails to guard its essence and so ill weather can attack the Center.

Therefore the sages, even when people could not see, would dare do no wrong. Even though in an honorable place, they dare not self-profit. They act in accordance to circumstance, happy with their share. Even if rich and lofty, they do not give in to lust. Even if poor and inferior, they do not go against the law. In this way there is no outer brutality and no inner disease; how can one not be cautious in these matters?

Commentary by Master Gān Liǎo:

In modern times, when people attempt to improve their lives and health, the biggest difficulty, the greatest hurdle that they face, are diseases of the Heart. This issue is defined by the Post-Heaven Yīn, which is the obstacle standing in between my conscious Heart and the realm of the Dào and virtue. This is what obstructs me from reaching and connecting. It resembles the impenetrable Yīnshān (阴山) mountains of inner Mongolia; it is like an impassable turbulent ocean, obscuring the Xìng from the Mìng, concealing my destiny.[2] As if divided by a vast gulf, a dark abyss, the Xìng and Mìng cannot acknowledge each other. The lead and the mercury cannot mix, no matter how sternly I heat them. So how can we ford the three thousand raging rivers? How can we traverse the huge Yīnshān mountains and navigate the rough seas?

Heart diseases need Heart medicine, which are revealed in the purity contained within the texts of the one

---

[1] Hún (魂) and Pò (魄) are the immortal and mortal souls, according to classical Chinese theosophy.
[2] Xìng referring to Natural Character; Mìng referring to fate, destiny, or Heaven's command.

hundred diseases, offered in chapter 5, and the one hundred medicines. We must observe the small to know the big. Truly, it is a sagely medicine when the physician administers Heart medicine for Heart diseases, resulting in the Heart becoming open and clear. With one taste of it, the patient always wants to take more; they follow the correct way of cultivating truth. Because of this, cultivating the Heart is the commander and chief of therapy as it brings along with it the cultivation of Xìng and Mìng. It bridges the gap between the Post-Heaven and the Pre-Heaven.

With treating and curing the Heart, the internal realm becomes clear about virtue and shines brightly through the fog. The Yīnshān mountains naturally disappear, the impassable seas and rivers dry up. The Xìng and the Mìng can see and complete each other. If you can obey this immortal recipe, everyday chew on it carefully, slowly swallow it and take it into your Center and Heart then in the end you will achieve a great accomplishment.

Otherwise, you will waste the essence of lead and mercury. Your Will, even with its high and lofty intentions, will flounder. In reality, the body is at a crossroad, stuck. Even through diligent practice, you will be walking blindly. You lose the upper levels of virtue, and the foresight it brings. The great day at the end of our lives is then inevitably blockaded. In the end, all your hard work is just a dream. These texts are like the nimble hands of the sagely physician that can excise evil from within and cure the human Heart. Every flavor is against a disease, every medicine can remove the problem by its root. We wish that all people use this medicine.

Good medicine, even though bitter, can nonetheless quiet our disturbed Heart, bringing clarity to the Xìng and Mìng. We become as refined as the sages of old. If you want to be a student of the Dào, how can you refuse to face this harsh reality of the Heart? The author wants us to use this medicine daily, to swallow it and transform our acquired Xìng and thereby vanquish chronic disease. Old habits extinguish and do not propagate, our character becomes peaceful, and successfully we enter the excellent realm of cultivating our inner virtue – the truth.

Gān Liǎo, Sìchuān.

CHAPTER 10

藏言

Zàng Yán

The Concealed Words

*"To the accomplished student of medicine, please take note;
contracting a disease is a hardship for the human being,
please use these words to treat the disease which has not yet formed!"*

Liú Bèiwén

From beginning to end the physician searches for Center, the place that drives us and moves our relationships and interactions with the world at large. Deep within, imbued in our Xìng, the human being has *Concealed Words*. Yáng ☰ within Yīn ☷, these words represent how we engage with our Center throughout our lives ☳. While not spoken aloud ☲, they are the springboard for our view of reality. For some, these words are released with their final breath, for others these words remain secluded within. For us, we reveal them with Xīnfǎ. They hold the inner truth for each individual; a truth that completes the human being, and allows for a fulfilled life.

Concealed words can be *good* or *bad*. Using the mind, our clever intellect often nurtures the Wounded Warrior, justifying and rationalizing actions, thoughts and practices. So we now leave this behind and contemplate with our Heart. When bad words hide within, people adopt a negative view of life. They tend to be difficult to get along with and their interpersonal relationships are often dysfunctional. When good words are contained in the Center they act like a guiding principle, like candlelight in a dark room. Too often these words are not acknowledged as the individual does not *put* them there intentionally. Over a lifetime they are written; given, nurtured, matured and fertilized. Through Xīnfǎ the physician discovers these words by traversing the many layers of habit, culture and society that form and instruct their human Heart.

The One Thread of Life is steadied by good words and destabilized by bad words. Thus, by revealing what is written within the Xìng the physician can come to terms with their own words. If bad words are found, they are transformed before the final chapter; the physician lives without regrets. This is the Lost Heart of Medicine ☷.

The Heart is considered the Master of the human body, a Master that must be nurtured.[1] This is the root of generating spirit. When we come across a disease that cannot be cured, this is always due to a malnourished Heart, and without this residence, the spirit begins its Separation from the physical body. Many diseases cannot be cured with manual therapies, drugs or herbs. Only diseases that arise from external factors, such as wind, cold and heat, can be successfully cured with external medicine.

When the seven emotions have caused internal injury, however, one must adjust the Xìng and stabilize desires. One must cultivate virtue and goodness, thereby staving off calamity. When the two residences of Yīn and Yáng offend and collide with each other, then one must remove, repair and reconstruct after the turbulence.

The many books on medicine talk specifically of herbs and prescriptions, yet many are without efficacy. The essence of medicine is in its spirit, understanding it and making it transparent and brilliantly illuminated. This is not in the realm of herbs or drugs. One must be flexible with medicine and not rely on one material method as a cure for all.[2]

During their career, a physician encounters numerous diseases that have not been cured by any medicines or therapies, Chinese or otherwise. Often these diseases are outside the scope of external medicine as they are disorders originating from deep within the patient's Heart and cannot be addressed by substances from the material world. Flexible in their approach, the physician looks up from their prescription pad and searches for the root of disharmony.

---

[1] "The Heart is the Master of the five Zàng, and so it controls the four limbs and the flow of blood and Qì. It reveals its vast ability of knowing right from wrong as it enters and exits the doors of the hundred affairs. Therefore, expecting to traverse all Qì under Heaven without first attaining the Heart and Center, is akin to expecting to hear music without ears, or enjoy articles without eyes. One's tasks certainly cannot be accomplished!" *Huái Nán Zi Yuán Dào Xùn* (淮南子原道訓), Seidman and Jaensch translation.

[2] Commentary on Medicine, p. 4094-2.

Liú Yuán talks to the emotions of the Post-Heaven Heart in a compassionate way, telling us that we are not at war with ourselves; our emotions are not something toxic or dirty. Rather, we rely on them to exist, to move the vessel and create relationships with the outside world through our daily Separation. If, at the same time, we can cultivate ourselves and accomplish Center, recognize our likes and dislikes and bring them into line, we become even more efficient and effective in achieving our purpose. Emotions are necessary, but being *emotional*, or being over-run by our emotions often leads to poor decision making. In Liú's terms, our emotions can then bring about our untimely demise by distancing us from the Heaven principle within, our Xìng. Balancing the movement of Separation and Unification is part of this cultivation. Rather than movements in conflict– Yīn struggling with Yáng–these apparently opposing directions flow together, like rippling from a spring beneath the mighty cliff. Free from mountains of obstruction, the human being can honestly read what is written in their Hearts and then *live* more of their lives.

> *When it comes to the fairer sex and the blood and Qì are moving during menses, if she consumes raw and cold foods or has an inharmonious Heart and Xìng, she frequently becomes angry and annoyed, sometimes furious, depressed and bitter. The entire gamut of this negativity leads to Qì and blood stagnation, resulting in the formation of clots, menses pain and masses in the body. If this situation is allowed to linger for too long it becomes very difficult to treat and she feels like she lives a ruined life.*
>
> *One cannot and must not ever make the mistake of trying to treat this condition like one would treat carbuncles. Never use a treatment that aims at scattering accumulations. One should not use this method. Rather, one must protect and nurture her. One must make her feel at home in her body, that her body is precious. Make her believe in herself, in her Center, one hundred percent, and caution her about the repercussions of doing evil.*
>
> *When I see this type of disease, immediately I tell the patient that they must reflect upon their intentions. This disorder requires Xīnfǎ as its modus operandi. Once this is established and on course, a great doctor can assist with the application of medicinals. She must be guided to understand that all deeds are to be overflowing with benevolence and virtue. Carefully enlighten her that it is through her thoughts and deeds that she*

will find her destiny and via this connection Heaven protects her. Help her cultivate virtue and become full of goodness. With all actions she must guard the true principle of Heaven. Heaven will then silently assist her to a complete recovery. When the physician treats her, all of these details must be taken care of and cautiously applied. The results will be self-evident. If her Heart is directed towards goodness, this becomes a great accomplishment and virtue.[3]

All too often in medicine the physician reaches a conclusion from a set of signs and symptoms, which forms the sole foundation governing the application of treatment.[4] In the case Liú has just described, Western medicine may reach for the oral contraceptive pill or a sedative, Chinese medicine may reach for Chái Hú (柴胡) *radix bupleuri* or Xiāng Fù (香附) *rhizoma cyperi*; both responding and treating the patient from the turbulent reflections of the Outer Water Circle. *Seeing* hormonal irregularities, they regulate or sedate. *Seeing* Qì and blood stagnation, they scatter. While these strategies may lead to a brief amelioration of symptoms, the reason *why* the body has become overwhelmed is overlooked. Good intentions guide the pen that writes the prescription, as the patient is in distress with a condition *very difficult to treat, and she feels like she lives a ruined life*. At the Heart of it all, however, is a weakness in the Center. By either stifling or scattering Xìng instead of nurturing it, regardless of intention, harming the patient is guaranteed and the virtue of medicine is lost.

Liú Yuán teaches the physician to talk to the patient's Heart, hear and know her words and convince her of her own goodness. Healing comes from within the human being and will be determined by her engaging cultivation and discovering her own potential. The patient has already started the journey by seeking help from her physician. Caring for her from the depths of their Heart, the physician does not simply *me-dictate* her, prescribing

---

[3] Commentary on Medicine, p. 4104-1-2
[4] "...in 1713, he was not at home when his wife fell ill. Local officials were rushing to deliver a shipment of military grain rations to the storehouses by year's end and Yan was assigned to assist with the project. In his absence, the doctor misdiagnoses Ms. Shen as afflicted by upsurging internal fire, invasion of wind and stagnation of phlegm. Accordingly, he treated her with drugs to purge, subdue and dissipate these pathological manifestations. But when these remedies provoked convulsions, the household dispatched a servant to ask Yan Chunxi for instructions. A glance at the prescription convinced Yan that the doctor had misdiagnosed Ms. Shen's illness, giving her drugs that were not only ineffective but would positively 'hasten death'...it was obvious that his wife's illness was rooted in depletion, not in excess or invasion...Yan rushed home in the deepest dread." Y. L. Wu, *Reproducing Women: Medicine, Metaphor, and Childbirth in Late Imperial China*, University of California Press, Berkeley, 2010, p. 2.

another drug, pill, herb or acupuncture point and then she is out the door to make way for the next in line. Rather, the benevolent physician sees the lost Heart of medicine right before their eyes, the patient revealing it with their words.

The Concealed Words are often only revealed to the individual in the last stages of life. A personal experience of one such moment will be shared here. A modern sage, teacher, father and husband, when on his deathbed spoke these words:

> "If I could do it all over again,
> I would spend more time with my family..."

These were his Concealed Words, spoken from deep within his Heart, hidden within his whole life. Being concealed in the Center of Xìng, they are elusive to human Heart as it searches for something *more* to life; something to fill an inner emptiness, more ink on the page. Craving these Concealed Words, the Wounded Warrior looks out instead of in. Desires, likes and dislikes assume control and cloud our perception, until Xīnfǎ flows through us, revealing our Concealed Words. The sage above found words filled with goodness, and these had driven the rotation of his life from beginning to end. Too often, however, what hides from sight undermines the person, with cruel words reflecting outward into their health and attitudes. Circumstances have placed them there, yet these circumstances are not what define the human being, who is only defined by Xìng. Thus, our Concealed Words can be transformed through Xīnfǎ to follow the compass from Xìng to benevolence before it is too late.

Through cultivation techniques such as the meditative practice of *Gazing at the Aperture and Gazing at the Subtle* (discussed in chapter 8), the physician clears the cloud of confusion created by the human Heart. Unobstructed, the Dào Heart reveals its words; those of goodness are treasured, while words of evil are transformed. Virtuous words calm the One Thread of Life and the Wounded Warrior who clutches it. Beautiful internal words manifest in our well-being, self-esteem and the vibrancy of our relationships.

The momentum guiding the brushstrokes that painted the patient's Concealed Words is a gift from their forebears. Their natural ability to work with the Inner Fire Circle and its discharging of internal Fire was determined by their parents and ancestry. Regardless of what was given, even words full of selfishness such as *I want more...Oh, why me, myself and I?* can all be overcome with an upright Heart and the script re-written. When the physician arrives here and then assists their patients, family and friends to achieve this same recognition, *this becomes a great accomplishment and virtue.*

> *The Xìng is without action while the Heart has recognition. The entirety of human activity relies on this ability of the Heart to recognize and differentiate. In the realm of the Xìng there are no sounds, smells or any stimulus from the outer worldly domain. If there is nothing there, how is it that we can nurture it? When we speak of the Heart and Xìng we are talking about the pure void, the true principle of Heaven and the divine spirit within. Xìng is pure oneness, while all that floats and goes astray with emotions and thoughts in melancholia or merriment, this is what we call Heart. Both are within our Center.*
>
> *Nurturing upon the vast Qì of the universe requires this void. In order to nurture this Qì of the void, we must first relinquish the Heart. Then we enter into the dāntián. If we can dwell here without movement for one hundred days, the essence of Pre-Heaven distils, condenses and coagulates within us. Then we know ourselves, adding clarity to the skill of nurturing Xìng.*
>
> *Through meditation and actions filled with virtue, the flood-like Qì of the universe day by day replenishes and accumulates in our Center. We are rejuvenated by our consistent nurturing of stillness. Any thoughts going astray and into disarray are relocated back into the harmony of our Center, manifesting on the outside with our restrained words and actions.*
>
> *Even the slightest impropriety is not indulged, and so the spirit becomes resolute in dāntián. This resolve permeates throughout our entire body. We have a pure face and flowing back, the proper posture. Without words it replenishes the entire body. Our brilliance and honor start from here. Nurturing dāntián and cultivating virtue in each and every action and reaction, we cultivate the inside as well as the outside. The root and branches are all nurtured. From beginning to end, virtue is accrued and the Heaven principle is full. And so Pre-Heaven Qì accumulates in the Center and is reflected on the outside.*[5]

In the end when breath and time are short, the veil of conscious illusions disappears and the inner world becomes apparent. As the grip on life weakens, the Wounded Warrior relinquishes its apparent control and the

---

[5] Additional Questions, p. 3952-1.

Concealed Words slip from the lips. As the physician and patient have both reached a sagely accomplishment with their Xīnfǎ, earlier in life they read their words, transformed them and defined their purpose from Center. They became a proper parent, a proper child.

> "If I could do it all over again,
> I would spend more time with my family..."

These are words of goodness, a reflection of his role as a father and husband, the most sacred of relationships: the father to his children, the husband to his wife. This is the Heart of the practicality of Xīnfǎ, its essence. In our lives, *human(e) relationships* are the stage where the principle of Heaven plays out, thus philosophical constructs transform into practical endeavors. Heaven principle within the physician should be reflected in all of their interactions, with themselves, with others and with the environment.

Being a father or mother, a son or daughter, a husband or wife, brother or sister, friend, teacher, student, physician or patient, are all reflections and expressions of our connection to Xìng. Being clear and yet clearer about virtue, the physician is a son or daughter and loving one's parents is the proper role of the human being. Not secluded in the wilderness, the physician lives their life through the appropriateness of their relationships in society, each one of which being an expression of Xìng. Emotions discharged from the human Heart had their seed in the Dào Heart, but being clouded by the Wounded Warrior, this virtuous momentum is twisted into likes and dislikes. In turn, this dichotomy plays out before the world in the functionality of relationships. *To cultivate our relationships is to cultivate Xìng.*

> *Heaven does not have two principles; the sage does not have two Dào. Of the Dào there is only one. The body has a Heart, a Xìng and a destiny, with the principle of all these aspects being the Dào of human relationships, which must be utilized daily. Everyone has this and can practice it. There is no other Heaven principle that sits outside of these relationships. It is manifest in the practical application between me and myself and those around me. Outside of this, where is there any sage, Yellow Emperor or Lǎozǐ?*[6]

---

[6] The Huái Xuān Pledge, p. 3714-1-2.

Human relationships are the practical expression of life and relationships *take time*. *Giving time* to relationships is not measured in minutes but rather how much we are *present* in them that defines their goodness. A *bad* father, ignorant of his Concealed Words, who abuses his wife and child, may sit at home all day spending many minutes and hours ruining the family's Center. Thus, it is not an *amount* of time that reflects propriety or impropriety. Spending *time* in a relationship means spending time being *appropriate* within that relationship. How much is one a father? How much is one a husband or wife? A son or daughter? How much is one a physician? All of our relationships, both Cardinal as well as how we relate to our surroundings, demand application from Center.

Conditioned by modernity, people have come to believe that human relationships are *two-way streets*: from point A to point B and back again.[7] *I'll love you if you'll love me...*Reality teaches us, often painfully, that this is a ridiculous notion; proven by the time we fell in love as young people, only to find that it was unrequited. When we love someone, it is not because they love us in return. When a mother loves her daughter, it is not because of, or reliant upon its reciprocation. This is not a two-way street regardless of contemporary social perceptions. *I'll love you if you'll love me...*is a construct of the human Heart invented by Wounded Warriors; an agreement of youthful folly, a contract to a relationship. Instead, true relationships start in our Center and radiate outward to everything and everyone. A radiance not determined by outer disturbances, just as the sun shines upon the Earth regardless of the blankets of cloud and rain that may obscure it from us.

One's Concealed Words are instrumental in facilitating one's understanding of relationships. A good mother loves her daughter regardless of her child loving her in return. This is a *proper* mother who has words of goodness concealed within. The physician will love their brother and that is it, for *the Dào of human relationships must be utilized daily*. Yet we relate to everything, not solely our family members. While composing this manuscript the authors had to relate to their reference material and typewriters. The tree, the apple, the couch, the car, the handbag; in order to experience these things people must *relate* to them with a movement from within extending outward towards the material.

---

[7] Two-way streets are necessary when considering the *give and take* discussed in chapter 4, but this relates to our respect and understanding of the sacrifice made by the living world for our survival. Human relationships are somewhat more complicated, whilst simultaneously facile.

These material engagements do not reflect the importance and elegance of our human relationships, yet we must be mindful of them as they can be the source of much fatigue and suffering.[8] Vital relationships are weakened by overt material ones.

> "Some call it magic,
> the search for the grail,
> Love is the answer,
> and you know that for sure,
> Love is a flower, you got to let it grow..."
>
> John Lennon

In order to fulfill their Xìng, the physician and patient must be the *most* son or daughter to their parents, the *most* father or mother to their children, the *most* sister or brother to their siblings, the *most* wife or husband to their partners, the *most* student to their teacher, the *most* teacher to their student, the *most* friend to their friends. And that *mostly* covers it, and is the practicability of realizing the full potential of Xìng. By stopping only at this ultimate goodness and compassion, the physician and patient become clear and yet clearer about their virtue.

Mòzǐ (475–220 BCE) and the Mòhist school (Mòjiā 墨家) advocated universal love: love everyone's parents as you would love your own.[9] In one sense, this sentiment has merit. Understanding that each and every human being is at Heart the same, with the same potential for goodness, necessitates our universal respect for others. Universally *loving* everyone, however, as one would love one's own family does not follow propriety. Hence, the critique of the Mòjiā by Confucius and Mencius, who articulated the propriety of the Cardinal Relationships as being most valuable.

To illustrate this failing to understand and observe this propriety, *parents* want to be *friends* with their children. *Wanting* their offspring to love them, they spoil them to win their affection and the propriety of this relationship is derailed. Strict adherence to what is proper is a *rule* and people often resent rules and being told what to do; free spirits and non-conformists who *want* what they *want*. Yet to function well the body *needs*

---

[8] "Brooding about sensuous objects makes attachment to them grow; from attachment desire arises, from desire anger is born. But a man of inner strength whose senses experience objects without attraction or hatred, in self-control, finds serenity...all his sorrows dissolve..." (*The Bhagavad-Gita*, 1986, pp. 37 & 38).

[9] "...according to Mohist doctrine, love should have in it no gradations of greater or lesser love, whereas according to Confucianism, the reverse is true." Y. L. Fung, *A Short History of Chinese Philosophy: A Systematic Account of Chinese Thought from its Origins to the Present Day*, ed. D. Bodde, The Free Press, New York, 1948, p. 71.

to drink water, eat good food, get good rest and breathe. These are rules also: lest we forget. A parent must follow what is proper for a parent and a child must follow what is proper for a child. A husband, wife, brother or sister; they must all follow what is proper.

Liú Yuán describes these relationships ☶ as the definition of Heaven's principle ☰ in the human vessel ☵. This is not a custom ☲. In the 21st century people are told that a good parent is *X Y Z*, while in the 20th century it was *A B C*. These are the trends, fashions and whims of fancy of the Post-Heaven dichotomy of Yīn and Yáng. Wading through this with Xīnfǎ, the physician seeks the Lost Heart of Medicine along with the lost Heart of everything, investigating truth from folly to find the path to the Center. Customary knowledge, social trends and political correctness reveal their lack of constancy; they are not timeless. A wife is to be treasured always and children are to be nurtured at all times. Timeless.

> ...One of these mornings,
> you're going to rise up singing,
> Then you'll spread your wings,
> and you'll take to the sky,
> But until that morning,
> there's a'nothing can harm you,
> With your daddy and mammy standing by...
>
> George Gershwin – Summertime

Since the Sòng dynasty until recent times, the eldest daughters of poorer families had their feet painfully bound to prevent natural growth (called chánzú 缠足). The gentry of this epoch *favored* women with small feet and dainty movements. In the not-so-distant past, those who frequented China could still see elderly women hobbling down the street, victims of the tide of social norms, culture and tradition. Shortly before the Sòng dynasty, during the Táng dynasty, women who were plump were *considered* (by Wounded Warriors) to be attractive, while now in most of the mainland, women are *preferred* to be slender and pale.[10] STOP! Stop.

Appropriateness relates to the Heaven principle; it is not man-made or *preferred*, not *a puppet on the string of society*. In Chinese medicine for too long, this inference has been buried by Wounded Warrior physicians. Our contemporary medical textbooks, along with the Classics, and indeed

---

[10] "That soul, I say, herself invisible, departs to the invisible world–to the divine and immortal and rational: thither arriving, she lives in bliss and is released from the error and folly of men, their fears and wild passions..." Plato, *The Trial and Death of Socrates: Four Dialogues*, Dover Publications, Inc, New York, 1992, p. 80.

the book you hold in your hands, were all composed in the midst of societal unrest and the authors' *relationship* to this. With Xīnfǎ, however, we can approach each and every word, Concealed or visible, from Center.

> A confession of Ni Baochun, deputy director of the Shanghai Second municipal Hospital. He readily acknowledged having ignored and ridiculed Traditional Chinese medicine, an "unscientific" attitude which he attributed to his education in American and British missionary schools and later in the United States. There he had become imbued with bourgeois and imperialist attitudes so that he neglected his own language and culture, coming to believe that only Western medicine had value. After liberation, he reported, his ideological consciousness had slowly been raised to the point where he was now beginning to grasp the significance of Party policy and appreciate the value of traditional medicine. In a tone of great humility, he acknowledged all these past errors and pledged his readiness to learn from traditional doctors, as "a small student to ask for their instruction." Finally, since this was now seen as an ideological problem, Ni stressed the need for studying Marxism-Leninism, Dialectical Materialism and "the advanced theory and experience of the Soviet Union". These may seem the antithesis of the ancient herbals and acupuncture needles of Chinese medicine but, from 1954 on, the compatibility of Traditional Chinese medicine concepts and theories with "the modern theories of the great Pavlov" was a common theme in medical writings. More important for China's modern physicians, both became touchstones of ideological reliability.[11]

Even for physicians, life starts at home. When taking an honest look at family relationships there are often many convoluted agendas at play. Manipulation and disrespect reveal a disconnect in both close genetic ties as well as interactions with friends and strangers. None of these distortions relate to the Dào Heart, but are reflections of a cloudy internal horizon. Our relationships become a microcosm of social fluctuations, all of which are led and directed by numerous Warriors licking their Wounds.

Examining the timeless within relationships, we start to discriminate and differentiate between a chaotic worldview and the clarity of Xìng. Any discharged thoughts still festering from their wounded origin are immediately encouraged to realign with Center, while thoughts reflecting the goodness within Xìng are embraced and exercised. Mankind sees the

---

[11] R. C. Croizier, *Traditional Medicine in modern China: Science, Nationalism and the Tensions of Cultural Change*, Harvard University Press, Cambridge, Massachusetts, 1968, pp. 169-170. When the Chinese Communist Party took over, opinions and customs had to change overnight. This quote is a poignant example.

unity of the myriad things and becomes one with Heaven. Loneliness and isolation belong to the stars and desert sands.

> "To be surrounded by a million other people,
> yet feel alone like a tree in the desert..."
>
> Michael Franti

All human interactions reveal relativity, with differing amounts of Xìng being spent depending on circumstance. If based on clouded judgment and old wounds, people reveal their greed, desires, likes and dislikes, melancholia or merriment. Xīnfǎ necessitates that each thought be measured for propriety (in line with the Dào Heart) or the alternative (habitual movement of the clouded human Heart) in relation to each kinship or object. Once measured, the kind Heart of Heaven principle (*tiān lǐ liáng xīn* 天理良心) is then put into practice.

Becoming a powerful momentum from within, the force mobilized by a positive acknowledgment of Xìng is often seen clinically. For example, a couple attends with fertility concerns and in their medical history we discover that they both smoke cigarettes. We articulate to them the issues surrounding this habit and the ramifications this choice has on the cells, which, though small and seemingly insignificant, materially define the chalice holding Xìng within future generations. All the rationalizations that we offer fall on deaf ears as they cannot hear past their arguments and beliefs. The following month they discover that they are pregnant and from that very day the smoking stops. Not one withdrawal symptom is felt, not one complaint. Some*thing*, from some*where*, created this change in them. It was not their physician who had been bantering and gently berating them during each and every consultation, but rather, suddenly *their life was not about them*. What was proper instantly became common sense thanks to a storm that cleared away the cobwebs. The eye of this storm is the Center, and regardless of the torments of the fray, the couple will not smoke again, they are now a mother and father and have something important to hold onto. Without a conscious directive they have transformed what was written on their Hearts.

The relationship between husband and wife is different to that between parent and child. Each has its appropriateness, and contemplating this is a part of Xīnfǎ cultivation. The patient learns that when weighed down with childlike ignorance, they mistake their emotions, desires, fears, greed or guilt for themselves; it was always the outer or stimuli that *made* them so angry or upset. Then, with Xīnfǎ, they look honestly at their reactions and find that they have nothing to do with the changeable material world, and everything to do with their connection to Center.

Further elucidating this, a father may not have fulfilled the definition of that title; he may be reminiscent of our example earlier, the abuser, the lout. As a child and adolescent, his son will react to him according to the framework of his Inner Fire Circle. Hatred, anger, fear, disillusionment, anxiety and shunning all come to the fore. Fire is leaking, like ancient dragons. This is a two-way street. *Since you are a bad father, I will be a bad son.* As an adult, however, this child is no longer. He sees that his reactions to his father were based on a deep fear that he would one day *become* his father. This was *his* own fear, which was not the fault of anyone but himself. It was not even his *fault*. Once recognized and the folly of youth washes away, the ache leaves his Center and what is left is gratitude and forgiveness. *I will be a good son regardless of you being an improper father, because **I** determine my benevolence.*

Being proper means coming from Center, with the Wounded Warrior no longer dictating actions and reactions (angry, sad, shouting, sad, disrespectful, sad, guilty, *sad*). Reflecting the Dào Heart without fears and desires, likes and dislikes, the physician and patient become pleasant people to be around. Locating this lost Heart, they spend the rest of their lives living. Separating in order for life to circulate, they stay united with Center. Overcoming the boundaries between *who they are* and their *true selves*, their relationships transcend time and space. For example, when a husband's life ends after many years of companionship, his partner is physically separated from him: yet there is still a bond, a unity, in spite of the physical Separation. Familial bonds of husband-wife, parent-child, brother-sister, are all stronger than death. The to and fro of our two-way streets stops when someone dies. *I love you, you love me, but now you are not here...*when the Xìng are closely knitted the Two become One and the relationship is constant, undeterred by Yīn and Yáng: life and death.

"Mother... I am finally coming to be with you..."

Uttered by a sage in his last moments.

Sometimes this is only revealed at the conclusion. A lifetime of being clouded by the mists and fogs of the Wounded Warrior hampers the ability to leap this hurdle from emotions to belief. We get angry and emotional with *our* family due to *our* fears and desires. We dwell in the shadows of two-way streets, dark and dank. Awakened to the dawn of a new realization, *there is no other Heaven principle that sits outside of our relationships*; we understand the true unity of kinships. The patient feels the love of their partner, even when they are not kissing them. The physician loves their father even though he has passed. After a lifetime together when one partner passes, the other will soon join them. A non-physical bond draws them together. While appropriate for husbands and wives whose relationship is horizontal in time, standing side by side, those of parents and children are vertical in time, as illustrated by this story.

> A calligraphy master was commissioned to write something to hang above the entrance to a family's house, to bring prosperity to everyone therein.
>
> The master wrote:
>
> > Grandfather dies.
> > Father dies.
> > Son dies.
>
> The family was furious, asking how the master could have written such a depressing statement, a curse! Taking up his brush again, the master wrote:
>
> > Son dies.
> > Father dies.
> > Grandfather dies.
>
> This is a curse, he said.
>
> Zen proverb.

Vertical and horizontal relationships have their appropriateness, which is often misunderstood. People often emotionally engage with other emotionally charged people in a horizontal relationship, as they perceive emotions as *being* life. Thus, the more emotions are discharged, the more alive one feels. Through the necessity of emotions and desires in order to survive outside of the womb, it is almost inevitable that they occupy a prominent role in life; *I desire therefore I am*. Seemingly we are alive *because* we desire and yet desires have Apexes that defeat the Center. Inside the womb, the baby's Heart is a pure reflection of the Dào and returning to this peaceful Heart is the path of *alternating vertical and horizontal relationships*.

The physician knows that the relationships that cannot be changed are the father-son, mother-daughter vertical relationships, as children are the physical result of the parent's linking Xìng. All other relationships are changeable. For example, that of a husband and wife is horizontal with both partners mutually assisting each other to become Centered. If the husband starts shouting, his wife immediately contemplates Center and changes the relationship to a vertical one. She is the teacher, finding a way to help him back to Center. For a brief moment their relationship changed from horizontal to vertical. Returning to himself, the husband understands his mistake, allots his black beans and the relationship returns to horizontal. If the wife engages in a horizontal relationship when her husband loses his temper they will both start yelling. Looking in the mirror at such times, they quickly see their reflections.

Relationships between friends and siblings are also horizontal, yet if person A loses their Center, becoming inappropriate and then person B becomes unbalanced, like a see-saw they too lose their Center. Hence they engage in the warfare of emotional dichotomy, likes and dislikes, on the battleground of Yīn and Yáng. The physician and patient, along with teacher and student, maintain horizontal relationships as long as both parties are Centered, but when either is off balance, the relationship must become vertical.[12] Through sorting their good from bad, they realign with each other and with benevolence, assisting each other along the path of Xīnfǎ. Although engaging during a time of Separation, by finding an element of Center they are united with the world around them, not just observers of it.

Two become One when we understand that through relationships we join as a whole with the other person. Husband and wife join as one whole. Parent and child join as one whole. Siblings join as one whole. Friends join as one whole. This is living to the fullest, without Wounded Warriors whispering, exaggerating Separation and feeding fear, guilt and greed; all of which are left gently by the river bank. When the Center of each person in the relationship is harmonious they become one unit; rather than a two-way street it is a flowing river. Each drop is different, yet they move together. Negative Concealed Words disrupt this flow as they stir the Wounded Warrior into a defensive stance, ready for the fight for perpetual sorrow and disappointment. Instead of fighting, we need the gōngfu of yellow and black beans to find our own enlightenment in Xìng.

---

[12] In these two instances, the relationship can only change in one direction, from horizontal to vertical. The role of the teacher and physician is to assist the student and patient. If the student and patient are Centered while teacher and physician are not, they then need to look for another teacher and another physician. The patient cannot treat the physician and the student cannot teach the teacher. While they can be friends, when it comes to treatment and teaching the relationship must have one direction.

> The samurai was furious. He shook, got all red in the face, was speechless with rage. He pulled out his sword and raised it above him, preparing to slay the monk.
> "That's hell," said the monk softly.
> The samurai was overwhelmed. The compassion and surrender of this little man who had offered his life to give this teaching to show him hell! He slowly put down his sword, filled with gratitude, and suddenly peaceful.
> "And that's heaven," said the monk softly.[13]
>
> Zen story.

The samurai then understood that the domains of *Heaven* and *Hell* are ones we create for ourselves with our internal clarity or disorder. Liú purposefully emphasizes the internal principle over external fears. In this way we are good from within and become proper regardless of *the slings and arrows of outrageous fortune*. Being proper in a relationship does not mean always being *nice*. Sometimes, for example, it is necessary for a teacher to be strict with their student and if coming from a point of Center, the teacher would be acting appropriately. Spoiled children may need sternness to restore harmony, yet were the parent to submit in the name of being *nice and loving*, the child would become internally abhorrent, deprived of refining propriety. The role of the teacher and the parent is to make the student and the child flourish.

> As an example of a clear window into our learning, while driving my three year old to a play date with his very best friend from pre-school, he became upset that we had taken the small car and was insisting that we go back and take the big one. We were already halfway there, so I continued driving, saying that I would pick him up afterward in the big car. Arriving at his friend's house, he refused to go in and would not budge unless we went back and drove in the big car. So I apologized to his friend and we went home. Once home again, he realized that he had missed his play date and he had *really* wanted to play with his friend. So he spent a long time crying. No matter how hard I tried to convince him, when we were at his friend's door, he would not listen.
>
> Yaron Seidman

A fascinating aspect of human character is illuminated by this story. Despite

---

[13] Feldman & Kornfield, (eds), 1991, p. 296.

wanting to go somewhere and in spite of reaching this destination, *life is not lived*. Regretting it in the end, whispering it with our last breath, along with our tears. The physician uses Xīnfǎ to address this before their patient gets to the end, and being proper, they do not miss *their play date*; we live life to the fullest. Passed then from parent to child, this becomes a heritage of positivity that transcends time, as evident in the very last paragraphs of the last book of Liú Yuán's Huái Xuān compendium. These final words were written by Liú Bèiwén (劉棍文), his eldest son. In the photo of the lost tomb at the start of this book, the gravestone behind Liú Yuán's belongs to Liú Bèiwén.

A distinguished scholar in his own right with great perspicacity, Bèiwén had ample filial piety and included this commentary on the work of his father. With these last pages, Bèiwén talks about the Five Hearts, in a chapter called *Learning the sages' capacity for forgiveness* (xuéshèng rénjú liáng 學聖人局量).[14] We include his work here after starting from the first page, studying step by step and arriving at these Five Hearts. Stilling the Waters with cultivation and understanding propriety, we become a reflection of Xìng.

One: A Compassionate Heart (dà cíbēi xīn 大慈悲心)

Feeling compassion for others is benevolence (rén 仁). Benevolence is the human Heart. It is the good Heart of Heaven's principle (tiān lǐ liáng xīn 天理良心). People must first have benevolence and only then can they cherish all affairs, only worried about knowing mankind's good and evil. With each word and each action one is only concerned with offending others.

As for the importance of human relationships; loyal, filial, friendship, brotherly and sisterly bonds, not bearing a thought of deceit with not a single thought of laziness or recklessness, what extra explanation is needed? One is benevolent and then they are called compassionate. This manifests initially in one thought, and then in all thoughts, initially in one affair and then in all affairs. This sequence should exist in any tolerant Heart. What is called 'inflicting no injury upon insects and vegetation' is bringing Xìng to fruition in order to cultivate the human character and the character of all things. This is assisting creation, and is the root of all relationships.

---

[14] Commentary by Liú Bèiwén, p. 4109-1 to 4111-2.

Two: A Vast Heart (dà guǎngdà xīn 大廣大心)

Vast refers to quantity. The ancients said, 'When one has a large quantity, one starts having good fortunes and blessings'. When quantity is small one harbors narrow mindedness, seeing the principle yet not understanding it, our temperament agitated, knowledge stopping at ourselves. We do not know that there are others, our stopping point is flawed and we are not concerned about harming others. Self-assured and not utilizing goodness, self-centered and not forgiving people, self-smallness and being intolerant.[15]

For one to have good measures from morning until night, one must reflect back and criticize oneself. In every word and every action one's only concern is to join with true principle, to not hurt others; so we examine ourselves in every moment. Even though others may be angry with me, scold me and treat me unfairly, I will pay no attention. I will not stop and engage them, but at home I reflect and ask myself, 'Has any shame been introduced into my Heart?' If anything unjust has been added, I weed it out, and ignore further taunts. In all human relations, from the great relation of ruler and parents, to siblings and friends, when it becomes perverse it has no impact on my Heart. There is no need to further explain this.[16]

Three: A Convenient Heart (dà fāngbiàn xīn 大方便心)

What is 'convenient'?[17] It is being agile in affairs, courageous and just. Humans get along with each other and must co-habit this world. They mutually interact and welcome one another, and this falls under the Five Cardinal Relationships. There are differences between seniors and juniors, great and small, superior and inferior, intimacy and remoteness, virtuous or not.

For example, one serves the monarch or parents with only utmost and whole-Hearted respect; our thoroughness is absolute and we cannot speak of convenience. In other relationships like those between siblings and friends, the kinship may be close or far, some being virtuous and some not; one

---

[15] The Wounded Warrior mentality.
[16] Internal resilience is needed in relationships, otherwise they become a two-way street. *My* appropriateness is *not* dependent on *your* mood or disposition. In this way, the relationship can more easily come back to Center.
[17] Fāngbiàn (方便): Can mean convenient, suitable, easy or helpful.

cannot view them all as being equal. Serving an older brother, loving a younger sister or trusting a friend, one must first cultivate their own Dào. Then we can love others, respect them and not deceive them.

Being like this for a long time without compromise, we ignore it if they say good or bad things about us. We stop only at fulfilling our own Heart, our own Dào; seeking our shame-free Heart. If someone has a task at hand, as long as it is not contrary to true principle, my good Heart will do the labor for them. With all my Heart I will help their winding road result in a good outcome. This is the Dào of convenience.

However, affairs have difficult and easy, circumstances have good and bad, situations change constantly. Even though we say 'convenience' one should always deliberate the reason and good sense of the phenomena. One cannot act upon all situations indifferently. For example, to save a person who has fallen into a well, one should not jeopardize one's own life by falling in also, thereby humiliating their parents. Thus, the ancients advised, 'If one is able to do it, one should exhaust one's ability to do so. If one's ability cannot do it, then one should still use one's Heart thoroughly.'

These words describe a relationship between our affairs and true principle. When from early morning one cultivates virtue in their simple body, in each word and each action, each step and each pace, despite our difficult affairs being many, their body feels convenient in the evening. This accomplishment is simple and easy to practice. As long as one pays attention and is not lazy or reckless, they can feel convenient and at ease in all situations. For example, when they walk on the street and come across a rock or tree obstructing the way, they will remove it as they are worried that it will obstruct others.[18] As for difficulties like hunger and cold, they are only worried that others will suffer under them. Having enough to eat, being safe and warm, along with all such positive realities, one is only concerned that others will have enough. On any given day, under any circumstance, there is no place that they do not feel convenient and at ease. This word 'convenience' literally demonstrates the two words: benevolence and righteousness.

---

[18] *Throwing oneself into difficulty and hardship for a noble cause: this is one medicine.*

Four: A Great Purified Heart (dà qīngjìng xīn 大清淨心)

What does 'purified' mean?[19] *One sees money and desires it not, sees lust and loves it not. In our thoughts or affairs we do not follow our desires or contradict the true principle. We are law-abiding citizens, diligent in our profession. We cultivate our Hearts and contemplate human life with each and every step; it is all part of our destiny. 'Heaven loves mankind' is reflected in human nature through the kind Heart of Heaven's principle. With each of my thoughts I never depart from Heaven's Heart. In each affair my body attaches to and acts upon it, no matter if it is for morals or justice. I elect one cause of action that is in accord with true principle.*

For example, if I work as a merchant I focus my Heart on learning this art, diligently without slacking, industrious but not excessive, honest and never greedy. I focus without scattering, examining each thought, not losing even one bit of Heaven goodness. In this way, no matter the situation, I can make a living and pass my days. Relying only upon the Heaven within me, my actions become a habit.

The human Heart goes astray endlessly, so one cannot conduct themselves as they wish and go unchecked. As long as one does not suffer hunger or cold and is able to provide for his family, one has enough. This then becomes a beautiful realm. As for the wealthy and famous who also accumulate goodness and virtue and then are blessed by Heaven with riches and good fortunes, I do not begrudge them their possessions and accumulations and do not allow my thoughts to go astray.

And sure enough, as I intentionally withdraw my interest in wealth and glory, I constantly eradicate stray thoughts and so over time this becomes the rule. Then no matter if I am poor or in difficulty, with a calm Heart I keep on going. In this way an ordinary person can curb their selfishness. They force themselves to study the method of purification. If an educated person cultivates their intentions and disciplines their temperament, returns to benevolence and righteousness and is kind to everyone under all circumstances, then in this way any vulgarity they had within naturally disappears.

External actions follow propriety, and after some time of cultivation, good and evil emotions completely vanish. We attain

---

[19] Qīngjìng (大清淨): Means peaceful, quiet, tranquil and purified of illusions.

a calm Heart and clarity in our actions. This accomplishment encompasses everything from beginning to end, from the roots to the branches. The sage does not act or think of righteousness in order to appease the Dào; at no time do they think of themselves, whatever high salary or position may be available, this is where their Dào comes from. The words 'pure Heart' represent aspiration to the sages and virtuous people, guarding one's actions and conduct and not being lax, These words speak of the Heart's emotions being like Water, adapting naturally to any circumstance. This is the natural state of the human Heart, yet we can find this nature only with effort.

Five: A Gentle Harmonious Heart (dà róuhé xīn 大柔和心)

Harmonious speaks of a kind friendship that extends everywhere. Its noble aspect is the cultivation of joy, anger, sorrow and happiness, all of which are regulated by the Center. It is reaching the Dào of all under Heaven. The profundity of Heaven and Earth act equally upon all generations and all people, yet it is only a sage who reaches the ultimate state of harmony.

Next to that one speaks of the Five Cardinal Relationships, each having its own Dào and place. Kindness is present and friendship is prevalent. The ties of friendship do not deviate from this. The harmony of these relationships one cannot do without; this must be explored to the fullest extent. Next to that, being without tolerance means being without benevolence. Being without courage means being without righteousness. Being careful and cautious, one evens their Heart and calms the Qì. They worry about hurting others, about spoiling affairs, about causing disaster.

Through embodying modesty and being compromising with affairs of great unfairness directed at them, which are too much to bear, orchestrated by hateful and offensive people, they pass it by in silence. If at home there is great competitiveness or anxiety, with great vigor they soften and calm it down, bringing relationships back to gentle harmony. It is the so-called 'using generosity and lenience for teaching, not reporting the non-Dào, this is the realm of the noble person'.[20] The meaning of 'lenience'

---

[20] This is a quote from the Doctrine of the Mean, kuān róu yǐ jiāo, bù bào wú dào, jūn zǐ jū zhī (宽柔以教, 不报无道, 君子居之). *Lenient and soft is used for teaching, not dwelling in tyranny, this is where the noble person resides.*

must not be associated with negative connotations such as being lacking in goodness, being weak or ambivalent, as this would bypass its real meaning.

Whenever a person cannot endure humiliation or tolerate rejection, it is because their blood and Qì are stiff and unyielding, their emotions are agitated and explosive. Therefore, they must soften their Qì in order to follow true principle, making the emotions harmonious in order to become compatible to others. Only then can kinship and friendship extend everywhere and all actions will then be without disaster.

These Five Hearts are found in the canons of Buddhism and Dàoism and their principle is not different to the Dào of the Confucian sages. The words and actions of the sage do not fall outside of this scope. The Four Masters and Six Classics and the discussions of great people of virtue also do not fall outside of this realm. However, common people disregard this principle and place it in a low esteem. They see it as impractical and laugh at it to the extent of heresy, completely shutting it out.

This state of confusion has arisen because they have no entry point to learn the teachings of the sages and the virtuous. I often teach our schoolfellows about these Five Hearts. It is teaching the sages' capacity for forgiveness and tolerance. One must first possess the understanding behind these Five Hearts and put their principles into practice. Only then can one gaze at the virtuous, to the sage and to Heaven.

What a pity! The ones who follow these Five Hearts are rare. Today it is looked down upon as out-dated. I have no choice but to present it to you in this book as if giving of one's own family transmission. My late father taught people his whole life and his teachings were very rich. They all revolved around Xìng, emotions and the art of the Heart, all to be carried out daily in human relations.

The preceding Five Hearts seem as if they are words from the schools of Buddhism, Dàoism, and Confucianism, but in reality they are universal true teachings. Now, because we have printed this book explaining medicine, I especially attached these words at the end. People of the past said, 'When treating a disease one should treat the formless'. This is the principle of the Five Hearts. If one can apply the substance of this principle, where can there be a disease? To the accomplished student of medicine, please take note; contracting a disease is a hardship for the human being, please use these words to treat the disease that has not yet formed!

Written respectfully by the son, Bèiwén.

These Five Hearts are the Hearts of Xīnfǎ, revealing how to *treat* the Heart. Through this cultivation the physician and patient reach places that medicines could never access. Opening the door, they read their Concealed Words and transform them into a reflection of the Dào Heart. By calming their Wounded Warrior, they find Center and Xìng. Once they have done this for themselves they can then help others do the same, with harmony rippling out into the world. One such transformed soul, a father and a teacher, whispered at the end:

"Can I leave like a gentleman?"

The last words of a great man, which led him through his entire life, trying to do what was proper; being a proper father, a proper son, a proper brother, and a proper friend.

"We are rejuvenated by our consistent nurturing of stillness."

Conclusion

塵埃落定

Chén Āi Luò Dìng

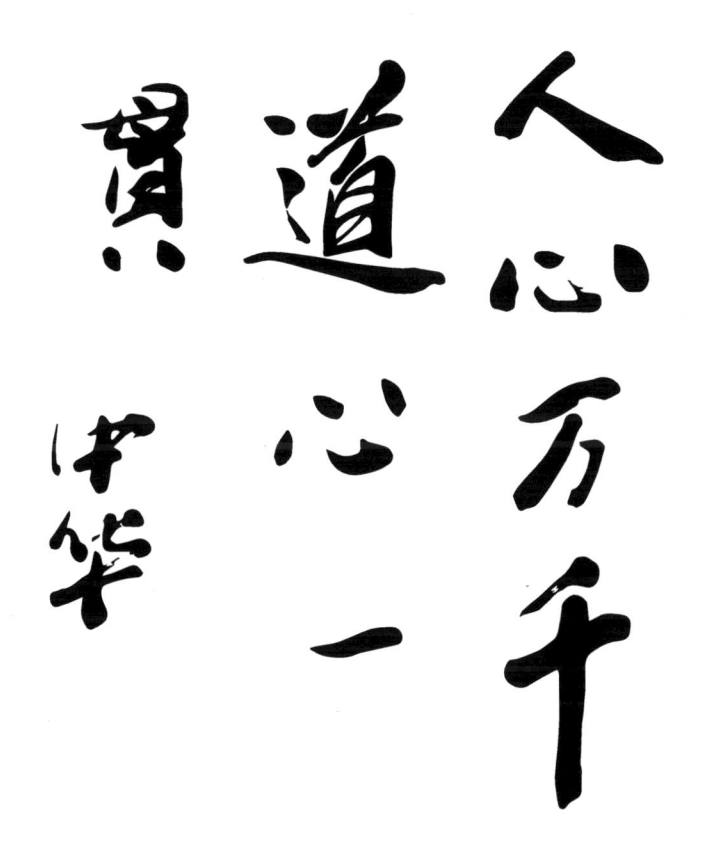

人心万千
道心一

The human Heart has endless variations,
while the Dào Heart has One principle penetrating all.

Chén Zhōnghuá

And so, Liú Yuán becomes an eternal teacher through both his words and his lineage. A true example of the prosperity of propriety echoing through the ages, his great grandson to this day follows the path of goodness, teaching one and all about benevolence and kindness. The ripples of this impulse wash out over the world from humble beginnings in a small town in China. Timeless.

Medicine has a pure Heart. Taking time, the physician offers this purity to the patient. From the Outer Water Circle to the Inner Fire Circle and what is Concealed within, every word, herb or acupuncture point directs more life into the vessel ☲. And that is it. The human being has an innate yearning for something more, a void the physician and patient fill with benevolence. Suddenly, loneliness vanishes. Physical sustenance is precious, yet not more so than the profound experiences between human beings. Born into the world of Yīn and Yáng without likes and dislikes, the baby joins harmoniously with their loving mother and father. Growing up and maturing, life's dichotomy gradually intensifies and the individual becomes characterized by circumstance, complicating the bonds of relationships. How easy it is for the Heart to break, and yet still the person strives on, driven by something deeper than their Wounded Warrior.

As the folly of youth is left by the riverbank, the human being looks in the mirror and sees the Dào Heart reflected. No longer looking outward, they look in and see life through the myriad relationships. Sunlight penetrates the vessel, vanquishing the shadows and the Heart is clear and yet clearer about virtue. Only now is the physician born, as they have found their Lost Heart. They graduate from being a skilled technician and begin their journey as a true healer. The patient is welcomed into a safe haven; out of the gales and torment, they enter the calm eye of the storm. Through knowing their words, the physician opens the curtains, and it is a wonderful day. Spring is so fresh, Summer so warm, Autumn so tranquil and Winter so cozy. Centered, physician and patient then engage their relationships, which are defined only by Xìng: absolute goodness. One yellow bean is a great accomplishment.

Like Shí Yīn Fū with one bag on the right, one on the left and one in the Center, the physician looks at the patient in their completeness, not one of us have been left behind, all are imbued with Xìng. The myriad pieces of medicine and symptoms are observed as they to and fro with the winds of change and season. Leaves are shed in Autumn, contemplated in Winter and then reborn in Spring, yet they are always connected to the roots. Growth and decline are the movements of Yīn and Yáng while the constant thread of life is only defined by the quiet rotation of Tàijí. So the physician starts each day by drawing an unadorned circle.

From here they uncover the true principle of treatment, moving into action from Xìng and out into benevolent medicine. The segments form the whole, the patient's life a curve of the One Thread of Life. Accepting the past to work in the present to give to the future, every thought, emotion and action comes from Center, and is directed at returning one and all to this same place. Not defined by the convolutions of society, politics and culture, we stop only at being proper in each moment; a proper parent, a proper child, all through the perpetual gōngfu of sorting good and bad. Thus, the Heart becomes full of life.

No matter how turbulent the past, *still* we must live. The physician recognizes internal confusion and so gently they plant a seed of goodness. When nurtured, this seed grows into an unshakable self-worth, and the patient becomes the physician of their own relationships. Seeing anger, resentment, fear and sorrow as reflections of imbalance rather than personal affronts, the family returns to Center.

The complications of life simplify as the physician embraces their role, assisting the patient back to Center to find their Lost Heart. And that is it! Thereafter there is no need for medicine, as life is being lived. Nothing is Concealed within as we approach our work and relationships with an open and kind Heart. Daily we cultivate warmth within the vessel with Xīnfǎ and the rotations of Unification and Separation. Now is the time for giving to our patients, allowing them to take the very best from the present; becoming who they truly are.

And the teacher returned from the mountain, river and the canopy, well rested from his sleep and his journey. Arriving at the little schoolhouse, he found all his students waiting for him...

學生: Teacher! Where have you been?

老師: I have been across the fields and river and into the mountains.

學生: Teacher! What are we going to learn today?

老師: The most important lesson of all. You will learn how to be yourselves.

Bibliography

Adler, J. A. 1999, 'Zhou Dunyi: The Metaphysics and Practice of Sagehood' in *Sources of Chinese Tradition*, eds W. T. De Bary & I. Bloom, 2nd edn, Columbia University Press, West Sussex.

Arnold, C. February 11, 2013, 'Effects of Stress can Persist for Generations: how your grandpa's rough life might make you more anxious' in *Scientific American*, accessed February 2013, from http://www.scientificamerican.com/article.cfm?id=effects-stress-can-persist-generations.

Bol, P. K. & Kirby, W. C. *China: Traditions and Transformations*, Harvard lecture series, accessed 2012, from http://www.extension.harvard.edu/open-learning-initiative/china-history.

Burnett, F. 1911, *The Secret Garden*, Puffin Books, London.

Cave, N. 1989, *And the Ass Saw the Angel*, Penguin Books, London.

Cheng, M. C. 1995, *Master of Five Excellences*, trans. M. Hennessy, Frog Ltd, Berkley.

Chin, S. F. S. 2004, *Nei Jia Quan: Internal Martial Arts: Teachers of Tai Ji Quan, Xing Yi Quan and Ba Gua Zhang*, 2nd edn, ed J. O'Brien, Blue Snake Books, Berkeley.

Cleary, T. 1991, *The Secret of the Golden Flower: The Classic Chinese Book of Life*, HarperCollins, New York.

Coelho, P, 2007, *The Witch of Portobello*, HarperCollins, Sydney.

Colgrove, L. 1941, 'Theosophy & Initiation' on *The Theosophical Forum*, Theosophical University Press, April forum, accessed 2012 from http://www.theosociety.org/pasadena/forum/f18n04p275_theosophy-and-initiation.htm.

Cort, J. E. 1995, The Jain Knowledge Warehouses: Traditional Libraries in India, *Journal of the American Oriental Society*, accessed 2013 from http://www.jstor.org/discover/10.2307/605310?uid=2129&uid=2&uid=70&uid=4&sid=21102078372297.

Crean, T. 2007, *God is No Delusion: A refutation of Richard Dawkins*, Ignatius Press, San Francisco.

Croizier, R. C, 1968, *Traditional Medicine in Modern China: Science, Nationalism and the Tensions of Cultural Change*, Harvard University Press, Cambridge, Massachusetts.

Dawkins, R, 2006, *The God Delusion*, Bantam Press, Great Britain.

Eknath, E. & Kobbe, P. (trans), 2006, *Dhammapada: Buddhas zentrale Lehren*, Random House/Goldman, Munich.

Falkayn, D. (ed), 1977, *Creating a New Chinese Medicine and Pharmacology*, Foreign Language Press, Peking.

Feldman, C. & Kornfield, J. 1991, *Stories of the Spirit, Stories of the Heart: Parables of the Spiritual Path from Around the World*, Harper Collins, New York.

Fingarette, H. 1971, *Confucius: The Secular as Sacred*, Waveland Press Inc, Illinois.

Foer, J. S. 2009, *Eating Animals*, Little, Brown & Company, New York.

Fung, Y. L. 1948, *A Short History of Chinese Philosophy: A Systematic Account of Chinese Thought from its Origins to the Present Day*, ed D. Bodde, The Free Press, New York.

Furth, C. 1999, *A Flourishing of Yin: Gender in China's Medical History, 960-1665*, University of California Press, Berkeley.

Gibran, K. 2008, *Kahlil Gibran's The Prophet and The Art of Peace*, New illustrated edition, Duncan Baird Publishers, London.

Giono, J. 1996, *The Man Who Planted Trees*, trans. B. Bray, The Harvill Press, London.

Goethe, J, 1984, *Goethe: the Collected Works, Faust I & II*, trans. S. Atkins, Princeton University Press, New Jersey.

Goleman, D. 1995, *Emotional Intelligence: Why It Can Matter More Than IQ*, Bantam Books, New York.

Greene, B. 2000, *The Elegant Universe: Superstrings, Hidden Dimensions and the Quest for the Ultimate Theory*, Vintage, London.

Hesse, H. 1973, *Siddhartha*, Picador, London.

Hoff, B. 1982, *The Tao of Pooh & The Te of Piglet*, Methuen, London.

Hóng J. S. 2006, *Chen Style Taijiquan Practical Method: Volume One: Theory*, eds Z. & H. Chen, Hunyuan Taiji Press, Edmonton.

Huang, H. 2009, *Ten Key Formula Families in Chinese Medicine*, Trans. M. Max,Eastland Press, Seattle.

Jaensch, T. A. 2001, *"..."...deep beneath the layers..."..." - TCM history in the Shang & Zhou eras*, Point Specifics, Sydney.

Jaensch, T. A. 1997, *Yì Shén (意神) Remember the Spirit,* Self-printed and self-bound, Sydney.

Juhan, D. 2003, *Job's Body: A Handbook for Bodywork*, Barrytown, Station Hill, New York.

Jullien, F. 2008, *In Praise of Blandness: Proceeding from Chinese Thought and Aesthetics*, trans. P. M. Varsano, Zone Books, New York.

Jullien, F. 2007, *Vital Nourishment: Departing from Happiness*, trans. A. Goldhammer, Zone Books, New York.

Koyczan, S, 2013, *To This Day*.

Lau, D. C. (trans), 1963, *Lao Tzu: Tao Te Ching*, Penguin Books, London.

Leavitt, F. 2001, *Evaluating Scientific Research: Separating Fact from Fiction*, Prentice-Hall Inc, New Jersey.

Leunig, M, 1990, *When I Talk to You*, HarperCollins, Sydney.

Liang, Z. T. 1997, *A Qin Bowei Anthology*, trans. C. Chace, Paradigm Publications, Massachusetts.

Lo, V. & Stanley-Baker, M. 2011, *Chinese Medicine: Chapter 9 of The Oxford Handbook of The History of Medicine*, ed M. Jackson, Oxford University Press, Oxford.

Mandela, N. 2010, *Conversations with Myself*, Farrar, Straus & Giroux, New York.

Marinelli, R., Fuerst, B., Zee, H. V. D., McGinn, A. & Marinelli, W. 1995, 'The Heart is not a Pump: A Refutation of the Pressure Propulsion Premise of Heart Function' in *Frontier Perspectives* – the Journal of Frontier Sciences at Temple University, Philadelphia, Fall-Winter issue, Volume 5, number 1.

Miller, B. S. (trans) 1986, *The Bhagavad-Gita – Krishna's Counsel in Time of War*, Columbia University Press, New York.

Murakami, H. 2003, *The Wind-Up Bird Chronicle*, trans. J. Rubin, Random House, London.

Musashi, M. 1974, *A Book of Five Rings*, trans. V. Harris, The Overlook Press, New York.

Nietzsche, F. 1973, *Beyond Good and Evil: Prelude to a Philosophy of the Future*, trans. R. J. Hollingdale, Penguin Books, London.

Plato: *The Trial and Death of Socrates: Four Dialogues*, 1992, Dover Publications, Inc, New York.

Porkert, M. 1974, *The Theoretical Foundations of Chinese Medicine: Systems of Correspondence*, Massachusetts Institute of Technology Press, Cambridge.

Robinson, K. & Aronica, L. 2009, *The Element: How Finding Your Passion Changes Everything*, Allen Lane, Camberwell.

Rose, J. 2005, *Music of the Human Heart may hold clues to Healing*, accessed March 2013 from
http://www.npr.org/templates/story/story.php?storyId=4510912.

Rosen, M. 2004, *Sad Book*, Walker Books, London.

Schmieg, A. L. 2005, *Watching Your Back: Chinese Martial Arts and Traditional Medicine*, University of Hawai'i Press, Honolulu.

Seidman, Y. 2002, *A Voyage Through Humanity: Poems of the Heart. Up the River*, USA Hunyuan Taiji Academy Inc, Connecticut.

Seidman, Y. & McLaren, T. 2012, *Hunyuan Fertility: Conception, Babies and Miracles*, Hunyuan Group, Inc, Connecticut.

Shannon, D. 1998, *A Bad Case of Stripes*, Scholastic, New York.

Shirreffs, S. M., Merson, S. J., Fraser, S. M., & Archer, D. T. 2004, 'The effects of fluid restriction on hydration status and subjective feelings in man' in *British Journal of Nutrition*, Volume 91, Issue 6, June.

Silberstein, S., Mathew, N., Saper, J., & Jenkins, S. 2002, 'Botulinum Toxin Type A as a Migraine Preventive Treatment. For the BOTOX Migraine Clinical Research Group' in *Headache: The Journal of Head and Face Pain*, Volume 40, Issue 6, June.

Silver, B. L. 1998, *The Ascent of Science*, Oxford University Press, New York.

St Augustine, 2004, *The Confessions*, Hendrickson Publishers, Massachusetts.

Sternberg, E. M. 2009, *Healing Spaces: The Science of Place and Well-Being*, Harvard University Press, Cambridge.

Unschuld, P. 2000, *Chinese Medical Ethics and atient/physician relationships in ancient China*, Lecture 15th April, University of Technology, Sydney.

Versluys, A. 2012, *Elementary Aspects of Canonical Chinese Medicine*, Lecture series, October, Sydney.

Waley, A. 1996, *Confucius: The Analects*, Wordsworth Editions Limited, Hertfordshire.

Wáng, Q. R. 2007, *Yi Lin Gai Cuo: Correcting the Errors in the Forest of Medicine*, trans. Y. Chung, H. Oving & S. Becker, Blue Poppy Press, Boulder.

Wilson, E. O. 1929, *Biophilia: The uman bond with other species*, Harvard University Press, Cambridge.

Wu, Y. L. 2010, *Reproducing Women: Medicine, Metaphor and Childbirth in Late Imperial China*, University of California Press, Berkeley.

Wu, Z. X. 2009, *Seeking the Spirit of the Book of Change – 8 days to mastering a shamanic Yijing (I Ching) prediction system*, Singing Dragon, London.

Yoshikawa, E. 1971, *Musashi*, trans. E. O. Reischauer, Kodansha International, Tokyo.

Yuán, L. (劉沅) *Huái Xuān Quán Shū* (槐軒全書) *The Complete Compendium of Huái Xuān Philosophy*. The original version compiled and printed in 1905. Please contact the Hùnyuán Research Institute for Chinese Classics for more information on the original text.

Yuán, L. (劉沅) *Shí Yīn Fū Gōng Guò Gé* (石音夫功過格) *Shí Yīn Fū and the Ledger of Good and Evil*. Chéngdū Shǒujīng Táng (成都守經堂) Chéngdū Guarding the Classics Printing House, 1922, Chéngdū Nán Mén Sān Xiàngzi (成都南門三巷子) Chéngdū Southern Gate, Third Alley.

APPENDIX A

石音夫功過格
Shí Yīn Fū Gōng Guò Gé

Shí Yīn Fū and the Ledger of Good and Evil

Original Chinese as edited by Liú Yuán (劉沅).

石音夫功過格傳

宋時，有一人，幼喪父母，流落群丐之中，不知己姓名，人亦不知其姓氏，因衣服藍縷，求為傭工，人不之雇，又身常凍餓，體復羸弱，因此朝夕乞食，往往飯不能充。自念人皆有父母居食，我何獨無，但天既生我為人，耳目口鼻心思，都與人一般，如何又者般窮苦，必定是我前世造了許多罪孽，所以今生才者般受苦，常常自恨，無有分文，無有力量，可以作些善事，培補前世之罪過。如此存心，歷有年所，卻怪總莫有一點好機緣，也無有人哀憐他窮苦，自家也無法，隻好將就乞丐度日。

一日行至太白山前，遇一道人，在路旁獨坐。此人見他形貌，與眾不同，便俯伏在地叩頭，要他指引一條生路。那道人道："你問生路，是問生死之生，還是問長生之生，或問生意之生，生人之生，萬物之生？"此人道："望道長指明，哪樣生意難做，哪樣生意易做？"道長道："你是願做易的，還是願做難的？"此人道："我願做難的。"道長道："那生意之生是難做的，譬如時至三四月，米價將貴，你買四五十兩銀子的米，到後來，米價昂貴，你才賣，可以賺得些利錢。你有本錢否？"此人道："沒有。"道人道："沒有本錢就難了。還有個難中易事，你去山中砍柴，挑到長街，賣些銀錢，可以養活身口。"此人道："打柴后有個出頭路麼？"道人道："命中隻有八合米，行盡天下不滿升。若單單生意之生就想有個出頭的路，不但你打柴，就是五湖四海許多大本錢客人，也不過混一生的口而已，豈能得出頭的路？"此人道："要如何才得出頭？"道長道："惟萬物之生，就得出頭。"此人道："更難更難。若論不殺生，方為萬物之生，雞鴨不殺，喂他何益？牛馬不殺，膠鼓何取？豬羊不殺，祭祀何有？若論不傷生，竹木不砍，柴薪何來？草林不伐，人宅無取。這真難也。"道長道："最容易的。雞鴨不損其卵，不傷其小，又不妄費，當用之時，取其大者而殺之，何得為殺？馬有扶朝之功，牛有養人之德，臨老自死，何必在殺，何得無取？竹木草苗，方長不折，相時方伐，何得無用？"此人道："這等看將起來，凡物當生旺之時，殺之方才為殺，至休囚當死之時，殺之不足為殺也。"道人曰："然。蓋生旺之時，乃天地發生萬物之時，不敢違悖天意。至乘天地收藏之時而取之，則用無窮也。"此人恍然曰："天地有好生之德，萬物有資生之心，凡事順乎天理人心而為之，勿逆其天理人心而行之，自然便是好事了。"道長道："你此言大有緣分也。但你此時片善未積，難以出頭。好好將你者個心腸實力行事，待你功行圓滿，自有出頭之日。你若恆心積善，則生死之生也在內了。你跪在地下，我與你取個名兒，叫做石音夫。"

石音夫跪而受教，待他起來，則道長已不見了。音夫大哭一場，仍然沿門丐食，思想我心常多亂想，如何可以作善？因之化些黑豆，化些黃豆，分作兩囊，一囊帶於左，一囊帶於右，又另做一袋帶於胸前，黃豆放於左，黑豆放於右，或日夜之間起了一點不好之心，作了一點不好之事，則取右邊黑豆一顆，投入袋中記過，若起了一點好心，作了一點好事，即取左邊黃豆一顆，投入袋中記功，滿一百日，取中袋內黃黑兩色豆來數，看功多過多。始而過多，繼而功過平平，久而久之，功多過少，至一年之外，隻見是功。日間行路，足不踐生旺之草；大小兩便，必遮蓋身體；途中遇虫蟻多處，避旁而行；瓜田不納履，李下不整冠；逢男人過，讓路，見女人過，遠避，決不回顧；路中拾得人貴賤之物，必候失者尋至而還之；晴雨寒暑，不怨乎天，山水險阻，不怨乎地；罵己笑己，不回人言，不恨於心。至行持兩年半，自覺心裡坦然，身子強健，就見了不識之人，也有一番愛他敬他之心。

陝西有一人名叫石心德，其家大富，隻生得有一女，其女名叫石音，自幼伶俐，因擇婿未能許人。是夜中秋之節，石心德夢神人告之，說明日有石音夫來，你可好好接待他，醒來十分驚異。次日天明灑掃門戶，安排迎接貴客，候至午時，並無客至，隻有一丐食之人至門。門夫報於石心德知之，心德想道："此乞丐有何好處，難道神人說的石音夫就是他？"也隻得留住他，且看更有人來否。候至夜分，並無人來，便與內人商議，莫非此人有些來歷。其妻道："可速出去問他來歷。"心德出來便問乞丐之人，你貴姓，何名，何處居住，看你形容異常，並非薄福之人，為何甘為乞丐？可一一說來我聽。石音夫道："小人川省人氏，合家逃難，至陝西地界時，小人年方兩歲，得一恩人，隨帶化食，十余年矣。恩人姓錢，並未問其名號，不期恩人身故，是我憑土埋之，所以不知宗派。欲作別樣之計，不得其門，仍然沿門乞食。兩年前遇一道長，與我取名，叫做石音夫，亦不知取此姓名何故。今在老爺貴府上，承蒙厚德，留住一日，不得不訴真情。"心德聽罷，默思石音夫者，乃我石音女兒之夫也，本要將女許配於他，惜乎同姓，不便稱呼，奈是神靈托夢，想必前生修積姻緣，亦未可知，乃向音夫道："看你這位英才，朝日乞化，也不是長久之策。為人在世，興家立業，方才算個漢子。若漂漂蕩蕩，雖然快活，枉自混過光陰。我有一女，欲招你為婿，不知你意下如何？"石音夫道："萬萬不可。小人一身，尚且難養，不要說出這樣折福的話。"心德道："婚姻配合，乃前生修積，何為折福？"遂將夢中之言告之。音夫方悟道長命名之意，方才應允婚事。夫妻配合，就住在石家。

石音夫也不以為得意，與石音小姐，時時講些功德事，又時行好事。常見岳父，小斗放出，大斗收回，石音夫苦苦勸之不聽。又見岳父，小戥放出，大戥收回，音夫又苦苦勸之，亦不聽。勸至多回，心德反大怒起來，罵這無志之人，生成討口之命，趕他出去，小庄上住，不用在此擾亂我的心事。石音夫便同小姐至小庄上，住了數月。音夫嘆道："原來我岳父大富，從這兩斗兩戥致的。但我受他恩重，豈肯忍心等他墮落？"日夜不安，要把岳父勸轉，此心才甘。次日半夜，扒將起來燒茶吃了，坐到天明，夫妻二人，又去看看岳父岳母，又勸戒一番。不知心德，惡事已滿，上界命火雷二部，要燒毀他房屋，將心德震死，以罰其罪。那天神因見音夫在此，恐怕震動於他，一時未施雷火。音夫一心要勸回岳父，故久留不去，一連住了兩三日。那晚夢一老翁，告音夫道："你岳父惡貫滿盈，雷火將及，你早早躲避為妙。"音夫夫婦同夢，醒來大驚，念己夫婦，受了心德恩惠，實實不忍，同跪在塵埃，當天拜謝道："上天譴責，乃自造之孽，理當如此。但凡民音夫，定要勸轉，倘若岳父，再不肯為善，石音夫情願替死受報。"他夫妻誠心禱告，暗中早已感動神靈，心德未知，反疑音夫顛狂，猶然不改惡念。忽然一夜夢中，見冤鬼無數，都來面前，要拉他去見閻君。心德心中害怕，醒來出了一身冷汗，也有幾分懼怕，然尚不改悔惡事也。

那石音夫，平日陰功浩大，所以在心德家中，那些鬼魔，都不敢十分侵擾。一日心德出外閒游，見一條蛇在地下，用腳踢開，想要踢他往路旁去，不料那蛇竟咬他一口，那都是惡鬼變成的蛇，因石音夫朝夕隨著心德，所以雖被咬傷，卻不甚痛楚。那心德因女婿在家，常說修行作善，公平正直之言，心中大不快樂，即吩咐叫他，各回庄上去罷，音夫隻得回去。那時冤惡之鬼，見音夫去了，一齊都進宅來。那夜心德，被蛇咬處，十分痛楚，如刀割一般，忙忙叫人快去叫女婿來。石音夫夫婦，不時到了，心德腳又不痛，心中暗想："莫非我女婿，果然有些好處？如何他一來了，我的腳就不痛？"心裡思量，口裡卻不好說出。他才去，腳又痛得甚緊。心德又忙發人去趕他轉來，腳又不甚大痛。此時音夫也不知其故，心德道："賢婿你可搬將回來坐，不要在小庄上了。"音夫道："回來到不妨，隻恐怕不合岳父的心事。"心德道："我如今諸事要聽你的話了。"音夫道："岳父須要改了秤斗的事，我才回來。"心德道："你必定要我改那些東西，是何緣故？"音夫道："凡人存心正直，自然神欽鬼伏，心懷欺詐，必定鬼神譴責，此乃一定之理。岳父做了欺心之事，安能免災難之來？"心德點頭道："是。"音夫又把他夫婦替他禱告話，說了一遍，心德聽了，也自知他被蛇咬傷，音夫來便不痛，其中定有緣故，即吩咐家人："將斗稱戥子，一概打毀。從今後，任從賢婿與我安排便了。"音夫道："叫家人上街，買備肉菜，設些桌席，將歷年借錢借米的賬主，一概請來。若還了頭的，還不起利息的，將借約退與他；窮了還不起頭的，也將借約退還，分文不要；

或不能嫁娶，或有緊急事，幫他幾兩銀錢去用，任他慢慢做來相還；目前無吃無穿的，周濟谷米，勸他做個好人；往常侵佔人田地，一一各還邊界；早年強要人家所愛的物件，逐戶退還。"心德一一依從，自此人人稱贊。

心德行之數月，心德也覺精神清爽，身體安和。一日有一醫人來借宿，心德蛇傷之疾，請他醫治，拿點末藥一擦，即便好了。次日起來，任隨游走，全然不痛。心德善根發現，恍然大悟，說道："我今得賢婿指點，昔年所為之事，果然錯了。想人生在世上，活得幾百歲，何不行些好事？"自是越把女婿看得甚重。

那時有一僧人，不會化錢糧，專要化富家。他說貧窮的錢米，來得苦，故不忍化。來至石心德家下，叩化修橋的錢糧。心德道："你看此橋，所費多少？一例有我結緣，不必去化他人。"僧人大喜，即日起工，工完之日，約計費一千八百錢糧，刊碑名叫獨善橋。

又一日，一僧名念和，師徒二人，欲修寺院上下二殿，師要化富家，徒弟道："不論貧富，隻要他人肯自己發心，不必強勉於人。"師傅來至心德家募化，心德發心，一例包圓修成。念和見他大發慈悲，滿心歡悅，速回動土興工，問徒弟道："你的錢糧如何？"徒弟答道："我的還早。"師笑道："你能有多大臉面，就想化起。實不瞞你，我的有了。"徒弟道："師傅先修上殿，待我慢慢化銀修下殿。"念和道："說過的話，不要反悔。"不數月，裝修佛殿齊整。念和大是得意，徒弟也不慌忙，三年然后成工。

誰知那念和罪惡多端，因與佃戶婦人有情，上殿后開了一條私路來往。那一夜睡至半夜，婦人要改手，去到茅廁出恭，茅廁板斷，婦人落下糞坑，念和隻得點火來看。婦人落在坑裡，爬起發嘔，叫高照些火，我才看見。那僧一時隻顧婦人，不想那火燒著廁房，一時心忙手亂，摸滅不及，又不好喊人來救火。那婦人一身是屎，又回去不得，又怕驚動人來看見，二人嚇得痴痴站著。即時大風暴起，將大殿燒得干干淨淨，隻留得徒弟所修下殿一向。當時心德聽說燒了上殿，夫婦悲淚嘆道："我去了九百五十兩銀子，方才修整齊備，今片瓦不留，這番功德何在？"不數日，天下大雨，即日平河大水，連獨善橋也打倒了，一磵不留。心德聽見，夫妻二人，傷心痛哭。石音夫知道，走來勸解，心德道："我一個家財費完，隻剩得田地房屋，方才做起來兩宗功果，今日一宗不留，叫我如何不悲？"音夫道："但提一言，岳父可以自知。先年你余積的錢，如何起得這樣快？"心德聽見，不覺著了一驚，豁然省悟道："這是奸狡詭計，瞞心昧己之錢，拿來做功果都是枉然的。也罷，丟了去罷，也不嘔他，我庄子上，年中還有些余剩，自己肉食酒菜，淡薄些兒，慢慢積來，又做功果。"音夫道："功果也要做些。"心德聽說此話，心中暗想："女婿之言，說做功果，就說做功果，如何說出也要做些？

其中必有緣故。"於是設備酒席，請女婿正坐，然后請教說："前日做功果也要做些之言，是何緣故？"不知音夫修積多年，心無一物打擾，慧悟日開，不垢不淨之中，豁然見天地之間，莫非一理貫通，何事不知，無微不照，當時應道："岳父所問，是單單做功果，還是想要積德，還是想要行善，還是想要修行？"心德道："有不同麼？"音夫道："大小不同，深淺不同，輕重不同。即如人借我物件，用壞，還不起我，就不要他還；借我銀錢，還我不起，即不要他還；我若借人銀錢，必要還他，不欠來生之債，此為積德。不背地說人是非，不揚人惡名，不破人好事，不助人暴氣，不使人弟兄不和，不使人父子不睦；勿圖小利，勿無故殺牲，勿成就人殺牛，勿因他人做不好事忍口不行勸解，此為行善。無錢不可強為，強為不成功果。有錢修橋鋪路，培補寺院，裝修佛像，刊刻善書，隨施便是功果。若修積，全憑心上用功夫，起了一點好心，他人不知，我自知之，起了一點惡心，他人不知，我自知之，善事可作，惡事莫為，方為修積。"心德道："你是如何用工夫？"音夫道："說我的功夫，也容易。我做三囊，盛黑豆一囊居左，盛黃豆居右，一囊居胸前。或時起了一點惡心，做了惡事，即將黑豆一顆，入於胸囊中記過；或時起了一點善心，做了一件善事，即將黃豆一顆，入於胸囊中記功。至百日滿，取胸中囊豆來數，看功多過多。始而過多，繼而功過兼半，久之見功不見過。"心德聽了，毛骨悚然，不覺大驚醒悟，嘆道："此乃盡性之功，致命之學。我當年讀書也曾應試幾次，雖無功名之分，而書中道理，亦頗明白。這等看起來，我雖讀聖賢之書，何嘗體聖賢之道？我情願學你所做，縱不能做出去，也不枉今生為一個人，就死也甘心。"即把囊袋做起，帶整停當，時刻檢點，不敢放曠。

那日出外游行，心德行至木橋上，板橋不穩，一歪幾乎失腳跌倒，急忙尋個小石頭塞穩，恐怕驚跌后來人。音夫道："岳父何不拈黃豆記功？"心德道："此小事耳，何足為功？"音夫道："此不但存一點好心，且已行出了好事，何得為小而不記功？"心德遂悟道："看起來絲毫是功，則必絲毫是過，故子思曰：'戒慎乎其所不睹，恐懼乎其所不聞，莫見乎隱，莫顯乎微，君子必慎其獨也。'"音夫常常細看他岳父，看他做事。那一日見岳父，站在河岸上小便，尿滴水響，心德聽了著驚，轉身來想，此事穢污水府，即取黑豆一顆，入於胸囊中記過。又一日，見他人牛，將食他人禾苗，心德即忙趕去，牛已下田，食了幾兜禾，速牽來拴著，才叫牛主牽回，他又往禾苗家，告主人道："我牛吃你禾苗幾兜，帶得一碗米來賠你。"苗主道："莫說吃了三兜，就吃一半，他自然會發起來，哪個要你老先生賠？"遂以禮貌恭恪送回。即取黃豆一顆，入於胸中記功。音夫見岳父功夫如此，滿心歡喜。

一日有一僧人，來至心德門首，盤腳坐下，一言不發。心德恭恭敬敬，向前拜問，那僧照心德一杖打來。心德道："老和尚，何必發怒？但要化甚麼東西，隻要我家有，無一不從。"僧即大聲應道："打開生死路，跳出鬼門關。"心德道："何為生死路？"僧應道："出家念佛生死路。"心德道："何為鬼門關？""紅塵便是鬼門關。"那知心德行善有年，心地已早開悟，微笑問僧人道："你和尚出家幾多年？"僧應道："自從出家不計年。"心德道："可曾有了道行麼？"僧應道："若言大道在眼前。"心德道："拿將出來我看。"僧道："玄機豈得凡人見？"心德道："一目照見病肉團。"僧人聽見，著了一驚，毛骨悚然，不敢起來。心德道："你兩眼紅赤，必有心病，其心中定有不遂之事；兩眉枯燥，心多過慮，傷肝動氣，而心中多有報仇之意；面黃唇縮，脾土失養，想是斷酒肉之故。此非僧家之本分也。但你身從何來？幼年出家，乃遵父母之命，無可奈何。至於中年出家，忍心丟別父母而不供養，則天倫有虧；歸之深山，亦如木石而已，有何功於世？隻要人肯修積，何論出家不出家？觀你之顏，知你修道，猶如飲食也。'人莫不飲食也，鮮能知味也'，此之謂也。"僧人慢慢跪將起來，低頭倒身下拜，叩謝而去，行至中途，嘆道："善哉善哉，今若不遇此人，豈不誤了我生平大事？"心中機謀怨恨，一例丟了，且去看我父母還在否。及去看時，還在人家營工混食，心中大喜，即回來寺中，與師傅商議，要把父母接來寺旁居住，取些田轉來，自己下苦耕種，量了本寺租子，餘剩拿來供養父母。父母餵養牲畜，做出來的錢，餘積安葬父母，不佔寺上一文錢。師傅想想要不依他，又想此我孝道徒弟，況此天倫大事，我們如今想來，也還有虧，若不肯要他父母來住，我徒弟怎麼甘心？想起同是出家人，大齊做些好事方妙，不如許他接來供養罷。僧因此得接父母，寺旁居住，克盡孝道。又常募化十方，修崎嶇之路，造來往之橋，路邊草木砍光，途中瓦石挖平，造河船以渡行人，買物放生，做棺槨，免尸骸之暴露，措衣食，周道路之飢寒。錢量費完，又邀眾會助銀，日修功德，夜無欲念，睡至半夜子時，靜坐片時，覺此心渾然，無一物打擾，行之久久，心地明白，每日虔誠潔淨，焚香三炷，朝西四拜，如此清修，行之數年。忽一日靜坐，瞥見佛光萬點，照眉目之間，陡覺心中，如光明境，身輕神爽，得了正覺。

有一道人，聞得心德行善，就想來騙他，來心德門首化緣。心德將米一升，用茶盤端出來，道人手抓七粒而去，心德即著人去，趕他轉來，那道人入門來，不言不語，跳在方桌上，盤腳打坐，不言不飲食，一連餓了三日。你道他如何餓得三日？原來預將牛肉，做成丸子，放在身旁，時時偷吃幾顆。心德見他坐了三日，飲食不進，也大奇怪，便去問道："仙長來此，弟子有大緣法，望乞指示。"道人道："你要內丹，還是外丹？"心德道："何謂內丹？"道人道："內丹不傳於和尚，搬運水火，醍醐灌頂，三百六十日，身輕飛體而去。"心德道："外丹如何？"道人道："外丹不傳銀匠，燒鉛煉汞，升出丹來，點石成金，點銅化銀。"心德道："所費多少本銀？"道人道"三百兩本錢，可以升一丹。"心德道："到有，但誰去採藥？"道人道："我與你去。"心德暗想："有道之人，心無私欲，則心廣體胖，容顏必然舒展。看此人一片郁氣，待我問他。"便問："仙長，帶有丹來麼？拿點我們用用。"道人說："沒有。"心德道："仙長從前，必定煉來用過，至今想也不多年，還是有的。"道人見他問在著跡處，心中著急，不覺失色。心德知他是假，便說道："為人在世，命中隻有八合米，行盡天下不滿升。你前世不能修積，所以今生受苦。內丹既可三百六十日成道，你何不為？看你一片浮氣，肉身尚不能保，何為修道？外丹既可以點銅成銀，何必用他人資本？你與師傅學道燒丹，定有一點金丹與你，未必你師傅折了本，一點都舍不得與你。況神仙不離忠孝二字，皇王之恩，父母之恩，俱不報答，托身空門，假作仙術，謊人銀錢，自作罪孽，后來作何結果。你尚不回頭麼？"那道人聽了，汗下如流，忙跪伏在地，請心德指點。心德遂將音夫來由，自己事業行持，敘了一遍。那道人心中，恍然悔悟，想起歷年行為之事，自己放聲大哭。心德道："你哭為何？"道人道："我這兩年，聽得實信，說我父母俱亡，弟兄都死，我假作道行，抱憾終身。今日聞善人之言，不得不傷心也。"即行拜謝而去。走到中途，見一小僧，年方二十五六，跪拜於地道："佛門難修，願從道門，乞師傅指教。"道人道："我幼時也想修道，故去出家，誰知錯走門路，被人引入迷途，誤了我大半世，幸得一恩人指點，不論儒、釋、道三教，俱從孝、悌、忠、信、禮、義、廉、恥中做成。天宮豈有不孝悌之真宰？洞府本無不忠義之神仙，我如今生不修，以待來世，焉知我后世，是人身不是人身？必要歸家盡道，方得取你。"小僧想道："我師傅將我歲半養成人，隻少懷胎十月，衣食飽暖，教育多年，此時百不求人，一旦私逃遠別，忍心而不供養，此中有犯天條，自造罪孽，焉知墮何地獄？"一時良心發現，恨不得就見師傅。於是拜謝道長指點之恩，急急歸家，一見師傅，雙膝跪下，兩眼流淚。師傅見了徒弟，一手扯住，淚如雨下，師徒二人，嚎啕大哭。見者問其來由，都發傷悲。六年未會之師徒，一旦相聚，兩來都有依靠。覺得寺中光景，恍然更新。以后小僧出外，必然稟明，預定歸家。久之明心見性，講經說法，竟成了一個大禪師。

且說那道人歸家，哪知他祖父使心用計，專務害人，損了陰騭，一家大小，被瘟疫收盡，並不留三尺之童。無奈隻得尋個靜所，記功記過，不履邪徑，不欺暗室，積德累功，慈心於物，正己化人，矜孤恤寡，敬老懷幼，受恩即感，有怨則忘，不信方術，不訕聖賢。絕不認恩推過，亦不嫁禍責惡；不棄順效逆，不背親向疏；不心毒貌慈，不左道惑眾；不輕慢先靈，不違逆上命；不以灶火燒香，不以穢柴作食。隻是利物利人，修善修福，日行陰騭，夜定心神，常時學作詩文。平旦之時，調神定氣，用明燈七盞，焚香七炷，朝北七十二拜，誠心念誦北斗真經。如此久久，遂覺心地超明，自知後世因緣，立些功德濟人，後來得了真人之位。

昔人有言："修行何必在出家，行止動靜理無差。但求時刻心無愧，九州大地盡開花。"此之謂也。又有一人，自幼勤學，連考數次，不得入庠，心中就起修行的念頭，父母也隨他去。中途遇一道長，拜求指點修行的路，情願與你為徒。道長道："你貴姓何名？"答道："小人姓白，名玉開。"道長道："修行要有恆心，非一日之功。"玉開道："實在不反道。"即發下誓來，就隨道長去了。

道長暗想："此人到有些善心。"不免指示他迷路，說道："我道家亦是五倫為重，才得成正果。雖有內丹，講起搬運水火，醍醐灌頂，五氣朝元，箭穿九重鐵鼓，黃婆引入洞房，會合三家結嬰兒，十月懷胎，真氣還元，見本來面目，諸般玄論紛紛，這都是修成了道的，說的玄妙。雖是這樣說，並非一個凡體做得來。若說外丹，燒鉛煉汞，採取真土，覓冰加炭，八卦神，申文進表，文武火功，七七修煉，離宮出火，巽門進風，震卦加炭，乾方煉出丹來，點銅成銀，點石成金，服能化身，這都是修成道了，天仙等，比喻身上的道理。就是仙家，個個都有妙法，其中也沒有幾個做得來的。仙家尚有做不出來，何況凡民？修道實在的功夫，總要從一心做將出來，到得心花開放，自然妙用無窮。"

白玉開聞言，深深拜領。道長暗想，等我試他一試，看如何，道："徒弟今日收拾起程，我們要去也。"玉開問道："往哪裡去？"道長道："到終南山去。"玉開道："有幾多遠？"道長道："走五六年就到了。"玉開道："幾時回？"道長道："永不回也。"玉開道："這樣說起來，師傅去，我不去。"道長道："你莫非要反道不成？"玉開道："我父母在堂，如何久遠丟得？"道長道："你去便去！"就回去把玉開幾掀掀推倒在地，長條條睡起。等玉開跁將起來，在自己天井中間，父母即忙扶起，扯住兒大哭。父子娘兒，一齊傷心。隻見胸堂上有張帖子，上面有幾行字，說道："心上如石頭，心下就有德，久之自然成道也。"此乃暗暗指石心德三字，叫他尋師也。他如何猜得出。這玉開自從道長指點，分別之後，再不聽旁言外術，異端之說，要從心上做工夫，隻是不知如何下手。想來想去，又到一寺上去。見和尚罵徒弟，開口就是傷他父母，心中大不快樂。把他經典一看，上面說的是孝悌忠信，禮義廉恥。那和尚又叫徒弟燒火做飯，做慢了些，師傅就與他一頓打，將父母亂罵。玉開心中想：

"這和尚口念經典，出言太過，此處不是修行之所。"又回家來，存心修積。不期兩年，父母雙亡。至葬后，子女婚配明白，誰知妻子又死。以后出外訪道，走了數月，並未見有行善之人。

忽一日聽說有一齋公，即去拜他。見他朝夕吃齋念經，與他同住兩三月，他卻行事詭曲，用心過分。外面名頭似善，心內比那不吃齋、不念佛的，還狠些。他弟兄二人，同一塆坐，哥坐上屋，他坐下屋。他把下屋中堂上壁，裝做神龕，不留門戶，閉塞上屋人出入之路。他哥本分，就左邊橫屋地基，等他侄兒修造橫屋五間，急切要豎房子，他佔地基，不肯折倉，定要做兩截分過。玉開苦苦勸他，他再三不依，丟了木魚，出外合掌拜天，咒他侄兒，口口聲聲叫他死亡絕戶，陷得侄兒，隻得在外看基立房子。玉開看此處亦不是修行之所。

忽聽人說，有一位石心德行善，慢慢訪來。訪到石心德家中，心德迎將進來，鞠躬深揖，待以上賓，正言相敘道："尊客容顏甚粹，然舉止動靜非等閒，其心必有修行路，想是雲游訪地仙。"玉開見心德出口成詩，心中大喜，答道："弟子白玉開，不遠千裡而來，拜求指點修行之路。"心德見玉開至誠，便留在家中，與他說些行善之法。玉開見心德翁婿，所言所行，無一點欺妄之事，心中依戀，滿心歡喜。三人同志修行。久之，玉開把心德、音夫二人行持的工夫盡得了，也不忍遠去，就買些藥材，開個藥鋪行醫。有錢來的，也發藥；無錢來的，也發藥。德行既高，藥也越發靈了。不論大小病症，藥到即除。心德翁婿二人，常去觀看，見玉開時時改過自新，得善則拳拳服膺，始焉或有違於頃刻之際，繼焉則見無違仁於終身之間，心中日見光明，外則體態雍容，安舒自得。心德見他做到了這樣光景，二人滿心大喜。

一日三人閒坐，外面人來報道："不知何處來的一位遠客，要來請見白先生。"此人學問甚大，上知天文，下識地理，中辨人才，三教九流，無所不通，也修積多年。聞白玉開名字，特來討論賢否，考自己得失如何。玉開聽說有遠客，急去迎他進來，四人相見答禮，分賓主坐下。茶畢，玉開道："尊客貴姓何名，有勞貴步。"此人答道："小弟姓李，名元亮，行游天下九州，聞府上真修，特來領教。"玉開聽說，知他走錯了門頭，遂設宴款待，四面坐下。酒敬三巡，元亮開言問道："學道之人，總要有緣法，彼太公之遇元始，孫臏之遇鬼谷，湘子之遇洞賓，子房之遇黃石公，得仙家之傳度，真大幸也。"玉開道："先生何為出此言也！前輩先生，不知幾世修積，方遇真師，指點大道。姜太公、張子房，一代興王之佐，該有此番遇合。孫臏雖遇鬼谷，不能潛心大道，隻想求名，所以不得成為正果。今人片善才積，一功俱無，妄想仙家傳度。獨不思仙是何心，我是何心。倘我之心，果如仙家之心，自必仙家喜我，或來傳度。

然我心果如仙家之心，是我已是仙家面目，何必望他傳度。尊客自諒其心與仙心何如？"元亮聽了此番言語，自想已心有愧，不敢妄言，便起身問道："先生是如何行持？"玉開道："孝悌忠信，禮義廉恥，此三教聖人根本。大乘三藏經旨，無非教人如此，依此修悟，明心見性，說法化人，指引迷途，有功於世，自然成真矣。"元亮道："如何又有說的：學道之人，要結三緣？"玉開道："無晴無雨，不怨乎天；久晴久雨，不怨乎天；衣食不足，不怨乎天；謀事不成，不怨乎天。此為結天緣。山高水遠，不怨乎地；溝渠江隔，不怨乎地；不毛少產，不怨乎地；物不遂心，不怨乎地。此為結地緣。他富我貧，不怨乎人；他貴我賤，不怨乎人；他強我弱，不怨乎人；他伸我屈，不怨乎人。此為結人緣。"

元亮道："如何叫做功德？"心德道："功德不分大小，隨人貧富而作。家富提攜親戚，歲飢周濟鄰朋，裝修寺院，培補橋路，刊刻善文，俱是功德。"元亮道："何為又有不得成道者？"心德道："作此一善，自己恃他有功，即便喪謗那作善的，就說他是何等功德樣子。或遇有一利害事，心中又改變。過多功少，不能長久為善，所以難得成道。"

元亮道："常見世間男女，常常看經念佛，何以不成道？"音夫道："看經念佛之人，貪心甚重。他本念原不想成道。"元亮道："拜佛之人，焉有貪心？"音夫道："你去查訪拜佛人，二三十歲拜佛，不是為妻子不遂意，便是為丈夫不遂心。四十前后拜佛，不是為子女不遂意，便是為家道不遂心。五六十歲拜佛，不是怕墮地獄，就是求后世富貴。其中豈無貪心？故曰他本念原不想成道。"元亮道："人生年幼無知，造下罪障，拜佛可以解得否？"音夫道："佛神無私，不因致敬而錫福，不以不敬而降殃。你若有過，任你燒錢化紙，看經念佛，不能解也。你想正直佛神，豈肯受賄？譬如你有不是，求教本方正直之人，買賄他歪枉為你，他直言說你的不是，且不肯受賄，況在於佛神。倘佛神受賄，反不如地方正直之人矣。"元亮道："孽障又如何解得？"音夫道："求人無益，當自解之。心孽以心解，事孽以事解。若知悔悟，時存好心，常行好事，慢慢自然解悟。"元亮聽說，駭然大驚道："真是有道之士！善惡辨得明白，出言合乎天理。"自知心高氣傲，都錯了，越是低聲下氣，問道："萬惡淫為首，我常戒淫。不知見人婦女，心中不敢思想，卻是美色不能便忘，奈何？"音夫道："見人婦女，尊年的，即如我母親相待；與我上下年紀的，即如我的姊妹而論；年紀小我的，即如我大女小女看待。自然一見即忘。"元亮道："惡由貪起，我常戒貪。見人暢遂順境，心中不敢圖謀。但是，一時難丟下，奈何？"音夫道："要知凡事有天命。天命我富貴，我要體天生成之意，多行方便濟人。如其貧賤，當思我德薄，所以福薄。那處好境的，不是自己今生心好，便是他前世有些修持。不然，便是他前人積德所致。然前人有德，也要他有好處，方才承受得起。不然，便中道折福了。上天豈有一毫差錯。所以作善的人，凡事都要反躬自責。"元亮聽了，十分佩服。又問："若作善又無好處，是何故？"心德道："凡事循天理而行，自是為人本分當如此。若預想福報，便是有為而為。倘久而無報，必生反悔了，哪得善心純熟。你看自古聖賢，造次顛沛不違仁，或為將相，如伊周，或為師儒，如孔孟，俱為萬世瞻仰。他何嘗想福報？隻是盡其在己而已。"

元亮道："請教眾先生如何行持？"玉開道："我三人每人做三個口袋。一袋裝黃豆，一袋裝黑豆，一袋作公。若有時起了好心，作了好事，即取黃豆一顆，入於公袋記功；若有時起了惡心，行了惡事，即取黑豆一顆，放在公袋記過。至三個月，取出公袋內豆來數，看功多過多。日夜時刻檢點，始而過多，繼而功多，久而久之，隻見功不見過。歷終身如一日，一息尚存，此志不肯少懈。"元亮聽得心中頓悟，說道："聽了先生高論，才曉得我從前事業，走了多少錯路。從今願拜為弟子。"遂依依不捨，一連住了數日，即做了布袋，照三人行持。欲歸家盡道，作詩一首，相辭而別。詩曰："幾番風過幾番波，船穩何愁浪影多。從今放過前灘去，穩坐舟中聽棹歌。"元亮拜謝三人歸家。

行至中途，遇十余年未會之窗友，名叫張秀芝，被二位官差扭鎖押解。元亮道："請問二位官差，解此人何處去？"差答道："往鄷都去。"元亮道："此人為何事？"差答道："現有牌上書一十三條，你可看來。"元亮將牌看畢，即悲辭而去。至自己家中，問其父母兄弟往那裡去了，其子道："公婆伯叔往張秀芝家吃四十歲生期酒去了。"元亮暗想："前十日已在路途撞遇，解往鄷都去了，今何又在家做生？我要往他家看看才是。"

不一時走到張秀芝家，果見大宴嘉賓，談笑不已。元亮見秀芝，端然在家，自己若像痴了。暗想見鬼之人必死，莫非我命當盡，即把路遇之事，對眾人敘明。眾人聽罷，啞口無言。元亮道："我在途中，秀芝友被二位官差解往鄷都，我欲阻止之，差即取牌我看，牌上寫道：'一條：反眼看父，惡語回母；二條：刻薄手足，親熱外人；三條：暗破閨門，私通寡婦；四條：圖謀人產，欺孤奪業；五條：妒人技能，刁破成事；六條：改路攔阻，埋茨傷足；七條：討牛不遂，用藥毒牛；八條：求果不遂，用藥殺樹；九條：砍柴被阻，放火燒山；十條：捕風捉影，假談利色；十一條：捏謗丑名，使人難洗；十二條：覆巢破卵，挖穴殺傷；十三條：順妻逆母，拋撒五谷。'"秀芝道："我害人物，人物不見報我。我又不害天地，與天地何干？他來報我。"元亮道："你不知天地生人物，即如父母生兒女。天地之恩，春發夏長，秋收冬藏，即如父母懷胎，生養，教育，婚配。天有雨露風晴，是天地之功勞，即如父母之於子女，誠求哭笑，乃父母之勞。你傷他人之兒女，他父母必然心痛。你害天地之物，天地豈不情慘？所以使鬼神報你。"秀芝聽說，即行走開，行至天井中，腳手踏地，做黃牛吼一十三聲，七孔流血而死。眾人一見大驚，各自悔悟，誤犯十三條者，便自痛改，常犯十三條者，速求懺悔。一人傳十，十人傳百，於是惡風變作善風，薄道化為厚道。元亮歸家，力行善事，感化一家，並親戚朋友鄉黨都是逢人勸化。父勸以慈，子勸以孝，兄弟勸以友恭，夫妻勸他義順，婆媳勸他親愛，妯娌勸他和睦。苦口婆心，總不辭勞。那些人見他至誠，都漸漸感化，作起善來。行之數年，一鄉之中，多是忠厚慈良之人。那元亮年逾八十，無疾而逝，此是后事不題。

且說玉開，將客送了，又來發藥，驚動多少遠州遠縣的人，都來取藥。其他無不是利人濟物的事。行之久久，心地開明，常覺天空地闊，神聖暗暗通靈，自知塵緣已盡，將赴仙曹。想當年原是石心德指引，特來他家一看，以作辭別之意。那心德功行已高，但他上年，大小秤斗，瞞心昧已之時，必要到地獄一遭。玉開心中明白，私想后來再救於他。來至心德家中，心德設席款待。玉開宴罷辭歸，不日端坐幾上，無疾而去。心德聞他死了，前去用棺木斂他色身，厚厚埋葬。

回家不久，話說那心德，早年行惡之時，去窮苦家討賬，那家無銀，就把他家男子漢，押到他家做活。誰知婦人在家無吃，忍餓不過，自己懸梁自縊而死。冤魂不散，變為男子，來心德家下做安童。有一醫生，來到心德家中，得急病死了。那安童說："我家主人，圖財害命。"眾人多有信的。過了幾日，便有人要去報官。又有一人說道："心德乃改惡從善之人，況他與白太醫甚厚，待白太醫不論錢米多少，白太醫何曾積得有錢。這事不可妄為。"安童道："我看著他拿藥酒毒死了，還不斷氣，又按倒在地，才打死的。"眾人聽說如此，恐怕日后連累他地方不得不報。

一報到官，發差去拿來一問，心德慌忙，答錯了話，說是他回去了的，不會在我這裡死的。安童死死抵住，那官即叫抬夾棍過來，連摧三繩，又打四十。心德當時夾死，又將冷水來噴，也不得活。抬出外來，一日一夜，心口回熱，用被蓋著不動，候他醒來復審。

那心德一魂到了陰司，冥官叫判官拿惡簿來與他看："因你作惡，暗計害人，曲死人命，該變作三世牛身。"心德一見，嚎啕大哭。冥官又叫拿善簿過來，把功過行持一一看了，便說道："你改惡從善多年，隻因此一番關系，人命的事難以勾消，罰你受些刑法，放你回陽。當益勵修持，再不來此地了。"

心德蘇醒之時，官又叫去復審。心德道："大老爺在上，看是何人，說在哪裡，何不拿來檢驗？何必屈挾小人。"太爺即吩咐下鄉檢驗，安童就指住是這個墳。等一挖開，乃是千年古墳，骨尸已爛完了。便喚白太醫家人問時，家人供說，原是自己得急病死的，與石心德無干，才把心德釋放。
那官員說道："這一場禍事，不與鄉保鄰裡相干，全是安童搬說起來。惡奴欺主，告人死罪，當得死罪。你回去，本縣自必依律治罪，決不寬恕。"心德心中暗想："此人乃是前世誤死之身，今日若不救他，冤仇難解。"又訴道："太爺在上，要開天地之恩，容小人訴來。這也難怪安童，他本是我的家人，是小人在路途遇著，見他衣食不足，引他回家做活，是我苦克他太狠。年幼孺子，一時狂言，誤害小人。望乞太爺開恩超釋。"那官聽說，心中大驚，想道："我常聞人人說心德大德之人，今日看將起來，果然不錯。到是我不能容察，屈審了他。"即將鄉保裡鄰放回。以律而論，奴害主，當問凌遲。若要執法，又辜負心德好念，隻得問個軍罪，赦他一死。
那鄉保裡鄰回來，個個大驚。安童是他買的奴，本是害他的人，他反救他。我們聽了一偏之詞，累他受刑，此心何安？議定各備禮物，登門叩謝。心德道："不關你們事。是我誤了你們受累，你反謝我，這就萬萬不敢。"一例不受，又設大宴款待，以禮貌送回。眾人心下，愈難解釋。又議道："有恩不報非君子。"不免約起會首，化些錢糧與他做供生齋。選擇諸山名僧高道，九日九夜，申文奏表。
石音夫因岳父功德日盛，數年前勸他娶了一房妾，生了一子。名曰石成金。此時已有六歲了。音夫也早生了二子，名喚石如玉，石如璋，年已十歲九歲。兩家人，內外俱存好心。夫婦妻妾，都相親相愛，毫無閑言。延請有德有品的人，教訓兒子。平日敬重師長，禮貌恭敬。兩家兒郎，不數年都入了邑庠。心德、音夫，越發勇於為善，地鄰親戚人等，凡與他翁婿來往的，俱感化向善，不殺生，不妄為，不說謊。也都教訓家人等，做些寬仁厚德的事。又數年，心德兒子中式本省鄉試。音夫長子，亦同榜中式。眾人見他兩個平生向善，也未嘗貧窮，家中依舊飽暖。兒子又成名，俱深信為善之美。鄰家有一人，姓鐘名一千，存心正直，作事惟憑天理，但不知修行之路。見音夫化轉心德，如此安榮，也學他二人行事。其長子亦入了邑庠，次子亦登科甲。后來音夫，年登九十，心德年亦八十有五，俱預知死期，先期沐浴，臨時冠帶，吩咐兒子輩，各遵行功過格，勿替他家法，端坐含笑而逝。鄰人等俱聽著空中音樂嘹亮，中堂中香氣撲鼻，逾一二時方散。后來二家子孫，遵行前人功德，多成進士，歷顯宦，為良吏，至今子孫，尚繁衍不絕。
看官聽說這兩個人，一個是乞丐出身，沒有分文，隻因他實心向善，后來富貴皆有。心德本是富人，隻因大斗小秤，存心不善，幾乎被雷震死。因聽信女婿善言，回心向善，長久不渝，亦轉禍為福，又得壽終。所以凡人不論貧富，隻要實心行善，天心看成。若說行善，便要窮餓，是天不顧善人，反任隨惡人富貴了，又何以為天。

世間有些不信善，不信神，任意妄為的人也在富貴。他都是前生修積得有些善事，或是他祖宗父母有些善事，方才得此富貴。然他任意妄為，不肯回頭，到得日久，把他前人積累及自己前生所積折磨完了，未有不遭慘禍的。上天原無一毫差錯。你看周家忠厚開基，出了多少聖人，享八百余年國祚，到赧王時失天下。秦國何等暴虐，也不曾將周家子孫殺戮，就如人活了八九十歲，無疾而終一般。

其余作惡之徒，如曹操、司馬懿等，他前世也有根基，奈他行事不端，僥幸而子孫篡得天下，一二世便受了強臣挾制，子孫俱被人殺戮。何況尋常百姓，有多大身家。

就是求名求利，也是人之常情。然必照著天理行事，所得名利，才對得過天地神明，子孫才得久享。若瞞心昧己，隻圖眼前，不顧天良，為兒孫作牛馬，反折了兒孫之福。不如那作善之人，心地干淨，就是粗衣淡飯，睡也安然，行也安然，生前為人敬仰，死后受天寵榮，子孫受享他的積累不盡。兩兩相形，孰得孰失？

就是出家僧道之流，多因幼年貧苦，方入空門養活。但父母若在，他割愛送兒子一條生路，心是何等苦楚。出家人，若長成之時，父母尚在，必要設法供養，盡其孝道。若父母不在了，也要燒錢化紙，盡其孝思。要知三教聖人，都沒有不忠不孝的。至於中年出家，亦如此行，方才可以燒香念經。

諸般惡事，惟有邪淫二字，須先除去了此事，方才講得作善。自來勸善的書，勸人戒淫的不少，不用我細說。

至於孝字，不但是親生父母，凡八母俱要孝敬。繼母庶母，更要孝敬。敬母所以敬父也。家庭以父母為主，凡父母所愛敬，都要愛敬。國家以君為主，凡君所喜的人，都要尊敬，是一般道理。今人曉得尊敬官府，不曉得尊敬父母，及伯叔兄弟，便是昏愚了。敬君要安分守法，能如石音夫、石心德所為，便是朝廷良民。且善德傳家，教訓兒孫成聖賢，為國家棟梁之材，豈非大忠。至於作官，念念不欺君，不虐民，尤為忠之至也。

功過格傳終

APPENDIX B

說百病崇百药

Shuō Bǎi Bìng Chóng Bǎi Yào

Explaining the 100 Diseases and Revering the 100 Medicines

Original Chinese from Master Gān Liǎo (甘了).

老子说百病崇百药

说百病

救灾解难，不如防之为易；疗疾治病，不如备之为吉。今人见背，不务防之而务救之，不务备之而务药之。故有君者不能保社稷，有身者不能全寿命。是以圣人求福于未兆，绝祸于未有。盖灾生于稍稍，病起于微微。人以小善为无益，故不肯为；以小恶为无损，故不肯改。小善不积，大德不成；小恶不止，以成大罪。

故摘出其要，使知其所生焉，乃百病者也。

喜怒无常是一病。忘义取利是一病。

好色坏德是一病。专心系爱是一病。

憎欲令死是一病。纵贪蔽过是一病。

毁人自誉是一病。擅变自可是一病。

轻口喜言是一病。快意逐非是一病。

以智轻人是一病。乘权纵横是一病。

非人自是是一病。侮易孤弱是一病。

以力胜人是一病。贷不念偿是一病。

威势自胁是一病。语欲胜人是一病。

曲人自直是一病。以直伤人是一病。

恶人自喜是一病。喜怒自伐是一病。

愚人自贤是一病。以功自与是一病。

名人有非是一病。以劳自怨是一病。

以虚为实是一病。喜说人过是一病。

以富骄人是一病。以贵轻人是一病。

以贫妒富是一病。以贱讪贵是一病。

逸人求媚是一病。以德自显是一病。

败人成功是一病。以私乱公是一病。

好自掩意是一病。危人自安是一病。

阴阳嫉妒是一病。激厉旁悖是一病。

多憎少爱是一病。评论是非是一病。

推负着人是一病。文拒钩锡是一病。

持人长短是一病。假人自信是一病。

施人望报是一病。无施责人是一病。

与人追悔是一病。好自怨诤是一病。

骂詈虫畜是一病。蛊道厌人是一病。

毁訾高才是一病。憎人胜己是一病。

毒药鸩饮是一病。心不平等是一病。

以贤愤高是一病。追念旧恶是一病。

不受谏谕是一病。内疏外亲是一病。

投书败人是一病。谈愚痴人是一病。

烦苛轻躁是一病。摘捶无理是一病。

好自作正是一病。多疑少信是一病。

笑颠狂人是一病。蹲踞无礼是一病。

丑言恶语是一病。轻易老少是一病。

恶态丑对是一病。了戾自用是一病。

好喜嗜笑是一病。喜禁固人是一病。

诡谲谀诌是一病。嗜得怀诈是一病。

两舌无信是一病。乘酒歌横是一病。

骂詈风雨是一病。恶言好杀是一病。

教人堕胎是一病。干预人事是一病。

孔穴窥视是一病。借不念还是一病。

负债逃窃是一病。背向异辞是一病。

喜抵捍戾是一病。调戏必固是一病。

故迷误人是一病。探巢破卵是一病。

刳胎剖形是一病。水火败伤是一病。

笑盲聋喑是一病。教人嫁娶是一病。

教人摘捶是一病。教人作恶是一病。

含祸离爱是一病。唱祸道非是一病。

见便欲得是一病。强夺人物是一病。

能念除此百病，则无灾累，痛疾自愈，济度苦厄，子孙蒙佑矣。

崇百药

古之圣人，其于善也，无小而不得；其于恶也，无微而不改。而能行之，可谓饵药焉。所谓百药者：

体弱性柔是一药。行宽心和是一药。

动静有礼是一药。起居有度是一药。

近德远色是一药。除去欲心是一药。

推分引义是一药。不取非分是一药。

虽憎犹爱是一药。好相申用是一药。

为人愿福是一药。救祸济难是一药。

教化愚敝是一药。谏正邪乱是一药。

戒敕童蒙是一药。开导迷误是一药。

扶接老弱是一药。以力助人是一药。

与穷恤寡是一药。矜贫救厄是一药。

位高下士是一药。语言谦逊是一药。

恭敬卑微是一药。不负宿债是一药。

愍慰笃信是一药。质言端悫是一药。

推直引曲是一药。不争是非是一药。

逢侵不鄙是一药。受辱不怨是一药。

推善隐恶是一药。推好取丑是一药。

推多取少是一药。称叹贤良是一药。

见贤自省是一药。不自彰显是一药。

推功引苦是一药。不自伐善是一药。

不掩人功是一药。劳苦不恨是一药。

怀实信厚是一药。覆蔽阴恶是一药。

富有假乞是一药。崇进胜己是一药。

安贫不怨是一药。不自尊大是一药。

好成人功是一药。不好阴私是一药。

得失自欢是一药。阴德树恩是一药。

生不骂詈是一药。不评论人是一药。

好言善语是一药。灾病自咎是一药。

苦不假推是一药。施不望报是一药。

不骂畜生是一药。为人祝愿是一药。

心平意和是一药。心静意定是一药。

不念旧恶是一药。匡邪弼恶是一药。

听谏受化是一药。不干预人是一药。

忿怒自制是一药。解散思虑是一药。

尊奉老者是一药。闭门恭肃是一药。

内修孝悌是一药。蔽恶扬善是一药。

清廉守分是一药。好饮食人是一药。

助人执忠是一药。救日月蚀是一药。

远嫌避疑是一药。恬淡宽舒是一药。

尊奉圣制是一药。思神念道是一药。

宣扬圣化是一药。立功不倦是一药。

尊天敬地是一药。拜谒三光是一药。

恬淡无欲是一药。仁顺谦让是一药。

好生恶杀是一药。不多聚财是一药。

不犯禁忌是一药。廉洁忠信是一药。

不多贪财是一药。不烧山木是一药。

空车助载是一药。直谏忠信是一药。

喜人有德是一药。赴与穷乏是一药。

代老负担是一药。除情去爱是一药。

慈心悯念是一药。好称人善是一药。

　　因富而施是一药。因贵为惠是一药。

此为百药也。人有疾病。皆有过恶。阴掩不见，故应以疾病。因缘饮食、风寒、温气而起。由其人犯违于神，致魂逝魄丧，不在形中，体肌空虚，精气不守，故风寒恶气得中之。

是以圣人虽处幽暗，不敢为非；虽居荣禄，不敢为利。度形而衣，量分而食。虽富且贵，不敢恣欲；虽贫且贱，不敢犯非。是以外无残暴，内无疾痛，可不慎之焉！

APPENDIX C

劉沅: 槐軒全書

Liú Yuán: Huái Xuān Quán Shū

Liú Yuán: Huái Xuān Compendium

Original Chinese quotations cited in
The Lost Heart of Medicine.

槐軒全書　咸滎敬書

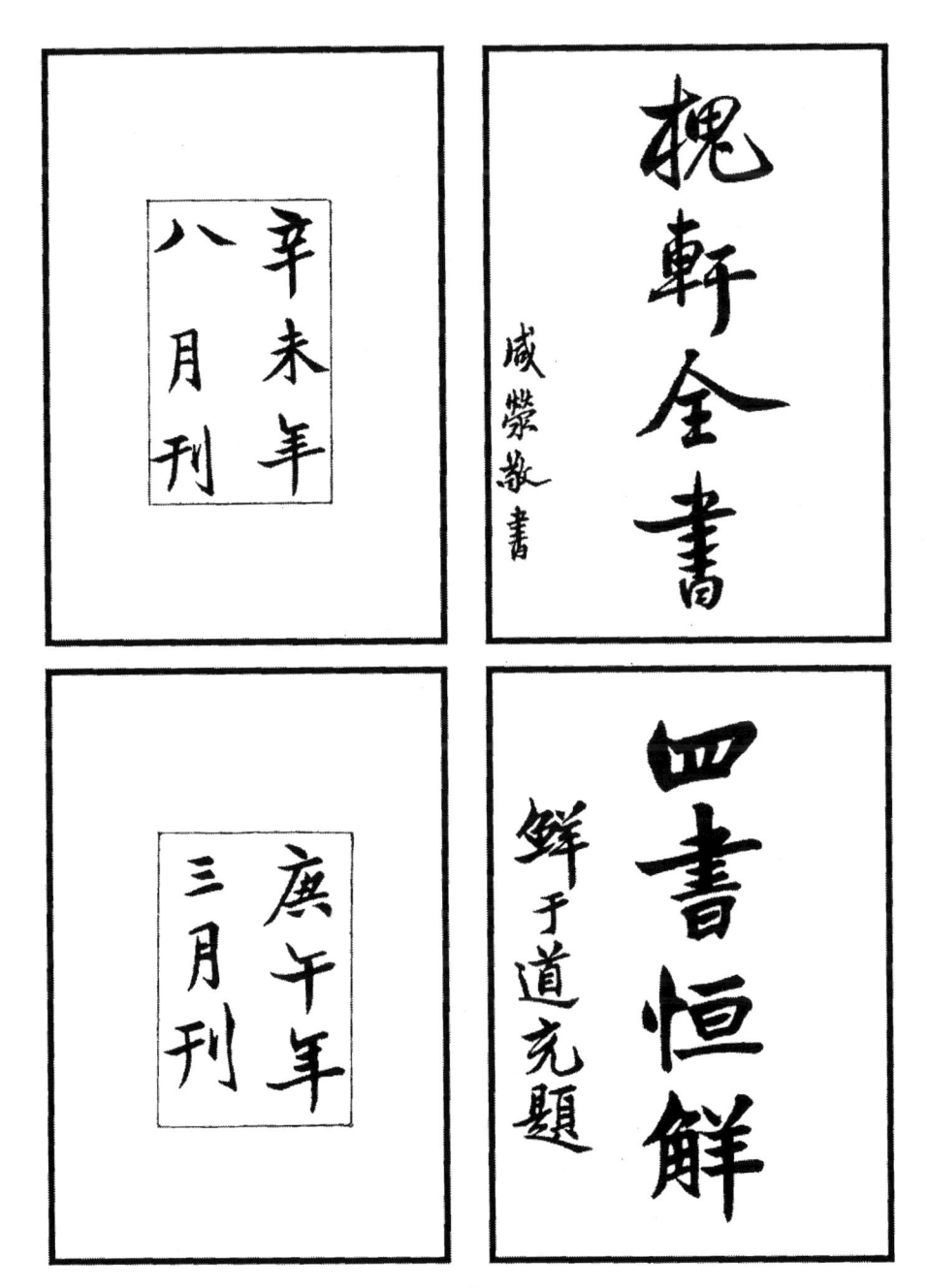

辛未年八月刊

四書恆解　鮮于道元題

庚午年三月刊

儒林劉止唐先生八十八歲肖像

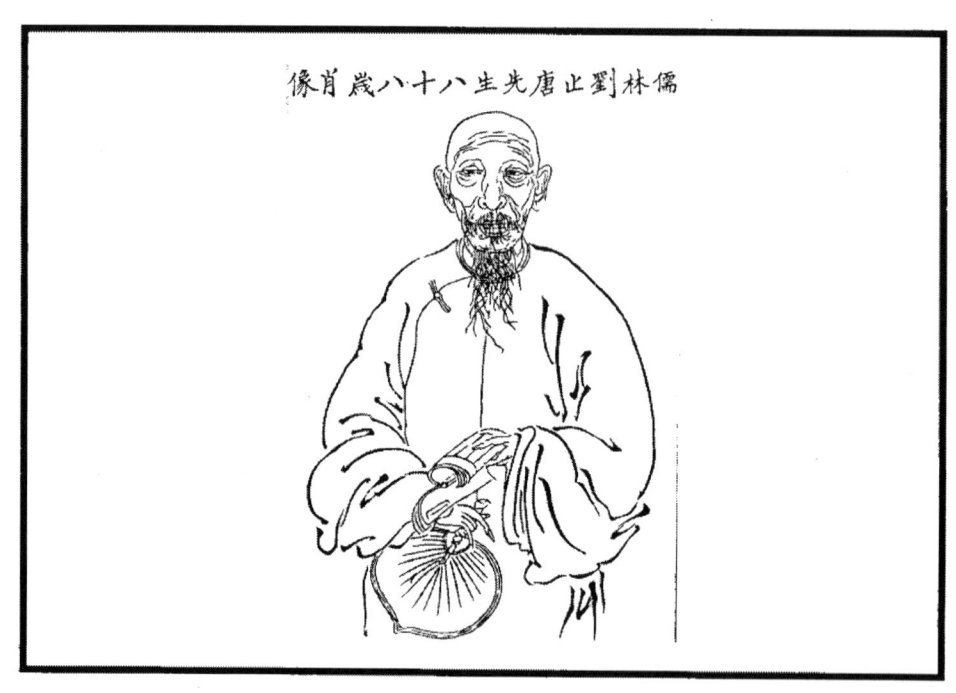

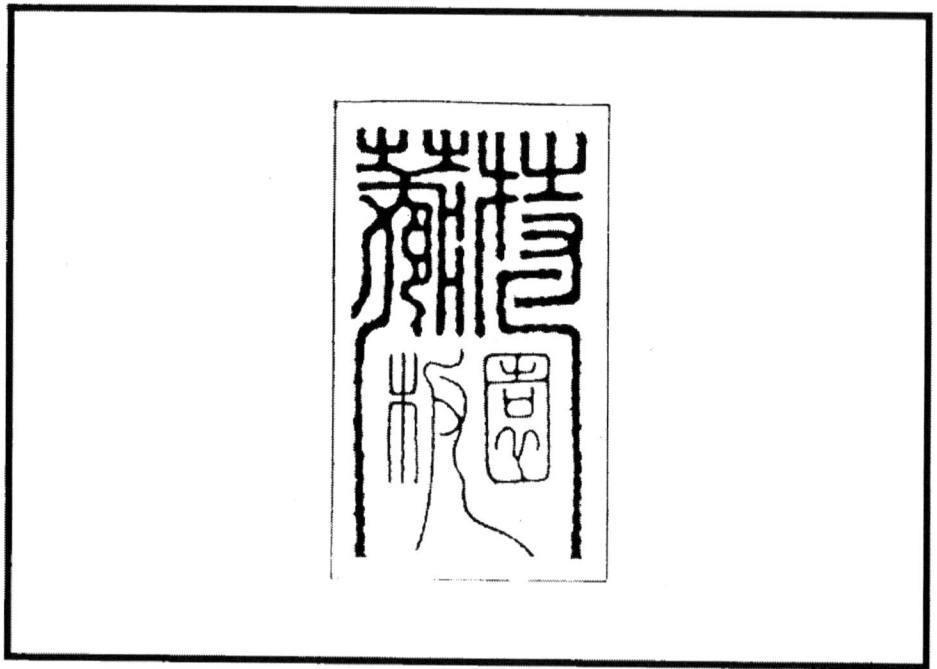

-2-

文不幾武斷耶

一朱子竄改誠意章原文增出明德新民章止至善聽
訟章又補格物章明德章四明字新民章數新字
止至善章數止字但觀其文亦甚覺天然之位置
然明德之功由止至善而入夫子故特以所謂
義第明德不易明須從誠意入手曾子故特以所謂
誠意章為首誠意必由致知故引淇澳之詩詳釋
其義誠意則是誠其所知所知之事無非所以明
德故能誠意則德可以明克明顧諟峻德引三書
而結之皆自明明夫子言明德二字原本古聖但

四書恆解　大學凡例　三峨西充鮮于氏特圓藏

須自密其功耳然何以言明明盖德峻必明而又
明始可造其極故引盤銘康誥無所不用其極言
無事不本明德而修齊治平悉該矣上文民不能
忘沒世不忘之故益明極即明德非謂明德新民
皆止至善邦畿以下又申明止至善之義蓋誠意
動察也止至善靜存也惟靜而有主乃動而能察
止至善如文王則動靜一原內外一致是所以引
為止至善者勸也緝熙敬止明德之本仁敬孝慈
明德之著靜而止動而宜所以聖人無思無為而
有以應天下之變也宋儒以心為性出於禪家心

未嘗可不存而存其心所以養其性但以後天之
心為性則難守心之久至於妙明洞徹而修齊治
平亦不能踐其功朱子因而補格致一章以為如
此而後可修齊治平也然聖人明德即是盡其
性即是身修矣性盡則人物之性而參贊化育
修己安人安百姓修身天下即平非明德矣而又
待講求新民之事耕稼陶漁之舜即恭己垂裳之
舜無兩副本領故心性之實不明即明德之全
功不知程朱之品學何可訾也而明德之學止是
僧流守心之功故解止至善為凡事知止於至善

四書恆解　大學凡例　四峨西充鮮于氏特圓藏

凡人於一事之來知其至善所在何以便能定靜
安耶定靜安亦止是知止後尚有美
大神聖境界夫子不過言明德之功以知止為要
耳下文故言物有本末事有終始知所先後然後
入道有方古之明明德於天下又從明德究竟功
夫從後說來歸本修身此等義理身體力行俱有
實際豈可臆斷哉
一朱子分十傳詁聖經然曾子實止有五傳因恐人
不知大學入手切要之功故特標誠意為首而反
復言之意即心也何以意誠而心猶不正故又言

講矣然古制猶可言焉古者大學之道其要在明明德蓋人受天地之中以生五常之性粹然者一太極之體我固有之故稱為德本虛明者也第有生之初所禀氣質有厚薄清濁之殊有生以後習俗變化有善惡是非之異而德因以不明以不明聖人示人以學惟欲人內外兼修明而又明以化其氣質之偏去其物欲之蔽全虛明本體而已然非宗守此心便以為明理散見於天下人之性猶己之性也而天下人之境遇情狀不同學者高談性命博究典墳而或不能施之實用則以民情未

四書恆解 大學 三 西充鮮于氏特園藏

克周知經濟無由盡善而學遂為偏寂之學矣大學之道己德既明推以及物與民相親相近久之乃有以盡乎人情之變而得其同然之理一旦得所藉手本成己者以成人而無不包而更親民以盡民也夫明德之量固無所不包而更親民以盡理人情表裏洞徹然德非易明功必有所由始人為萬物之靈得理氣之粹未生以前理氣之渾然者一如太極也迨形體具而理為固氣亦駁雜明明德者必當於先天受中之地收已放之心入虛靈之舍止而不遷其止維何人秉

天地之中氣以生百骸皆為後起有至善之地焉乃天命之性所含非一切血氣之倫可比名曰至善有生以後知識開而七情擾明明德者先求放心常止於其所知止於至善則心存而性乃可養故大學之道又在止於至善也苟不知止於至善則以明牽引外來之欲而憧憧往來心日以蔽德何以明入大學者果能知止則人心退聽道心虛含而后志有定向持守之久心常定而后天性日生天君常泰而后靜不擾靜久而后內無情欲之紛外無形骸之役安舒自得天下之事身世之緣雖無窮

四書恆解 大學 四 西充鮮于氏特園藏

也然果至於安則凝然有主湛然虛明凡事理之來必能審擇揆其是非而能慮矣慮則酬應萬事不至乖違而後然則止至善之功大學之道不當以知之為先哉夫天下事物無窮何以知止卽能慮能得蓋凡物必有本末凡事必有終始皆必自此心而窮究心止其所而至於安則靜自生明知本始而先務則易近道矣古之欲明明德於天下者不自天下求之也知天下之本在國先治其國欲治其國者知國之本在家先齊其家欲齊其家者知家之本在身先脩其身欲脩其身者

少年先從事小子之學曲禮內則所記及學記離
經辨志博習親師之事以束身於規矩十五而使
學大人之學始教之以全人之道其教徧於天下
而倡於天子故二說仍是一理毛西河謂小學乃
學宮分大小經無是說甚辨然朱子以幼學
為小學成人之學為大學雖古無是言於理亦自
無礙從之可也○德即天命之性明明德即盡性
之事後人因大學言心不言性中庸言性不言心
遂生出許多枝節不知德即天理惟人得之在未

四書恆解　　大學　　七　　　峨西充鮮于特圓藏氏

生以前渾然粹然本至虛明劉子曰民受天地之
中以生其語至粹中者何天之太極而人得之以
為德者也未生以前為先天德本純全故孟
子曰人性皆善有生以後有此形質即有嗜好日
與物接即有牽引之緣而所得於天之德日以梏
亡矣聖人教人許多禮法惟欲人全其所得之理
所謂復性之功也因不明而明之故曰明明德謂
明而又明內外交修動靜交養有許多功夫次第
周制以六德六行六藝教人由鄉學而升於太學
其德已是規模大就以保氏為師化其偏而歸於

中和夫子第約言之曰在明明德以功夫及門所
知且詳悉非師不授故但總括言之耳舊註因其
所發而遂明之特擴充之一義不足盡其本末之
功以有覺之心為天命之性故解為明德止曰虛
靈不昧不知性也虛靈不昧而心有覺者乃德
也即性也不可以為德也○親
民改親字為新盡因空談性命不能實踐倫常
故云然其意亦美然後世高言清靜空談性命及
一切刑名法術之為皆由不知明德之實又不能
次第深造故為偏枯之學若知道德即天理明明

四書恆解　　大學　　八　　　峨西充鮮于特圓藏氏

德是盡人合天則果能明明德措諸萬事一以貫
之尚何不克新民之有子曰為政以德譬如北辰
又曰修己以安百姓中庸曰盡其性則能盡人物
之性而參贊聖人無兩副本領天以一理運化萬
物聖人以一理貫串古今後人以心為性見僧流
守心即或靈通亦不能修齊治平故謂既明明德
倘有新民之學不知明德函天下之理聖人治天
下如運掌非能盡天下事物接乎其前皆灼知其得失
其心至明凡天下事物接乎其前皆灼知其得失
所謂坐照如神也且其心至虛凡天下一材一藝

四書恆解 《大學》 九 喇西充鮮子氏特圓藏

明明德者自明其德必於日用周旋與人晉接有一人之情狀親近焉而體察其是非擇其善者而從其不善者而改久久存諸中者益純得於聞見者日博以三隅反本物理人情而推之由近及遠由粗入細人情物理洞察其由然後可以精義入神其不曰取友而曰親民者為大學之地貴冑及俊秀皆與民相遠者也慮其封己自是或徒矜博識無當於人生日用之恆故云民字該貴賤一切人不是單指黎民從古聖王立教元子冑子與齊民同學於大學正為其生長深宮不

隨其所長舍己從人執兩用中所以垂拱無為也故明明德則全體大用已該無俟另求經濟試以聖人經籍及常人參考並證以日用言行求其至當則必知之不得徒苟同於先儒也然則言行雖者何大學之教所以儲大人之材無論元子適子習於貴冑未涉民間之甘苦必難圖治即凡為學者講明義理易實踐經濟雖聖賢之義理雖在書籍而必措諸實事驗諸物理人情恰合乎中天下之大民生風俗嗜好得失夢如安能盡為涉愿祇是心理皆同宮室衣服飲食人倫日用亦無不同

四書恆解 《大學》 十 喇西充鮮子氏特圓藏

中庸言中和非中無以為和亦不可謂中人秉天地之正其在先天天理氣所函粹然至善者與天地同受中者在此後天義未發之中者亦在此夫子故特為之名目示人從此入手三句蟬聯而下非平列三項也後人因三在字文法似平謂明明德之德即是天理天理純熟必由集義生氣有至德以凝至道故知行並進內外交修一時並到不過由淺而深功夫須漸次行來若德已明而不能新民是其德非全體之德即非大學之明明德蓋

知民間疾苦其在高宗舊勞于外爰暨小人亦越文王康功田功不遑暇食可見一斑惟周知物理愚夫愚婦有一能勝予之懼故其明德之功聖自聖而明明德於天下益宏且遠後世有志之君守道之儒少親民一段功夫故主術不洽於輿情而儒術貽譏於迂疎不知天理爛熟必從民情閱歷而來臨時處中皆由萬理周知之故此明德又在親民也〇德即至善也而心又曰止至善者何天人止此一理具於心而心有人心道心欲去人心而純道心必有動靜交養之功靜者動之本也

修己即可以安百姓安明德新民是一貫事德造其極則堯舜文武是矣其新民亦至善德有毫髮未明則新民亦不臻醇備大學之教非等後世詞章法術之學誦習之卽是一學問臨民之時又一學問其童而習之卽禮樂之事長而居業志聖賢之獸曰用倫常必踐其理天地民物研究其精所以壹是皆以修身爲本非如禪和子終日靜坐屏棄人事止求養得此心空空然而倫常物理仍昏昏然也故一言一行之善亦可謂德而此章言明德則以全體而言在明明德一句已了又丁甯

四書恆解　大學　士　西充鮮于氏特圖藏

之曰在親民在止於至善乃一定義理必如是始盡其說而文法順遞而下實非平列中庸天命之謂性三句文法正與此同其語亦似蟬聯而下然下單承道字說此單承止至善說相例卽明何乃以爲三平乎〇知止作知至善之理而止之亦無大謬但身外至善之理皆本身內心未虛明身未修德惟恃耳目見聞物物求理譬如磨磚作鏡欲別妍媸安能得其況天下之物非可一一盡知者乎夫子詰子貢曰女以予爲多學而識之者與非也予一以貫之正爲徒求諸多識必紛贖而

無所折衷耳如朱子說知知所當止之處卽可以定靜安試思如知子當孝知臣當忠而何以不能實盡忠孝此豈知之難乎中庸言學問思辨篤行而曰有弗學學問思辨蓋有不當學者惟當學則弗能弗措五者皆然非知之功則好惡亂其中利害奪其外心之內無存養之地果如此知止卽如此能定靜定靜能慮說又說能慮得總覺模糊不清聖人安知何從外求知孔子亦不能讀盡天下之書閱不敘人逐外求知孔子亦不能讀盡天下之書閱盡天下之事以此言知止與言格物一般徒使天下聰明人終身務博不從傍身養性實踐則明德不可明矣至善者存心養性之地天地之理渾然無名目爲太極太極天地之中也人身亦然夫子曰成性存存道義之門人身血氣心知多與物同而其靈於物者則惟中氣之元而天命之粹也人感父母而生實受天地之正理而生無天地尙無父母何有我雖有天地若無父母何有我故父母天地一也當未生以前受天地之中有其理地焉理氣之渾然者在此旣生以後氣散而理亦分寄非復受中之本然矣其虛明之竅仍在

四書恆解　大學　十三　西充鮮于氏特圖藏

血氣不能累私欲不能到空洞無塵故名之曰至
善明明德者收視返聽止於至善之地性命合一
天地同和久久純一則致中矣知止言其功定靜
安言其效然尚是第一層功夫若由是而有諸己
而充實而大化聖神猶有許多功面功夫亦易知止
則明明德之學便得即後面功夫在密文王之
曰允執厥中安汝止易曰洗心退藏於密文王之
緝熙成王之基命宥密孔子曰志仁無惡孟子曰
養氣不動心皆是此義乾坤若非靜專靜翕則不
能動直動闢此止之說也欲明明德者若不收放
心而止於其所憧憧者何所既極哉故曰知止而
后有定定而后能靜靜矣而形神猶有擾攘者乎
安矣而志慮有不清明者乎惟心靜而理明故
知止而入時解專向外說並而后字神理皆晦定
務而皆得此明之始事也定靜安慮得各字有實
之說實際不分明原前人之意恐類於僧流空空
靜安實然佛言真空不空何曾說人倫日用皆空
後世僧徒不得佛全體之功止以養虛靈之心為
禪卽通神通慧亦不能修齊治平先儒知其誤而

四書恆解　《大學》　十三

實不能出其範圍故靜心矣又當格物而此書之
義俱不分明夫禪家之守心誤在於以心為性養
其空空洞洞之識神而不知知覺運動之心非復
先天之本體故卽強制其心而不動天地民物之
事業實有所不能知豈知僧流守空乃告子不動
心之學非孟子之不動心也精一危微堯舜德全
愼於危微爲務防守雖勤陰私不淨明德全功以
於身猶不忘敬愼而後儒未知明德全功第以
之純孔子從心不踰矩罕有能及者由知止之功
不得其正耳禪以空寂爲性道以呼吸爲氣而儒
者又逐逐於事物大學之道安得不日益支離乎
大學之功敬靜以執其中窮究事物以博其理一
時並到知止而後浩然之氣可生純一之性可復
次第功效必一二身體乃知孔子十五志學七十
而後從心不踰孟子有諸己以至化神言之已詳
定靜安是知止初功尚未說到物來坐照之境也
○慮而后能得緊黏定靜安說蓋必知止至善之
地久久到定靜安境界則私欲漸少義理日明凡
事物之來是非易知乃可以得其理矣慮祗是審
察辨別之意書曰慮善以動卽此夫子曰苟志於

四書恆解　《大學》　十四

四書恆解 大學

仁矣無惡也緣求仁之功先要收放心而靜養至
定靜安時功夫已得大半孟子所謂有諸己時孔
子之三十而立顏子之如有所立卓爾皆是但由
是而充實美大聖神尚有許多功夫次第此特止至
善是明德始功知止至善宜先則雖未與
言凡事物有本末始終知止至善宜先則雖夫子
道一亦近乎道以結上文之意時解說慮而能得
太深似一慮即得不知德造其極物來順應夫子
所謂天下何思何慮者也知止然後
在所先末在所後何為本止至善是也

涵養有方明德之明漸開故能慮能得雖未必事
事皆當而已近道下交因即先後意推廣言之仍
歸到致知在格物物即是止至善時常常虛靜
不使物欲入來物欲少則心漸虛明智慧日生前
人但養有覺之心亦云源頭活水況得存心養性
之全功者乎○古之節承上先後字推開說言平
治修齊極大功能一一溯原歸到致知在格物仍
收轉必知止之意非謂大學之道欲如此必先
此也故下文即承之以自天子至庶人皆以修身
為本試思聖人治天下何嘗說我想治天下且先

四書恆解 大學

治國想治國且先齊家想齊家且先修身祇是己
德已明則推之家國天下自然身範端分證明綱
紀肅人心治夫子因言大學之道入手在知止至
善欲人先從此立本結之曰知所先後則近道謂
功由此始知命不惑從心不踰皆從此舉也
然止至善始為平常恐人疑天下國家平治
非只此圖功便可近道故又推言天下國家平治
修齊皆歸本於誠正誠正必先致知知何可盡但
能知止則可格物而養天性之明譜意似泛說先
後實仍收轉知止能得之義且前人不知德即天

命之性以空明妙了為性覺明明德矣猶不免難
以修齊治平又不知止至善即是存心養性實際
故於夫子之言不明而遂以為此節乃為學先後
之序不知夫子下文緊接壹是皆以修身為本身
修即德已明而功在止至善豈必事事而營之
在而學之乎格物司馬溫公張橫渠俱解作去物
欲二人朱子所服膺也而不用其說然按諸山格庭前
驗諸日用倫常物物而格實有難行象山格庭前
竹子七日格不出道理來亦天下人之公言不得
病其異於朱子也且格至也窮至事物之理作一

心正者乎應之曰然

附解心之發動處爲意意誠則心宜正矣而經又云修身在正其心豈心外別有意哉蓋大學之始教人窮理以致其知知其善矣卽於心之動處實好其善實惡其惡然止是於心之動處愼其獨知至誠意以愼其動則此身血氣之動處愼所獨知但旣生以後氣質之欲太多苟未能知止以養其源心之本體內含虛靈之用虛靈之用非可無也但而心不得其正矣心在先天渾然者卽是性是心之本體也旣生以後有此血氣之身卽有七情之擾而知覺運動之心非復先天渾然之心爲其緣

圓書悞解 大學 堅 峨西充鮮于 氏特圈藏

氣質而生故以爲身有所忿懥非心字譌爲身字也人身得天之理本無駁雜而身之氣以成形者厚薄清濁迥異所以有生安學利困勉之分明明德者明其先天之性而已性心之體心性之用不離體故惻隱羞惡辭讓是非人皆有之體心不離用故動靜存動察必心爲之但性本無爲而心有覺覺則動動則妄妄則僞而雜平旦之氣因而梏亡矣誠意者能制於動而無以養其清明之體則何質之心牽擾虛明之性而心不正矣心不正身何

以修故曾子特標明身字見七情之偏身所以不修而正心之功非徒省察克治可了必由致中致和久而能不動心然後有覺之心悉聽命於無爲之性自然非禮之來視如無見聽如無聞聖人所以清明在躬志氣如神者以此此謂心正而身修也知止誠意不動心朱子覺其不安故補格致傳謂必窮究事物之理乃可齊治均平然明明十六字爲聖學力持其心久久亦能不動然實告子之學而已故符離喪師安睡不動謂爲不動而范滔夫女亦能不動心久久亦能不動心也知止誠意孟子集義養氣之說在其中先儒

四書悞解 大學 堅 峨西充鮮于 氏特圈藏

德之功動靜交養本末交修博學於文約之以禮內外一時並到夫子告顏子爲仁仁卽明德爲仁卽明明德知止之功具焉其目在視聽言動制外所以養中養中方能制外戒其非禮卽誠意也致知不是事物之理盡知祇是日用倫常一言一行一動一靜必審其是非其功則學問思辨是也知之卽誠而行之是爲篤行行亦不但行事由一念以及於念必由一事以及於事事惡則克治善則擴充誠其所知而已故致知誠意不分兩事意卽心也而分言之則心是本體意是發動處誠意者

四書恆解 〈大學〉

能治其動矣至心之本體欲求渾然天理則非憤動可了故曾子又明正心之義道心理也人心欲也欲此心純乎道心無有人心非知止誠意漸造其極安能復還天命之性夫子三十而立七十而後從心不踰則人心莫非道心矣心純乎理則一念可以通於天命而此身之美大聖神上律下襲因之聖人之身不同凡人之身豈非由其心命之理哉前人第知心為身主不知心有後天天之分孟子言耳目之官不同於心之官人心氣質之靈道心即是德性故心正者身然後修知告之所以修而天下平亦不外此孟子曰形色天性也惟聖人然後可以踐形即此章心正身修之義而曾子謂夫子江漢濯之秋陽暴之發明聖人心象亦該此章特實踐者少故人心道心所由分與其所以合千古不明而孔曾思孟之言亦難以得其會通矣識者詳之

所謂齊其家在修其身者人之其所親愛而辟焉之其所賤惡而辟焉之其所畏敬而辟焉故好而知其惡惡而辟焉之其所敖惰而辟焉故好而知其惡惡而

四書恆解 〈大學〉

其美者天下鮮矣○朱子曰人謂眾人之猶偏也身修自反無惑矣而旋之於人之猶偏也故歷言五者之情好惡已陷於偏故偏惡類此則身不修故下莫知好惡直指之偏好惡已陷於偏以見莫知好惡之碩苗碩之姤生者引諺以明辟矣而不察其惡故曰身不修不可以齊其家偏身不修而言身不可以此謂身不修不可以齊其家誠一之

右傳之三章釋修身齊家

貫解上文言修身在正其心則正心之後身可以修矣而經言齊家必先修身似正心之外猶有修身之功不可以不釋也所謂齊家在修其身者非正心之後身猶不修特心雖正矣而心之見於好惡者或自恃其正而不加察則必有偏而身因以不修夫正心者當好而好當惡而惡一家宜其勸善而懲惡矣而未必然者自以為好惡之當而實已偏於好惡故身即不修家卽不能齊如一家之中宜親愛者多矣然親之愛之並其言行之失皆姑息優容則辟矣亦有素行不端勸懲無術為所賤惡者應然苟牽德改行固當不念舊惡即或一端可嘉亦應略短取長而或不然則於其所賤惡而辟焉若夫父母兄長之屬所宜畏敬也然事之以道

節謂之和中也者天下之大本也和也者天下之達道也樂音洛中去聲○喜怒哀樂情也其未發則性也無所偏倚故謂之中發皆中節情之正也無所乖戾故謂之和大本者天命之性天下之理皆由此出道之體也達道者循性之謂天下古今之所共由道之用也此言性情之德以明道不可離之意致中和天地位焉萬物育焉致推而極之也位者安其所也育者遂其生也自戒懼而約之以至於至靜之中無所偏倚而其守不失則極其中而天地位矣自謹獨而精之以至於應物之處無少差謬而無適不然則極其和而萬物育矣蓋天地萬物本吾一體吾之心正則天地之心亦正矣吾之氣順則天地之氣亦順矣故其效驗至於如此此學問之極功聖人之能事初非有待於外而修道之教亦在其中矣是其一體一用雖有動靜之殊然必其體立而後用有以行則其實亦非有兩事也故於此合而言之以結上文之意

右第一章爲全書之綱領溯其原揭其要明其本體而究極乎功效之全以明道不外乎性天人所以合而萬化所由生也

四書恆解 〈中庸〉 二

附解蓋自堯舜三代以來聖人之君相皆能有以維持乎民心而悉協於大道自周之衰聖化淩夷孔子明道以濟世而莫能尊羣言淆亂靡所折衷子思述祖德以爲此書大要本乎天理之正而踐乎人生日用之常以明道本無奇要在率性而已其實此章則其提綱挈領之詞也其言曰今之言道者紛然矣愚者卑高者誕而不究乎其得天之本然則道愈晦豈知人爲萬物之靈爲其得天獨粹而已天道至神然其陰陽五行之本渾然

然萬古不貳不息者爲天之主宰如人之命然是理氣之原人咸得之以生則謂之性天之於人性一而二二而一也萬物莫不統於天之性莫不賴乎人人獨得天之粹果能率天理而行措諸萬事無不宜卽謂之道但人之生也氣質厚薄不同形氣雜而嗜慾遂逹於道體天之心以化斯民在上則爲禮樂兵刑在下則爲表章師儒斟酌時宜上協天道修而明之則謂之教性也者道之所從生敎也者道之所由明其名雖三其理則止一道也者率性而該萬物人之所以爲人無論表裏精粗非是不立不可須臾離也若猶有毫髮之間人可須臾而離則是身外之物起之緣必非道也聖人敎人修道內外兼盡微特可睹可聞之地必愼其功卽所不覩亦必戒而愼之恐其失性而不足爲人卽所不聞亦必恐而懼之恐其獲罪於天所以然者何不覩不聞無迹而無聲響此亦一念未見於言行亦至微矣而忽見乎此且一念之動天地知之實莫不及防卽著於外實莫顯乎此故君子不以爲至隱微其幾甫動卽愼而察之善則擴充惡則克治

四書恆解 〈中庸〉 三

四書恆解 中庸 四 氏特圖藏

乃能不離道也夫天下之事物至繁則道之散見於天下者何可勝窮而君子修道但先慎獨者以天下之理皆本於性性即道道即性修道所以率性性不待於外索修道豈外吾身而修如人心有喜怒哀樂固應事接物不可無也然發於外而後有此名若其未發渾然在抱不參毫髮之私則謂之中中人不可得而見然果存乎中之本體則萬理咸備是天下之大本也本此中之本以行凡喜怒哀樂之發皆中其節則萬事咸理謂之和是天下之達道也性體如斯故君子由慎獨之和是天下之達道也性體如斯故君子由慎獨而精之極之於無聲無臭而有以全天命之本然則致其中矣本慎獨而發之極之於萬事萬理而有以協人心之至順則致其和矣中者天地之理萬殊所以歸於一本和者萬物之定理萬殊所以歸於一本和者萬物之定以散爲萬殊誠致中和則靜極而得天命之自然天地位焉動極而得率性之至當萬物育焉天地至神萬物至賾而位育皆在一性此所以修道者祇自全其天性而非求諸難能不可知也○人爲三才之主無人則天地之功用亦窮然人之所以貴者以其得天地之性也傳曰民受天地之中以

四書恆解 中庸 五 氏特圖藏

生所謂命也此語至精命字先儒作猶命令解是天自爲天人自爲人下文致中而天地位說不去且性本無聲臭如何命法語義亦窮張子云在天爲命在人爲性得之矣子思因當時言道者流入高渺特以中庸立說人性即天性此何等平常然至神至奇即在至平至常之中所以爲中庸詩曰維天之命於穆不已命字如秉質流行而不息高明無所不統然其生化於無窮而不息有箇主宰之理在易有太極是乾坤之眞精即天之命也惟此太極之粹天以之清地以之寧人以之命也惟此太極之粹天以之清地以之寧人以之聖本無二理故名曰道特分而言之不得不異其名以析其解子思言天有所以爲天之理是爲天命人爲天地之心獨得天命之全此之謂性既爲天之理則人果能率其性之本體而所存所發莫非天理此之謂道第人性雖即天性而受形其閒清濁厚薄氣化之雜不盡純乎天命則氣拘物誘遂失其本然人全己之性則心一天心道一天道或爲君相爲師儒因人之性而制爲禮樂刑賞裁其太過輔其不及修明大道使人各全乎天命此之謂教語意直截了當本無難解後

四書恆解 中庸 六 西充鮮于氏特園藏

儒紛紛議論不本諸天理實踐而求諸語言文字愈辨愈惑轉令本文塵封今愚但就白文口氣繹之其諸家論說難以徧摘老子之意言天地成形之先天地生者斥之不知老子之道本無名道之一字道在天地而天地未形之初天地非有又將何以名道夫子曰易有太極是生兩儀又曰大哉乾元固自後人名之而太極之平統之乎統天乾元萬物資始乃統天夫天也而有以統之乎統天非卽理非卽太極乎老子所謂渾成先天地生者非卽此意乎第天地卽太極太極卽天地自其未分未生生之意性所以存主之意其實一也此章為人性溯原故曰天命之性天所以生之理卽人之性而未畢宣其旨後人遂拘泥而不得其會通盡性至命之功其可緩乎蓋天之性命所以形言之則祇可言太極不可言天地自其已奠已形言之則可以言天地亦可以言太極前聖言之而一句其義無不該而全部中庸在是矣性字舊此一句其義無不該而全部中庸在是矣性字舊兼人物言蓋為下文育萬物張本及後文盡人性物性云云覺物皆有性故兼人物言然天之性至粹所謂乾元統天之氣氣也卽理也非凡理氣之

四書恆解 中庸 七 西充鮮于氏特園藏

成形成色者可比天命之謂性蓋指其粹然之中萬物之性理之徧者也人之性理之全者也先儒言理多不敢以氣言不知形形色色之氣則有粗有精而太極之眞卽氣卽理以理言理本無名無象著於形色而始有名象從其原言之則不得以其散著為本體也故仁義禮智信為五性然五性祇是一性之澄然在中者無貳無雜性之自然順應者悉得其宜是皆天命之本而非強以相赴盆其本無故曰率性之謂道也前人謂在天為元亨利貞在人為仁義禮智其誤愚已於周易乾卦爻言明之又云元亨誠之通利貞誠之復通復者陰陽循環消長之機一誠所貫義無大失而以元亨利貞分貼則難通蓋道理聖人已是說盡必另立名目以已意參之而按諸天理身心不合則爲臆說故愚嘗言凡言道必如王天下章所言諸身六句均一一符合方是大道稍有不合卽為偏駁也董仲舒春秋繁露以五行配五性蓋不知五性祇一性猶五行祇一太極鄭康成以木神為仁金神為義火神為禮水神為信土神為智宋儒

以水屬智土屬信於理未為大謬然以解此章性道惟人身之理與天同故中和如此此虛說性
字則為支離大文明言天命之謂性一句已了其即天命之意以起下致中和就現成性體說非謂
他曲說尚多茲不悉贅○道也者四句一反一正人人皆能作是觀下文致字方是學者修道以致
總以明性外無道外無人戒愼二句特舉所中和凡人一念敬靜一端合宜亦是中和然不可
覩聞以該覩聞是故二字從不可離生來既須臾語乎性之全體也且本節倘未說致中和功夫○
不可離則雖不覩不聞皆道之无周布瀰漫得不上文言中和之體用如此故學道者戒愼恐懼靜
覩聞恐懼○莫見節又申明不覩不聞必戒懼之存動察祇欲全中和之性量一致字中該括許多
故不覩不聞卽隱微卽是獨隱言其地微言其幾功夫在存理之極而渾然者天地同其廣大高明
己所獨知常人以為隱微故子思特地醒之曰莫覆載萬非遽六合非遜天地位焉矣忘私之極而當
見莫顯而以為君子必愼於所獨以其非隱非微然者萬物安其血氣心知益生益養仁至義盡萬
也故字從莫見莫顯生來語意相銜次第不爽若物育焉矣位育不必說到得志乘時聖人盡性而
四書恆解〈中庸〉八　　　西充鮮于氏特圖藏
日既常戒懼於此尤加謹焉則不覩不聞又何地合天無處不中和夫子不惑知命中也耳順從心
情可見故就四者未發以明愛中之始其理如是不踰矩和也推而言之孟子曰存心養性所以事
也不覩不聞倘不足為隱微則必其猶有可覩可天文王之德之純亦如於穆不已其中如是故止
聞之跡乎○喜怒哀樂節就性之本體而言以為仁止敬等和即如是中和之用中和之用祇
下文張本非謂人人皆有此中和之本性不可見全得一性字自事物言之則曰道前人競競辨動
性無不該故致中和則位天地而育萬物以文法靜體用恐人誤認究之動靜一原體用相資純一
言之則脫接者也以義理言之是復從天命之之至而靜固靜動亦靜動則中也和也異其名不異
推原其體段也人性之中卽如太極之渾舍故曰其致也靜則萬善俱含動則一以貫萬非實能致
大本發而為和如天生成萬物無心成化故曰達者烏足知之
四書恆解〈中庸〉九　　　西充鮮于氏特圖藏

關忠孝人紀之事可以能可以不必盡能者也若
夫盡性盡倫之事隱顯出處之宜聖人固無不能
之聖人所不知能可以不必知能者也然一一
物莫非道之所在則道之費自非聖人所能窮天
地即道也天地之大人猶有所憾者天地能生之
而不能養之能養之而不能教之必待人功輔相
裁成若非聖人為之君師天地有許多缺憾處人
猶有所憾非憾天地之難盡洽也侯氏
以問官問禮等語解知能已誤以覆載生成之偏
寒暑災祥不正解有憾亦誤覆載無偏生成有偏

四書恆解 〈中庸〉 芙[西充鮮于氏特圓藏]

其偏也氣化為之人事失其正而後然也人不反
求諸己而咎於天則以為天地有偏不知道在人
地本渾成無少渣滓特人物自駁雜耳故邵子以
為天地有盡時者不知道舊以體用分貼費隱
亦誤體固義用亦有隱如聖人精義入神義在顯
處其精當當出人意表便是隱此隱字不作幽深隱
闇解作精微解緣就道之全體大用渾括處言指
出費字實際無所不在實精微難測也及其至至
字非極至之至猶言充類之盡意焉飛戾天節承
上節作轉乃指出上下察以明道雖費隱然卻昭

四書恆解 〈中庸〉 毛[西充鮮于氏特圓藏]

著在耳目之前臨時臨事有當盡之理鳶飛魚躍
鳶魚之性得於天之自然焉鳶魚自適其飛躍即可
戾天于淵則于淵鳶在天而飛則戾之魚不知有
淵而躍則于淵流行品物皆可作是觀凡自天子
至於庶人道各盡其形亦皆如是觀
察是欲人實體諸身心不可遠求故下緊接造端
於夫婦盡道之費隱上文已詳此節原非複說作
含吐不盡之詞仍言費隱則為重複且拈花微笑
棒頭一喝竟作禪語虛鋒矣然佛言真空不空妙
有不有即費隱之意一切佛田不離方寸即上下
察之意儒者必非之亦為故相貶斥如青青綠竹
莫匪真如粲粲黃花無非般若吾道於鳶魚飛
躍之中便見天命率性然彼如般若吾道於鳶魚
於翠竹黃花之外別有真如般若則於道之全
言道無不在能全真如則一以貫萬無處非此理
之發皇耳究之物理止道之緒餘惟性為道之全
體佛言真如般若即是性但語不同耳僧流以知
覺之心為性則將謂心之所在即道之所在其失
非小羅氏所見亦止如此而又闕其言不知己之

所學亦與同也夫佛以虛無清淨為存養之法蓋
人心難制必虛無而後可以凝道又曰度盡衆生
方得成佛卽修道以仁而至德至道不凝焉者也夫
非言人倫日用皆虛無也廢人倫者西方夷俗之謂
國僧流廢人倫日用為其本鰥寡孤獨藉以養身佛有
妻有子奈何諉之渾然天理乃作棒喝語者豈不
知佛之眞如卽是以虛詞煽誘自謂妙明慧解所謂口
麼些子如是渾然天理人天性倫理亦作影
頭禪也愿代文人師之於聖人天性倫理亦作影
響參悟語又儒家之口頭禪而中庸一書尤今

四書恆解　中庸　堯☆西充鮮于氏特圓藏

子二就本文解之一切當辨甚多兹不悉贅末
節總結上文言道之賃隱如是而實昭著於日用
之間是故君子之道從日用切近行之卽如夫婦
至親至近狎而易玩然天命之性人倫之本卽起
於牀笫之間君子愼獨修身正內正外陽教陰敎各得其宜
婦而果盡其道則正內正外陽敎陰敎各得其宜
天地之陰陽和而風雨時品物章而萬民育皆是
理也語氣是從上兩節總括指明尤為親切有味
造端夫婦義理包孕無窮易之為書也乾坤父母
而生六子三男三女斡造化之綱維而坎離實括

四書恆解　中庸　堯☆西充鮮于氏特圓藏

其樞分之為五行散之為萬物蓋不可以言語窮
而人身受天秉地以成性命則尤其精焉者也夫
子曰一陰一陽之謂道道本天地為人父母
此性命之根極於陰陽者其理精父母為受生之
父母者其氣全賢愚之所以分人物之所以異天
地也夫婦道則誠其身以及父母之胎育其
亦安能知致功之法奈何亦曰戒懼愼獨存養其
天命之良推極乎泛應之當久之而在抱形
神精氣無弗與天地相通則人身亦具太極二氣
流行無間而萬化一元相孚人也卽天也中庸一
部皆言此理此第略而言之

子曰道不遠人人之為道而遠人不可以為道 此言下
其則不遠執柯以伐柯睨而視之猶以為遠故君子
以人治人改而止
求道之方不遠人道卽人理之所以為人道止自全其為人之理耳詩云伐柯伐柯
其則不遠執柯以伐柯睨而視之猶以為遠故君子
以人治人改而止 朱子曰柯斧柄則法
一寸有半脫邪視正視睨視伐柯也車人為車柯
伐之柯也引詩言人為柯其則非外此柯之理以
則猶遠惟道卽吾身外之事所謂非道去人以為
乎為人非強別以身事人所以為人也盡其心而

忠違道不遠施諸己而不願亦勿施於人 道不遠下二句解忠恕之義言為道必本於忠恕也

右第十六章申卑邇通於高遠之故而卽子言鬼神以明在一誠者天之道誠之者人之道人之究通乎天地家庭之際至性感乎其一端也夫子不嘗云乎天地間形形色色莫非道之所寓也主宰之變化之令人莫可端倪則鬼神之為也神之為德其盛矣乎何以明其盛也凡物有形皆宜其有聲可聞而鬼神視之弗見聽之弗聞則可見神之為德其盛矣乎何以明其盛也凡物有形皆理天理無聲無臭成形成象而始有可指名人為迷誤而談講學者紛紛斜斜結矣不知道止是天庸二字作此書乃此章忽引子言鬼神講章遂用附解子思本因異端言道多涉荒渺故特述夫子中本合一莫能載莫能破者豈外人倫日用哉

四書恆解〈中庸〉 吳氏特圖藏

乎夫此陰陽之靈固一氣耳而宰氣者理之妙者神氣相須如環不可以兩分故氣之所在卽神之所在而氣以變化不測鬼神卽神之所在而氣以變化不測鬼神卽敏之名神卽鬼發舒之處鬼神之在天者如斯此鬼神之正所以在天為星辰在地為河嶽萬古而不朽也若夫散而為萬物皆分陰陽之精氣皆有鬼神然梏於質習於汙駁雜之氣多清明之氣少鬼遂與神分途矣此章言德之盛專就鬼神之正者而言子思曰中庸之道至卑至邇卻通乎高遠如詩言和妻子宜兄弟父母其順此中感通不秉此陰陽卽莫不秉其靈而謂鬼神與人相遠靈也一陰一陽之為道而鬼神者陰陽之靈人之天地之心獨得天地之菁華者何卽陰陽之

四書恆解〈中庸〉 吳氏特圖藏

祭祀而觀之鬼神非邀人以媚享也然而人心之肅不能自昧感發於天命之性自動其悽愴惕之心莫或使之而若或使之天下之人皆齊明盛服以承祭祀洋洋乎如在其上如在其左右則夫鬼神之體物不遺可概知矣故大雅抑之詩曰天人本無二理人心動繫乎天心天不可見也而神則可見神者秉天之理而鑒乎人心神之格思不可度思時時戒慎猶恐有咎矧可厭射而不敬乎夫鬼神無形與聲則至微矣而體物不遺則又至顯夫微之顯鬼神之為皆實理充塞之為也誠之不

四書恆解 中庸

平行動天地可也一言何以能動天地殼
子裏如物在人腹中豈有腹中之物而謂我不關
心者乎縣天地祇是一氣渾成流行不息其主宰
之者曰帝變化不測者曰神神之一字就天地言
之夫子妙萬物而為言及此章體物不遺盡之矣
則人而言則志氣如神聖而不可知之謂神盡之
矣若鬼之一字在天地則止是陰陽之靈之傳感
則由氣質清濁之偏兼山川草木飛走之靈在人
受氣化不齊是以變態雜出君子體天之道合天
之氣以天之心裁成一切帝謂可以贊通中和敬
來為民捍患禦災所以為不朽之人者亦往往有
於萬彙此書已詳言之而降龍伏虎役鬼驅神自
之矣若巫覡邪術等不知中庸之道而專就鬼神
求吉凶者豈足語於此哉夫子不語怪神而又曰
某之禱久祭神如神在繫易於大人固曰與鬼神
合其吉凶矣不為道何以知鬼神為道而遠人又
何以知鬼神止中庸耶
子曰舜其大孝也與德為聖人尊為天子富有四海
之內宗廟饗之子孫保之撑敬惟德動天而引子言
聖人之孝蓋無愧於父母即無愧於天地也故
為聖人則已全其大孝尊富饗保又以其遇言之故

命
者培之傾者覆之鄭康成曰林質也篤厚也栽植
也故天必因其材而篤焉故大德之生物必得其
應勤人以修德故天必因其材而篤焉故大
者也詩言大德之人必得其效之故詩曰嘉樂君
人受祿於天保佑命之自天申之盛鄭康成曰憲憲興
助也嘉樂詩作假人臣王也又引子言大地之事以證之故
詩言成王之德宜民宜人皆有德無不受命而體中庸之德
者也故天必受命所以通乎天也受命受天保佑之
德者必受命

右第十七章承上文誠不可揜而言庸德可以享
天心無非一誠之所貫注而凡有中庸之德者可

四書恆解 中庸

知矣
附解子思言鬼神之德之盛一誠之不可揜凡天地
間形形色色莫非道之所在即莫非鬼神所在鬼
神陰陽之靈天地即陰陽之體中庸之德庸德也
而即天之所以為天故聖人全天之道德一天德
而天亦應之卑邇固通乎高遠夫子嘗言舜矣曰
舜其大孝也與人子事親承歡竭力皆孝而必德
造其極使吾親之身通乎天地乃為大孝惟舜也
德為聖人凡事天如事親事天者皆以
貫之而遇合之隆又盆逐其尊養之志尊為天子

皆不外乎修身為誠身上沿誠不可撅下
起天下至誠也

附解子思意謂觀於舜及武周本孝德以治世而夫
子歎美之且推其義以為治國在是則知道無二
理一家之繼述在是則即天下之典章在是要在身
體而力行之耳不觀夫子之論政乎哀公問政子
告之曰政真備於文武公文武之後今猶是文武
之天下文武之政布在方策無所不詳特未有如
文武者舉而行之耳苟有如文武之德者是文武
之人猶存矣則本身以行之政不難舉苟無文武
之德是其人亡矣雖方策昭然政亦難舉其故何
哉政乃先王之陳迹不難知而難於行苟有賢聖
之才則行政至易人道固敏政者也正如地易以
敏樹而文武之政為明備之休一王之舊於政之
中尤易舉行如樹中之蒲盧也特政非一人可行
欲為先王之政必得賢臣共治而知賢惟取人
必在君身身不可不修也修之惟在以道道者天
理而已凡天理之發見惟此不忍人之仁人人
皆有修道者以此仁心推之於萬事萬物即不患
天理之不周徧所以然者天地生生之理人得之

四書恆解 〈中庸〉

辛酉 西充鮮于
氏特園藏

之人不外修身而已是故君子知仁為道之本仁
者即能盡道道全而後身可修也不可以不修身
至於親者吾身之所自來有親而後有身能事親
而後可以為仁則思修身不可以不事親然事親
之道無窮事親之事不易知非賢人為輔安能知
仁與道一事親不可以不知人也人不難知而為
君者不能修身蓋於天與我之理未能瞭如故思
有天德之賢人亦莫能知故思知人又不可以不
知天也天者理之所從出人得之而為賢我得之
而有道知天則知人知人則有所以輔身要祇全

四書恆解 〈中庸〉

辛酉 西充鮮于
氏特園藏

以為性是人之所以為人者特其慈祥惻怛必於
父母之前先十分周至而後能推暨於民物故親
親為大親者吾身之所從出仁者吾身中之天良
無親何以有身不能親親何以為人果仁矣本此
而施之於凡事親能修其身以之輔身然後
而敬莫大於尊賢賢者能修其身以之輔身然後
行事各得其宜若夫由親親而仁民而愛物以漸
而殺由賢而師保也道有大小位有等級
凡節文度數皆由此而推禮所生也要而言之禮
生於仁義義以行仁以修道道重修身為文武

四書恆解 中庸

乎修身之事耳所謂修身之道安在天下之達道有五所以行之者有三君臣也父子也夫婦也昆弟也朋友之交也五者或以天合或以人合情誼相聯義理相屬智愚皆不能外是天下之達道也明五者而不惑爲知行五者而無私爲仁守五者而不懈爲勇三者天之所以予人雖偏全純駁不同而實人人皆有是天下之達德也以三德行達道其目似繁人人亦不易盡而要其所以行之者惟在專一不貳而已心一於理而不他始終其身而不倦雖資秉或有不同而有生而知之或困而知之或勉強而行之其所行者不同而及其積久自得而成此達道則一也惟其資不同而可同歸於成所以爲達道特用功之始不可以三達德爲患耳有人爲知不如人然知道之美而好學焉學之不已雖未必遽知道而見聞日闢識量日超近乎知矣或仁不及人然信道之眞而力行焉行之至久雖未必卽全天理而私僞日去義理日純近乎仁矣或勇亦遜人而知恥不如人爲因恥生奮

四書恆解 中庸

奮志不懈雖未必配乎行健而有進焉無退愈近乎勇矣三者非難爲之事而實致其功卽是修身則修身者豈不知斯三者耳知斯三者則知所以修身身者人之表而天下國家所待治也知所以修身則知所以治人知所以治人則知所以治天下國家矣治天下國家豈有過於交武哉臣嘗誦習而總括其政言之凡爲天下國家有九經文武固已備之矣九經雖何日修身也修身之學早裕於平時而修之功不懈於頃刻所以爲立政之本也二曰尊賢也尊賢以導吾身而出治三曰親親也親以廣吾仁而敬宗四曰敬大臣也大臣爲身之輔得其人而敬之體肅而權有歸五曰體羣臣也羣臣分吾身之職任推仁以體之恩周而情乃不隔六曰子庶民也庶民雖繁一以子視之則恩義無弗洽七曰來百工也百工至雜有以招徠之則獎罰無弗公八曰柔遠人也他國臣民無使有乖離之心交武之政其大要如此此何故哉治世不外於道卽吾身之理修身則道備於己而建其有極可以爲會極之本矣賢人道大

四書恆解 中庸

動靜云博厚所以載物也高明所以覆物也悠久所以成物也申言悠遠三者可以及博厚高明天悠久無疆者惟天地有餘而至誠乃能承天地之表著而有而變無為而成者諸身不見而章不動光輝不爍動而變化無所作為而如此者不見而章不動天悠久也悠久也皆一天地之道可物不測也悠久也皆一天地之道可以以此也不測者以此即生物也明也悠久也皆以其生亦無以此也不測者以此即生繫焉萬物覆焉今夫地一撮土之多及其廣厚載華亦無以此斯昭昭之多及其無窮也日月星辰今夫天斯昭昭之多及其無窮也日月星辰生物不測之自然也一誠之德自然而無所其也所以至誠配之不貳誠也一誠之至然而一言而盡也其為物不貳則其生物不測天地之道博也厚也高也明也悠久也以至誠配之不貳誠也天地之道不貳高明悠久不外一誠

右第二十六章承上而言自成之者可以配天也由至誠無息也因言天地之盛而以文王配天也由至誠無息也因言天地之盛而以文王證之

附解上文勉人自成自成則為至誠矣此章乃極言至誠之功用合乎天地以終自誠明下五章之義至誠何以不息人身有氣而後有質氣質人物所同天理人之所獨特有生以後駁雜之氣晦其天命之性而平旦之氣梏亡與人相近也者幾希矣

四書恆解 中庸

至誠盡其性則自有諸己以至化神一元之理氣充周浹洽心與天通氣與天合靜而渾然粹然動而因應無方雖猶是羣類皆有息絕之隙至誠體無論何時天理充溢凡物皆有毫髮間斷之隙乎此本心性內景象難以形容下文姑就不息二字擬議推言之夫天下之物惟有息則不能久至誠既不息矣以其功而言一日如此終身亦如此以其量而言一時如此千秋亦如此則久矣久則中之所積自徵於外徵則動靜云為皆有悠遠無

獄而不重振河海而不洩萬物載焉今夫山一卷石之多及其廣大草木生之禽獸居之寶藏興焉今夫水一勺之多及其不測黿鼉蛟龍魚鱉生焉貨財殖焉夫音振華藏韻並去聲卷平聲夕市若反卷區也華嶽名河南華嶽河南府華陽縣也振收也卷小也此也 鄭氏曰昭昭猶耿耿小明也振猶收也卷區也華嶽名上聲韻韻皆能吐霧致雨鱗甲黑色一二能橫飛者也嬰大者數圍細者如箸首尾似鼉鱗甲似魚足有長八十分而一鱗如鬚鈿似蜥蜴而大龍鱗甲能橫飛者秋分而入淵能昇能幽能明能細能巨能長能短春者鮋其所承山水天地所生物者皆天地所生也已蓋曰天之所以為天也於乎不顯文王之德之純蓋曰文王之所以為文也純亦不已○引詩而釋之

四書恆解 中庸

育萬物峻極於天言其蘊含太極之理足以充周六合彌綸天地而有餘也蓋天地雖大祇此至誠人身雖小亦此至誠之理萬物俱從此出在天曰太極在人曰性名異而實同至誠之人性量與天地相含眞有可以發育萬物之理孟子言直養浩然之氣則塞於天地之間夫子言大人與天地合德日月合明鬼神合吉凶先天而天弗違後天而奉天時皆謂其實有發育萬物峻極於天之理特無人造到聖人地步遂以爲虛誕耳向來講家就功用說以不言功用爲虛而無著且發育峻極功用而明其本體也下文優優大哉乃就道之著於功用者言日用事物何一非天以一本之理含宏言之總以明道無微不在蓋天以一本之理含宏是從心體無象可名中而想像指點言其在我之理氣足以彌綸充周若此語雖似言功用實乃卽生化而聖人心體如之上節是也天以散殊之理物物生遂而聖人之禮制如之此節是也舊說謂大而無外小而無間大槪亦是但於洋洋優優二字不恰切且語似混入費隱二字中費隱亦是此

章本原但彼言費而隱一而字特分顯微此處專言聖道之大不可牽混講家紛紛都緣萬物非聖人所發育下文又言待人而行遂以道爲仍指天地云聖人二字不重只重道字殊不顧上章來脈矣或疑爲之聖人有窮達何能發育萬物且下文何以又云待其人也張甄陶以上古聖人中古聖人分屬二節可謂支離不通而講家分一屬天地一屬聖人尤非語意故愚今一一清邊本文正義學者毋輕忽讀過其日待其人而後行何也上三節就現成說聖人之道如此但必有聖人之

四書恆解 中庸

人始可行聖人之道其字須要剝清若謂待人而後行則與上文誠卽道之得於己者如何又言至道以凝至道此義向來含混最不可不辨明蓋道德各言之則道者理之總名德者道成於己相絜言之則道是天地人所共之道德乃人秉受善性之德而此章至德兩至道字尤不可以他處槪此一名皆有道而此一行之美皆德而所云至德則純粹以精之德也孟子言集義乃能生氣意亦如此蓋凡人秉受雖云皆善而各有偏

重如質樸恭儉仁慈謙下皆德也得一亦云良士
全備更爲善人有人焉秉氣既淸善多惡少又加
學問變化諸惡莫作衆善咸歸是全德矣而猶不
可爲至德者仁義禮樂之事躬行實踐口無
擇言身無擇行善氣固已充溢於心矣由是而存
養性天次第深造致乎美大聖神之境一以貫
萬心通造化氣塞乾坤則至道凝於身焉蓋道之
至者天命之原萬理之總而德之至者氣質中和
涵養純粹及其既成功則道大之人即全德之人
當其致力則有一分之德乃可漢一分之道後人
四書恆解　中庸　篡岫氏特圖藏
罕造精微之詣但知德外無道而不解于思此章
之言至韓文公竟謂道與德爲虛位以闢老子道
德之旨不知道有君子小人德有凶有吉以道德
二字作虛字用耳至於言道德之眞則道即天理
之總名德乃人身之所得老子道德何獨不然五
千言不言神僊與夫子言悉皆純粹而後世怪妄
之徒誣指老子不解道德經之所云則妄爲之說
其謬甚矣且所謂神僊者即中庸之道德
非有飛昇變化奇幻之說世傳方士技藝皆戲幻
小術昧者即以爲僊法豈老子之敎乎至於聖人

之德日月合明鬼神合德其神明不測之用此章
所謂至道即自來所謂神僊而修養家言謂至道
陰八百德行始可求眞入道亦至德凝至道之
說也其所謂眞人即至誠之人所謂金丹即天命
之性特其書多寓言遂令學者迷亂而妄庸之士
從而穿鑿支離棄倫常抛妻子求長生鍊金石種
種謬遂爲誕不能禁人之毋求也惟知聖人即
斥以爲聖人非神仙是聖人之外別有神仙即
仙則力行聖學自可通乎造化如禹之平成舜之
四書恆解　中庸　夏岫氏特圖藏
端拱神化無方祇此至道自然之用而一切異端
可不辨而自明矣今姑略舉其槪以明道德二字
不可混而不講他未遑贅也故君子節細言修凝
之功內外交修本末交養然是詳盡尊德性敬存
天命好仁無以尙之所以正其原道問學窮究古
今折衷以求至是所以極其用
門博文約禮功正如此而字糢上折下看此句冒
下下四句淺深相承爲學問所以究德性之具德
散著於事爲學問所以究德性之散殊也內外一
原不可單指一爲在內一爲在外德性本廣大也

承上古之聖大道光華至此而盛三代因堯舜之
道而禮明樂備之規折衷至善莫隆於文武仲尼
去堯舜遠矣而祖而述之之精一執中外此別無
學放勳元德應久如親光華以之爲宗而傳述以
詔將來其淵源若此文武之道近矣存於方策世
衰教微時人莫知嚮方仲尼則憲而章之雖列
禮修齊治平之本末以教及門謨烈顯承禮樂詩
書之遺留著爲法則其表章如斯然則百王之矩
千聖之模不於仲尼集其成哉匪特此也天以一
元化生萬類而時有遷移理無二是仲尼上律之

四書恆解

中庸

冕帨西充鄧于特圖藏

焉至變之事宰以不變之運若有定若無定惟其
中而各得其宜自一言一動以至於出處行藏胥
是道也天地本水土合成而水善流行土惟安靜仲
尼下襲之爲至誠之理運以神化之能虛而不滯
實而能該一以貫之端倪莫測故莊敬端嚴未嘗
不神明變化悉此意也然則天地之機三才之撰
不自仲尼合其妙哉夫其德盛如斯果何以能然
也人本天地之心五行之秀特自狹隘菲薄滯其
神明昏其氣質於是人遂弗如天地仲尼不然以
生安之材殫修凝之道其性已全其天已定語其

四書恆解

中庸

冕帨西充鄧于特圖藏

曲成萬物有加無已之心辟如天地之無不持載
而納諸懷抱無不覆幬而予以生成也語其純粹
光明志氣充周之致辟如四時之錯行而一元往
復如日月之代明而並照不窮也蓋惟心性之內
理氣極於精瑩斯身世之行擬議不能遽罄人不
知聖人之所以爲聖曷觀天地之所以爲天地哉
夫天地無可窮究卽萬物可以徵之萬物至不齊
矣乃其生也養也並爲育而不相害昆蟲草木各
遂其天卽各成其類不聞氣化之有未周且其消
也長也道並行而不相悖生殺制化不一其施寶

各成其用不聞義理之有偏駁以其小德言之川
流不息派衍無窮無斁悉之弗偏也以其大德言
之敦厚其化包孕靡遺無一理之不含也合而觀
之並育而生生之意無窮並行而剝復之機有定
小德而見其一本之萬殊大德而見其萬殊之一
本此天地之所以爲大也天地如此而聖人之德
亦然則其體用功能之大又何怪其然哉○中庸
一書教人盡性以全天命應應說來至大哉聖人
之道章詳言修凝推及功效見非至聖不能至此
章乃表仲尼爲法首節言其道貫往聖學綜三才

次節形其在己之性量末節復言天地之所以為大以見聖人理與天合則取譬不為夸侈次第本甚瞭如講家未晰遂覺意多重複堯舜之前非無聖人經世之制至堯舜而始見端一執中性學虞書始肇故言祖述言其尊而親之意亦在其中述則承先啟後之詞也中之為憲表章其遺法文武賴以光大舉四聖人則凡聖人皆在其中不得因此菲薄他聖天道之妙在於時聖德如天而此言律天時則專就因應無方時中之用言也對

四書恆解 〈中庸〉 犖曬氏特園藏

水土句說有動靜互為其根之意水土句不易解蓋地者水土合而成者也其在先天水浮為陽土凝為陰是天地之所以摩盪其在後天水載氣以行土含精而育是天地之所以成質天水生之故法天下法地而曰律天時襲水土以成質子思不言上而言朱子謂兼內外本末精粗言是也天地之初生也水為土和之其奠位也土養之水生之故水土者天地之化機而人身亦然天一之水裕於稟受坤靈之德厚其生成其體以為德則水以發其聰明土以厚其安貞文王演易日習坎有孚惟

心亨夫子繫易曰至哉坤元含宏廣大非深明天地之與天亦烏知襲水土之真哉次節以天地覆載日月四時喻其意量云覆載特加一持字幬字九有深意言曲成萬物範圍天下其殷殷無已之心常若持之恐墜幬之恐漏勤懇肯乎天地是為聖德之本下二句又狀其化神之意四時遞功聖人有陽陽中有陰屈伸消長相間而後成歲功動靜太和元氣周流無間其動靜消長時止時行動靜不失其時其道光明亦如四時之錯行也日月代明則充實之光輝暢於四支發於事業渾然在抱

四書恆解 〈中庸〉 䨱曬氏特園藏

而神明煥發寒暑溫暖晦朔弦望之機皆自身而具前文所言形著動變化孟子所謂美大化神皆在其中後人罕造盡性之全功以為道盡於形色之間而人身中和位育之理莫得其實佛老之徒其高者廣設譬喻人鮮能知遂以為恍惚離奇不可以訓而卑者又益之誕妄並子思此章所言皆為荒誕矣安得不愷切言之日月者乾坤之精華天地未分則日月無象而真陰真陽之純一者統於太極天地既分日月成質而真陰真陽之互宅者其為功化動而生陽靜而生陰日月斡流行之機

動中有靜靜中有動日月妙生成之體人心之靈
通乎造化心陽精而孕陰陽精而陰陽氣不能無
命陰竅而孕陽先天義理之性所由寓由義浩然
之氣以復純一之心命立而性全性盡而命固陽
性之昭者實挾日之華而光照不窮陰性之縄
繩者實具月之精而循環遞映聖人之所以知周
萬物神化無方在我性命之理爲之即在天日月
之靈共之如日月之代明此其義也存心養性立
命事天之功不深造而得則天人合一之故總不
明而仲尼之德幾如精靈物怪不可方物矣萬物
之基不以爲嫌是不相悖也前人以道字承四時
之大無可言窮特就萬物之化生以見其功用如
日月說於上下二節承接之意不明子思緣天地
道則以生殺剝復之機言如物類之制伏人事之
消息不必盡屬生養然魁以爲生之地渝以爲長
並育如禽獸草木昆蟲各遂其生各適其性即是
四書堙解　　　中庸　　　臺山　西充鮮于圓藏于
斯下二句乃承出小德大德言其一本散爲萬殊
萬殊遝歸一本理本如斯結以此天地之所以爲
大也歎想不窮而聖人之德亦然以此爲發明上
交取譬之意川流卽川流以形其周浹叉各分明

敦化敦厚其生化之原朱子所解是也
唯天下至聖爲能聰明睿知足以有臨也寬裕溫柔
足以有容也發強剛毅足以有執也齊莊中正足以
有敬也文理密察足以有別也
而民莫不信行而民莫不說
洋溢乎中國施及蠻貊舟車所至人力所通天之所
覆地之所載日月所照霜露所隊凡有血氣者莫不
尊親故曰配天
四書堙解　　　中庸　　　臺山　西充鮮于圓藏于
右第三十一章申言小德大德之意見其本屬一
原實足見諸功業而結以配天週應天地之所以
爲大
附解子思意謂觀天地之所以爲大不外小德大德

四書恆解 中庸

華如是存心義理日以消亡猶晏然自以為能大抵中庸之道罕傳牟皆然矣豈知君子心性倫常全其天理盡乎分所當為無一毫求知之想哉故下文申言君子之道之實淡簡溫三句皆兼內外而言身心靜默倫紀踐行本無華飾安得不淡然靜養天機神明之旨趣無窮動循天理愧怍之情形何有故不厭內而存養省克不過去人心以全道心外而誠敬忠恕不過盡五倫以敎人紀以宰制無多豈非至簡然一理之中涵而萬事歸於溫五常之克盡而六合可以彌綸豈非至文溫有溫厚溫和二意盛德之至容貌若愚渾全之天圭稜悉化人之見之直無處求其端倪而實聽明內朗晰極精微在中者細緻精純博厚高明景象自喻在外者縷分條析表裏精粗克盡無遺此三句該括聖人德性許多境地在內非文字所能畢宣尤非空言所能彷彿也舊說以為下學立心之始講家從而影響猜摩令子思形容於無可形容之意不明且並字面亦多晦滯幾疑子思之詞不達本矣下文知遠三句乃教人以學聖之法而言遠本於近風必有自微可以顯學者知之則無俟求諸

四書恆解 中庸

夫天地以一元生萬物而太極中函理氣統焉是以動而無動靜而無靜氣之所行即理之所見而形形色色者莫非一元所發越也人身亦然有氣而後有此形形色色莫非天性也浩然之氣本乎天地而主宰吾身乃性命之原非黃冠養後天之氣可比其粹而為仁義禮智信理之元而氣之璞也其發而為喜怒哀樂性之流而氣之著也惟本天之氣無不中和故人性皆善惟本親之氣不盡粹美故情有不正聖人養其中和之氣於一身而與天地合其體普其正大光明之氣於百為而與天地

同其用氣之至純理即存焉故持其志無暴其氣
為初學入德之門而志氣如神為君子復性之徵
易曰乾以君之坤以藏之風以散之造化之氣純
一者其神流行者其化無可見諸見於風也知風
之自則知感被乎人物者悉本於至誠而流行於
周身者必有其原本凡物者悉本於至誠而流行於
自不容已矣公孫丑問孟子浩然之氣答曰難言
子思亦後儒罕踐其事故不明其說而時解第謂
如風庚風采之風自字不可通風字亦強矣可與
於一元後儒罕踐其事故假風之自以明理氣之散著本
詩猶是上文闇然日章之義潛雖伏而孔昭幾雖
闇而必謹故有德之君子內省不疚而一念之動
必加謹懷求其無惡於志然則君子之所以不可
及即在於此人所不見謂心曲也既不可見豈非
闇然既不可及卻又日章內省二句是舉現成君
子作式樣末欸其不可及二句重用功以起第三節舊說混而不明且內省二句承不見意來爾室屋漏人
複無味相在爾室二句承不見意來爾室屋漏人

【四書恆解】 中庸 壹 西充鄰子氏特圓藏

入德義即在三句中非三者即德知此則自盡修
德之功耳第二節乃教人以修德之要引潛伏之

所不見而相在嚴焉則人所不見天實見之矣倘
不愧句該括靜存動察許多功夫在內人心之靈
本乎造化天地之賴有人者此心耳心正而神鑒
之人道以全天道以合心偽而鬼臨之人道以失
物類以羣故聖人之學以畏天命為基此章示人
闇然之修特引相在一詩蓋必如此而後息息畏
天不敢一毫妄念此為慎獨此為無惡於志下承
之曰故君子不動而敬不言而信敬則不肆信則
無偽懷於不動不言則動言可知而不愧於不
徒空空敬畏神明已也近世言理者每以神明為
妄遂令學者任其意之所發無有顧忘而乃從而
告之規矩禮度其源不清盡思古聖人
之教人臨保旦明者謂何哉故此節為全章要緊
功夫是闇然之學正面文字舊說以淡簡溫三句
為為己之心而以此節為又言君子之戒謹恐懼
無時不然與上節一例看虛實淺深不明不知上
節祇言君子之不可及在人所不見處以見闇然
之自儆此節正言懷以神明謹於動靜下文乃言
其誠敬之效可以格幽明通上下如詩所云奏假
無言時靡有爭一心之精虎並無言說而有事於

【四書恆解】 中庸 壹 西充鄰子氏特圓藏

四書恆解 上論 上冊

明生於貴胄獨能了明義理戒殺戒貪戒淫戒妄皆聖賢之道也民雖夷人天良不殊感而好善者多數千年後尚沿其教調馴可治惜佛沒後更無聖賢繼而敎化之不能如中國黃炎虞摯接續以肇文明是宇宙之大憾也而竝佛化民之功沒之可乎哉後儒斥佛老不過曰廢人倫然攷佛本竺國刹利王子娶妻曰耶輸陀羅生子曰摩睺羅十九歲於檀特山中學道靜養十二年歸妻子復聚又四十九年卒未嘗棄人倫也番僧出家佛之前已有此俗至佛死後其民自以戒定不如佛多出

化導論於禽獸特生瞿曇氏以化之其人天姿高中國言語不通嗜欲不同天憐其地之赤子無人怪誕皆託於老子老子何嘗有是耶佛本西域與又曰吾師未嘗有一毫非議也而後世一切法術者老子與夫子問答皆中正之言子贊之曰猶龍必曰楊墨佛老楊墨之道孟子言之詳矣闢佛老者始於昌黎然闢道之徒可闢老佛不可闢也何誤將來更有不可勝言者試詳論之古今稱異端將避菲薄前人之嫌而令聖賢心學不明於世其之詰者故其雜世之心雖切而言道之旨未精今

四書恆解 上論 上冊

作老子傳詳其子孫以明老子非無稽之人夫子與之游稱爲猶龍蓋易傳稱龍德而隱之意後人以爐火黃白等妄說皆託於老子而謂爲異端老子嘗有是言廷十六字爲聖學淵源莊子載老子告孔子之言曰至陰肅肅至陽赫赫肅肅出乎天赫赫出乎地實十六字所本也何者天地以至陰至陽產萬物而人得其秀靈陽性本於天而陰質滯之陰命根於地而陽精寓焉性者天地之華而性情者陰陽命之變性命各正太和保合陰陽之純全者不見其分其在先天性情存已有此俗至佛死後其民自以戒定不如佛多出

常事李根陳元裴伓七百歲何疑於老子太史公人之流而第以其退年謂有神怪不知長年古人目老子爲異端矣老子長年博學人莫識其爲聖雜以方技之流奇幻詭秘皆託於老子於是人悉記家語史記所載無非道者後世妄爲神仙之說致不近人情其於老子也亦然老子與吾子言禮而效之又經多妄造竝撰許多神異意欲尊佛反宇收養穌寡孤獨非以出家爲賢也愚民不察從中國相沿出家由秦漢而後井地壞窮民多以寺家學道如營男子學柳下惠之意然非佛本意也

雜理欲消陰陽之互宅者難返於一故人心道
心一心也而有微危之分危者陰之流微者陽之
粹也惟精則必別其陽中之陰惟一則必守其陰
中之陽陰陽變化由於天地之交精一之者善也
天地之正易曰一陰一陽之謂道繼之者善也成
之者性也夫陰陽之變化無窮而天命之不二者
為性性者太極又陰陽則性命之本而造化之機
陽中更有陽至陰至陽則其精天元地黃之始也若
肅肅赫赫狀其象而名其精天元地黃之始也若
夫本天地卽互為其根之義而天地之生成人
至乎其為世訛病因道德五千言文義字知而學
老子者又偏於一端是以儒者因流而告其始亦
原天人合一之妙旨故夫子歎其猶龍易卦惟乾
象為龍以況聖人之德而老子如之其德可不謂
如古來薰心名利違棄禮法之儒言語文字非不
燦然可觀科第功名亦復儼然達者然內而心性
克復之功未踐外而日用倫常之德不修以是為
夫子之門人豈夫子之過哉是故老佛不外一性
聖人本無二心僧羽之流愈傳愈謬則誠異端矣

四書恆解　　　上論　上冊　　堯㘶　西充鮮于氏特圜藏

欲使天下無憎道之徒必盈天地間無一夫不得
其所無一人不明其性而後可然此登一朝一夕
之故哉故五性五倫之外無大道卽技藝百家有
益於民生日用者猶形下之正也惟害理蔑紀惑
世誣民及怪妄不經之類則異端也邢昺謂異端
諸子百家之書亦非諸子百家有可取者特必
以聖人中正之道為權衡耳

子曰由誨女知之乎知之為知之不知
為不知是知也
呼其名而告之言所誨女者知之否乎知之
是知也眞則力行之為眞知不知者闕疑以待問為
知之眞則力行之為眞知不知者闕疑以待問為
知之乎見之明而信之眞者卽為知之安而行之
可無遺憾矣知之似而辨未眞者卽為不知徐
而察之不必欲速也如此則得一善舉拳服膺而
知之分量未精故呼之曰由吾平昔誨女之理可
知之行不可偏廢子路勇於行求知之功猛奮恐

附解知行不可偏廢子路勇於行求知之功猛奮恐
功可徐徐漸進是卽求知之方也蓋恐其稍以疑
似相安故慰勉之誨女二字讀斷章意甚明子路
聞過則喜惟恐有聞非強不知以為知者前人誤
解不知句竟無著落是知也句是也二字神氣亦
輕明者當自辨之

四書恆解　　　上論　上冊　　㗺㘶　西充鮮于氏特圜藏

子曰不患無位患所以立不患莫己知求為可知也

其無如禮何也

附解事有精粗道無大小自天子至於庶人皆有各盡之道而能處之咸宜至大不易然聖人曰修己即可安百姓安性即可贊化育何也萬物之理已裕於一理盡其性而己修則天人萬物之理已裕原故能至明以擇眾善若泉陶耕稼之舜即可垂裳傳巖至虛以容眾善若漁陶耕稼之舜即可垂裳傳巖與求為可知夫子已示之也若不知養性修身實功而欲患此不患彼豈非空言無補

四書恆解　上論　上冊　宅飒西充鮮于圓藏

子曰參乎吾道一以貫之曾子曰唯參所金反唯上聲○一無二也

渭濱乃與商周豈能小而不能大哉自聖學罕傳不知修身不得不臨其才器而節取之此章夫子為門人言欲其自修實德以所以理誠於身而以之應事無不宜貫之之謂曾子果會其旨子出門人他子詢曰曾子以守約之學而曾子果會其旨子出門人問曰何謂也曾子曰夫子之道忠恕而已矣行實心日忠以己諒人心日恕要一誠而已
會子發子意以曉門人本末精粗在是矣
附解天地人無二理也在人日性在天地日太極言

其渾然粹然不可得而名象則日無極即太極也人受天地之中以生則太極之理全在此身聖人祗是全其天命之性故蘊於中則渾然粹然者如乾坤之靜專翕也其始靜養浩然之氣動審天地之成形成象也其由淺而深由勉企安行之以誠持之以息則凡人皆可作聖夫子自言十五志學七十而從心不踰孟子言有諸己以至化神其功夫次第非聖人不授非誠恆交致不能竟其功曾子從夫子久於窮理盡性之學篤行蓋非一日矣

四書恆解　上論　上冊　尖飒西充鮮于圓藏

夫子知其中之所存者已熟定不致疲鶩於外故詔以一貫謂天下萬變不外乎中天命之源已徹則萬事萬物以一理宰之而有餘耳曾子果能喻之應之遠而無疑門人學未深造安能知之曾子告以忠恕忠則實心行天理而不留隱憾恕則推心體萬物而不存偏私誠能如此久久不倦則至誠可以無所不孚至公可以無所不容而一貫之旨曉然無餘蘊矣書旨本明白易見講家多為影響揣測之談遂令聖賢實義類於口頭禪語艮可浩歎至一字祇是一理字但理有本末精粗散為

四書恆解 上論 上冊

萬殊者無窮歸於一本者有定中庸言天下之大本曰中中一之實也即天命之性也在天曰太極在物為理統言之曰道以其至真無二曰誠以其為天地生生之意所含曰仁人之秉天地之靈粹其先天則皆性也故虞廷但言心而未言性其後天則性雜於情矣故湯始別之曰性而不第言心大學言心不言性中庸言性不言心夫子言性相近孟子言性善語殊而義實一不實踐其功亦不能剖析如此章一貫竟說得十分離奇似言亦不乎達化窮神則自身之理不明即聖人之

後世禪和子拈花微笑棒喝虛鋒不知曾子以忠恕明之已是說得十分透切乃謂其移下一層說是不知聖人神明不測止是理極其精至於事天明事地察亦從忠恕入手行到十分二字簡易精微忠之久而極其誠恕之久而極其公至誠至公之不過一言一行何事不可格何人不可為乎二字淺言試問天下何人不可為乎萬姓不識神不外乎是陋劣儒家得禪家守空之學以後天識神為先天元性即靈通之至而不能修齊治平文人鑒之以窮理讀書為務有才智之明而弗知仁義

四書恆解 上論 上冊

之本故淹雅擅長而不能倫紀無忝所謂忠恕二字又安能時習深造且夫佛曰明心見性謂盡其心者知其性而非即以心為性也即心即佛專指天理之心而言知性亦如求仁即仁之語僧流失真以空明妙了為知性其智者已譏之矣景岑曰無量劫來生死癡人喚作本來人因一貫之唯有頓悟一家其明者亦誚之矣陳致虛曰曾子當年一聲唯誤了閻浮多少人故以後天之氣為浩然非文佛之本然以後天之氣為浩然亦非孟子之所謂儒者知誚僧羽之誕而忠恕所以一貫之故又不明是何異己迷途而笑人問津耶夫養浩然之氣以至於不動心此孟子發明孔子為仁之義也而以後天呼吸之氣為一元之氣則非仁人心也謂其為天命之性也而以知覺運動之心為天命之性尤謬蓋先天後天之義不明即存心養性之功不實養之學不深則雖欲求其忠與恕而心之私妄不除必不能至一貫之境哉佛之真者曰修宣於書君子安可以不亟求其故哉佛之真者曰修真空不空妙有不有非偏於空寂之道之真者曰修真養性入聖超凡非涉於幻妄因僧道流傳失實

四書恆解 上論 上冊 夏𪾔西充鮮于氏特圖藏

不可中輟致負夫子一片婆心也夫子之文章凡一言一動莫非由性而發第其迹顯著其事易求其得失精粗易見故學之深者因端以會其原即學之淺者亦即事而明其理可得而聞也夫子之言性與天道性者人之所以生天道者天之所以立在天爲天道在人爲性非有二也但非由博而約窮理盡性以至於命則無以知天之所以與人之所以合天而萬事萬物不外乎是在夫子未嘗不言而學者功力未至言之而亦不知故不可得而聞也語意全是勉人自造非謂夫子有所不傳已今獨有所得時解均誤或曰先儒皆言子罕言性天而子反之何也曰性者天之理而人心之良聖人敎人誠意正心惟欲其全性耳故窮理者窮其合於性否也致知者致其天理之明也凡一念之發一行之動合天理則善違天理則惡樂法度皆以維持人心之天理舍性不言而何哉第性之散於萬物者循其法度而修之可以盡過即可以修身性之本於天命者究其精微而踐之必由漸進乃可企於化神故子亦常言性與天道使人知萬事悉本於天理然而人不能盡曉則

四書恆解 上論 上冊 夏𪾔西充鮮于氏特圖藏

以實學未至不能强求其通也曰文明言夫子之言性與天道是夫子非不言乃言之而人自不明耳乃或以爲不言何哉

子路有聞未之能行惟恐有聞
善無窮而力有限賴勤恆以全之子路勇於義特表之以爲法

附解書曰非知之艱行之維艱又曰言之匪艱行之維艱故善恆有聞行者百無一二也子路實見得義理無盡而嗜之也切如饑渴之於飲食猶不足以方之此記者所以特地形容暢惕𢍰云如畫工寫物妙於設色憑空摹擬一氣嫁神颺勃勃不可遏抑之子路是矣充子路之量舜之聞善若決江河卽此而造也可覘哉

子貢問曰孔文子何以謂之文也子曰敏而好學不恥下問是以謂之文也
子貢文子名圉衞大夫諡文子貢好問又子貢之所宜急也故告之如此學以聞見言

附解古人諡以曾名非有大惡不被之惡名固宜子言勤長之意也文子素行不端子貢疑之固宜子言勤學好問故以爲文是以之云猶言如是已耳聖人取人之宏固不待言而策勵子貢亦在其中非第爲孔圉解圍也學問淺看若聖賢之眞學問則文

皆以粟十車列館門外每車一秉有五籔籔卽庾也是館廩之粟計十車有十五秉冉子以三分之一予其家頗確

子謂仲弓曰犂牛之子騂且角雖欲勿用山川其舍諸犂利之反駢息營反○子告仲弓以用人之道當發於鄙賤不拘資格如騂牛雖出於犂牛必爲宰時言取士不拘貴賤類多何氏文騂赤色角者周正中犧牲所用以祭也

附解朱子沿何晏邢昺舊說謂仲弓父賤行惡子故喻之張惕菴謂仲弓爲宰時子告以官人之道其識甚卓從之蓋周家鄕舉里選至春秋而法弊取人惟以名望寒賤類多屈抑子故曉之程伊川亦言聖人必不肯對人子說人父不善因仲弓父賤行惡古註遂誤解又張氏以家語爲不足信亦誤仲弓父卽賤而行惡子豈有斥擬犂牛之理

子曰回也其心三月不違仁其餘則日月至焉而已矣仁卽性也其心爲仁以生旅無窮故日仁先天之心純乎仁後天之心雜於欲克已復禮以全仁卽所以全其心之本體也簡存三月而更形其心與理合之時久所謂履空也日月至焉則亡無時之存

天理之存

附解明明說個其心三月不違仁是就後天之心而言矣蓋人得天地之心以生卽性卽孟子所謂仁人心也但此純乎天理之心在未生以前故

四書恆解 上論 下冊 六 唯西充鮮于氏特園藏

日人生而靜天之性至有生以後形氣拘累物誘緣之而生耳目口體所觸知覺運動之靈與物相引而天理遂以難純所以然者人得乾坤精氣而生先天純乎乾坤之氣體靜而無爲此性之所以無不善也後天非乾坤之本然性拘於質而爲命命乘乎氣而爲心心之靈乃雜於物誘而不能常存其天昊故聖人敎人復性不然心卽性矣而何復之云哉但復性之功非以義理之心養其浩然之氣必無以去氣質之陰而發其剛大之本體故孔門求仁博文以析其理約禮以存其誠而知止得止之功不能盡筆之於書也大學言明明德中庸言致中和而曰盡其性皆謂全此仁心卽可以無所不可周室盈禮法盡毀孟子乃指出養氣之功而其源則本於孔氏也後人見孔子未言養氣而孟子言之雖不敢謂孟子爲非卻不知我善養吾浩然之氣知心與氣之所以相關則知氣非後天之氣心亦非後天之心故黃冠導養不足爲養浩然而禪宗靜心亦不足爲求仁之功自宋以來儒者知聖學不外於心矣而不明心有先

四書恆解 上論 下冊 七 唯西充鮮于氏特園藏

四書恆解 上論 下冊

後天之辨故力辨禪宗守心而亦未免以心爲性
夫仁義禮智信五性也而實祇一性所涵其在先
天渾然在中者心也卽性也其在後天發焉而有
五性之一端存焉而無天性之渾成以心含陰氣
不能禁其無動於欲也性養活然之氣功深理熟
則心復乎先天之本體而渾然在中粹然無二靜
而萬善俱涵動而一私不雜心卽仁矣不然告子
之不動心非道卽原憲之克伐怨欲不行亦不爲
仁若此章言同也其心三月不違仁則言其養氣
功牟有諸己而天理漸多私欲漸少每靜存之時
實境因隱微難名藉三月狀之不然三月從何算
起日月至焉者候得而候失一日之內心有渾然
春夏秋冬各成爲一季丞著功用三月不違仁形
之一候一月之內心有渾含之大致其功亦非易
容其卓立之心體居然天理穩固正是三十而立
至子卽顏子以勵門人此章仁字蓋以全體之仁
而言也若一端之仁則雖常人一日之內亦有數
事而諸賢乃日月至於理爲不通矣

季康子問仲由可使從政也與子曰由也果於從政

四書恆解 上論 下冊 九

乎何有曰賜也可使從政也與曰賜也達於從政
乎何有曰求也可使從政也與曰藝於從政乎何
有與平聲○三子藉升斗以就學康子輕之而問子
明逵藝才其長欲其同升諸公也果見義必爲達事理
足應變

附解周制有官始有祿而春秋時士之無田者更衆
故有爲貧而仕之道孔門諸賢來學於魯卽藉升
斗以爲貧甘心權門鷹犬也三子仕於
季氏康子亦未以爲意從政之問其意甚輕夫子
極許之所以堅其意而欲其薦於公也如下章閔
子乃可以無需祿仕而不爲季氏宰耳三子惟冉
求之仕爲非甚矣讀書論世之難也詳見下章

子周遊二子卽無藉於微祿也前人不明此義以
由求之仕爲非甚矣讀書論世之難也詳見下章

求魯人終仕於魯由賜二子不久而卽反衛蓋夫

四書恆解 上論 下冊 九

子路季氏使閔子騫爲費宰閔子騫曰善爲我辭焉如有
復我者則吾必在汶上矣費音祕爲去聲汶音問。
閔子騫名損淡水名在齊南魯北境上費季氏之巖邑閔子
豈爲之私用故婉辭之如使同升諸公則不然矣

附解聖賢之仕所以行道上爲君下爲民而已爲貧
而仕者一官一邑其職易稱然亦必可以行其志
而無害於義乃可否則苟祿矣子路冉有仕於季
氏人多非之不知當時世官擅柄寒賤無由進身

四書恆解 上論 下冊 畢(呼)西充鞠于氏持圜藏

樂其與己志趨相同樂乎道而忘情於得失言門人學道者多然能純乎義理而無外馳時則甚難不知道在己而可以濟世亦何不可藏身時而用也則行時而舍也則藏此意惟爾知之則我之行藏惟爾共之耳至於夫子之道蟠天際地無所不可顏子尚未能之前人過高視之遂使人謂道高不免短命而聖人化神之道亦囿於氣數則誤天下後世不淺登故薄顏子哉蓋顏子得志亦可治平然必不能如夫子此章喜其同志欲其由此企於大成以為無加則非也觀下文子路誰與之問是方

子曰富而可求也雖執鞭之士吾亦為之如不可求從吾所好富厭〇周衰有德者無祿而士或無思之道哉行軍亦重事子恐其將以易心故教之非之道哉行軍亦重事子恐其將以易心故教之非子路如暴虎憑河者流也果爾何能使民有勇知

夫子自言用行舍藏顏子可與豈謂其已全有己

附解先王之世民皆得所有德則題周衰而選舉私士乃多貧求富一念非聖賢不能免然求之未必得而已失己幸而得之所謂不義如浮雲

者也但此非成德無以自持夫子特示以不可求若己嘗求富者然能蘇東坡曰如防盜者開門發篋示以無則廢然反矣誠善喻矣

子之所慎齊戰疾問之者皆反。幽明一理禍人一氣尤嚴敬畏故齊戰非得已疾為由生篤其仁孝慎何容已非第為得失死生也因當時三者多忽玩故記

附解夫子固無所不慎也而特記三者何哉自慎獨之學不講人以天為遠以神為妄凡祭祀之禮徒文而已豈知聖人心與天通道與天合然猶懍相在嚴對越未嘗稍肆也況常人乎兵者聖王不得已而用所以威不軌而昭文德春秋爭城爭地糜爛其民尚何慎焉疾之生也一由於七情之內傷一由於六氣之失調然苟正心修身起居飲食咸中於度則精神強固志氣清明自可延年卻老況時懷全受全歸之義安敢一息不謹也此記者特地教人之意

子在齊聞韶三月不知肉味曰不圖為樂之至於斯也漢書曰陳公子完奔齊韶樂在焉世業精專聖心相感聲容意象獨會其微所謂斯者音之元而道之精盛德天運人事合而備太和之蘊也肉味適於心口此之不知神與為化三月極言其久

附解後世樂教罕興此等文義遂多影響之談宋儒

四書恆解 上論 下冊 星氏特園藏

以三月不知肉味爲滯於物從史記加學之二字不知記者止是形容夫子心一於韶許久不能忘置耳凝滯於物謂膠固也若義理悅心忘肉豢之悅口乃是止理何爲凝滯豈由未知韶之所以至也天地之元寄於人心心德之至者與造化相函之而天心之太和則萬古虛明絕無壅滯人爲天地之心而氣秉陰陽質有拘滯聖人不能無藉食味別聲被色而生此形氣之所以不能盡侔於天地且也遭遇難齊雖以聖人盡倫盡制而堯水湯旱禹痛父四人倫之不幸一毫留憾隱微則被諸聲容即難與一元無心之化相似若韶之作也際乎成承禪讓本化神而宣暢豫由皇古以來適當無爲之候而舜自底豫後君臣父子夫婦兄弟五倫之際更無一毫抱歉故其樂宛然氤氳太和之氣而天人合一千載如新齊因陳氏韶樂獨精夫子德與舜符既篤嗜好既久而猶不知肉味固其所也矣必謂方學之乎斯之一言蓋言不能而味之無窮即天地奧妙備於人而著於韶者也後人既莫由覩韶之真又或未知子與舜心德之

四書恆解 上論 下冊 星氏特園藏

微則固不免髣髴而難肖冉有曰夫子爲衛君乎子貢曰諾吾將問之入曰伯夷叔齊何人也曰古之賢人也曰怨乎曰求仁而得仁又何怨出曰夫子不爲也衛人知之輒以拒晉而宋立輒入于戚實將并帝之諫敵輒所以拒如宋立公子魚於戚景泰爲之計非仁矣晉師既退輒迎亦不能決此權宜則聞夷齊之怨輒求無所忌憚奉晉竟然自兆時勢變古未得仁萬乘齊國卹求其仁得其心晏然心之所以不以國事實亦哉伊齊讓國事理國掩耳而諫而詳見附解附解稱兵拒父輒孰皆知其非冉有子貢何以不知且夫子曰亂邦不居以子拒父亂執甚焉子貢然於可乎本朝張甄陶據古註左氏辨證之其說甚長然猶有誤者今正明之按衛靈公叛晉從齊晉趙鞅與范中行氏構難齊衛助范中行氏鞅忿之魯哀公元年齊伐晉救邯鄲圍五鹿又會於乾侯救范氏魯亦同齊衛鮮圍伐晉取棘蒲二年夏四月丙子衛侯元卒六月乙酉趙鞅納蒯聵於戚相距七十日其入戚也使蒯聵八人衰絰僞自衛逆者告於門哭而入遂居之則知鞅以蒯聵爲餌聵衛實將吞衛夫子書曰于戚明鞅志不在趙鞅帥師明鞅之包藏禍心曰于戚明

四書恆解 上論 下冊 吳氏特圓藏

保全社稷也若顯然拒父倘得為孝衞多君子公論安在哉且夫子亦受其公養何也故予以夫子春秋斷之而補張氏之說如此子貢問夷齊止是要討出求仁不怨意以輒立非得已但其心若不忍忘父必不久據君位矣太史公作伯夷列傳因伯夷事蹟罕見特因夫子稱為賢人孟子以為聖人不可不傳故以孔子為主先言載籍極博必折衷於六藝而六藝尤以夫子為賢為聖信如許由等事是夫子既稱夷齊為賢人則誠賢矣而以所聞軼事言之殊可異焉所言夷齊叩馬一事不可信而歸結到伯夷之賢得夫子而名益彰事采薇之歌怨耶非耶蓋疑其與夫子之言不合見已作傳全是信夫子不信軼事後人不知其文義反以史公不信者為真亦可謂不善讀書矣詳見泰伯至德章夷齊皆以全父為重儲中子文叔齊全父之名說得甚好

而富且貴於我如浮雲

子曰飯疏食飲水曲肱而枕之樂亦在其中矣不義
而富貴者言以身示教欲人自得其樂也樂在性分自不因境而移富貴豈必卻之不義則甯貧賤矣
浮雲非實境也疏食也朱子曰飯食之也疏食麤飯

四書恆解 上論 下冊 吳氏特圓藏

附解時解沾滯夫子言似東方朔自譽非也聖人心如太虛於義理所在皆以誠應之而非有心也若非義之事即毫髮無能入心非強卻之彼自無緣得入當時學者於聖人亦知道義之美矣而涵養未純當察或疎有時外慕於不義之富貴故子曉之而言吾身自有真樂果得其樂雖至困亦在其中人世不常且本非真也飲食起居其事甚微然無常之詞非自詡也飲食起居常常如是故為至困之即於心有不安蔬水曲肱常常如是故為至困之其樂亦有得於己而精進鼓舞之意多夫子則與道為化而天機益溢之趣長固不能無分也

子曰加我數年五十以學易可以無大過矣假○易之為書廣大悉備然皆天地之理具於人身著於萬事者不得其原雖踐其實五十者圖書中土之義其天地之元而性命之本難窺天地之奧此章為門人上智者言欲其本然則心性倫常可假年而後可中之無大過日假年者易學也受人之本然則心性倫常可假年而後可見

附解天地之理皆吾身之理窮理盡性以至於命而後天理純熟施之萬事無不宜天地之理奚在一

-223-

陰一陽之謂道而太極則陰陽之蘊也動而無動
靜而無靜太極之體而動靜既形則陰陽遂分陰
陽迭運消長變化五行以昭五行以土為主其播
於四時著為萬物質之所區各有名象而元氣流
行如環不動則土為之樞土在先天渾然者無名
土在後天凝然者各給木火同居金水為朋以生
數言各得其五以成數言各得三五天五地十天
地之數已全天地之理氣渾合無間此所以生生
而不窮變化而不息人身一小天地也天地理氣
之全惟人獨稟故曰天地之心萬物皆備全而受
者全而歸止是完得先天太極之體太極在人日
性性者天地之命五也十也即數以言天地也不
敢自言法天地而曰五十也以學謙言之即數以窮理
可通天地之理以宰萬物之理耳而豈字之誤哉
或疑天地非常人可學不知天地止是一個誠字
止此一理萬古不貳故曰誠日誠者天地之聖人
果實之生意人能全此一理即為至誠之聖
人心如天地之覆載即為至善德者得此也誠者
誠此也人人皆有此理人人可為如大路然故曰
道以其為人人之所以生則曰性性者心之主心者

四書恆解

上論 下冊

吳 西充鮮于 氏特園藏

之命
也五也十也但非謂後天塊然之土乃先天一元
愚故不得已而質言之也尋常亦知受中中即土
數紛紛立義舍本求末於是夫子此章之義不明
易一書天人萬物之理備焉而數千年來理氣象
無非性氣質不得而累之萬物不得而淆之矣周
存有覺之心養無為之性馴至乎天人合一則心
性之用心純乎性先天則然心囿於質後天則然

四書恆解

上論 下冊

吳 西充鮮于 氏特園藏

九行交
易也
附解夫子祗刪定詩書至漢始出人尊為經當洙泗
子所雅言詩書執禮皆雅言也朱子曰雅常也執守
之文皆雅記義之文皆執記義之文也禮樂俱琴
瑟弦歌無故不離典墳師索記義以是誦習
周公所制時王之法當執而不違者常言以是誦習
講學時不過私以訓示門人至禮樂乃一王之法
夫子一介匹夫斷無私為刪定者不過當時王政
不行禮已凌亂夫子折衷是非以身為法間一
語門人孰是孰非使人循習今戴記所言其大略
可見也樂則因師摯等交遊私自告語喜其得
正人多未解動言夫子訂禮樂不知為下不倍之
義此章亦門人私記夫子教人之意非謂夫子自
我作古不遵王章六代之學各有詩歌而周公所

定用之閨門鄉國以淑性情者於日用尤切不可不講明而切究之書者聖人治天下之跡聖門無詞章博雜之學周制無鴻博文學之求則所讀之書自黃炎以降載道德而切身心者皆是也禮兼內外精粗大小之條春秋王制已豫人以禮爲煩苦否則嫌其樸陋子則身體以敎人故曰四方來學禮於孔子蓋非此無以束己而成德皆雅言也記者有得而歎憶之詞

葉公問孔子於子路子路不對子曰女奚不曰其爲人也發憤忘食樂以忘憂不知老之將至云爾涉反

附解葉公驚異夫子而問子路不對以深言或不能知淺言又不盡蓋亦愼重之道也故曰女奚不曰發憤學修身望天下若不言則人將高覗之否則誕置之非所以同人於道無窮聖心亦與爲無不必其未得蓋惟有得於心精進自不能已憤之至而樂生樂之深而益憤道無窮聖心亦與爲無一息倘存不能自已又何知老之將至耶此聖人極眞實語至平常實不易及蓋恆篤爲難耳憤窮

四書恆解 上論 下冊 羋州 氏特圜藏

○葉公問子路不對則啟其感子故曉以憤樂之功爲無異人也發憤求之勇樂得之深其至誠不息物累皆忘亦已見矣

附解祗此一理在天曰太極在人曰性其散見於萬事萬物者皆一理所充周也聖人生知不過氣質清明人倫日用是非之理自然而知天地之理何以在己己之性何以與天地萬物相通必由學而造至禮樂名物垂之於古驗之於今者尤當一體察參互考證返求諸身乃能得其會通究其精微當時門人情而目子生知子特告以實學信也非謙也學如不及猶恐失卽敏字註腳

子不語怪力亂神語怪以告人也人者天地萬物之物力重於聯亂生於神道主心失其正道反其常理而人必以怪生神道人不待問而語之則人必求其本也故亦不語

附解語告也前人或以語爲言又或以爲問亦不皆非也大易闡幽明春秋垂訓戒詩書存治忽怪力亂神子皆嘗言之若門弟子問尤必爲之辨之豈不告哉蓋怪生於反常能盡人道則怪自息春

子曰我非生而知之者好古敏以求之者也。好學者謂子生知而子誘之蓋學而不已乃至於聖古前人特書禮樂凡益於身心者皆是好學慕求實體敏速也

與前不憤之憤異祇是欣動奮發前人謂憤樂相反者太泥看憤字未知聖人深處

秋書怪皆使人修德以弭非奇其事而傳之也德
輕而後力重仁義治人安用力哉亂反常之至子
故不忍言神秉天命其鑒察人於幽獨之中而無
往不赫赫者君子以之修慝不一毫肆也然而神
必不應且降之殃世俗諂瀆鬼神矯之者又以明
神爲誣於是放情肆志無所不爲其爲害彌甚子
故未嘗不待問而告蓋人神一理人道盡則神饗
之非謂其恍惚而不語也易曰天且不違而況於
鬼神

四書恆解　上論　下冊　塞仙　西充鮮于特圓藏

子曰三人行必有我師焉擇其善者而從之其不善
者而改之諸於事其能擇則必自窮理中來也一行
一理順天理而天且可合何況於神若無德而神
且有如是

附解此章爲求師者言師不在人而在己果能自得
師即三人行必有之特患不自反求雖日與明師
相對無益也非竟謂師之可無擇而從此非平
日有學問思辨五者何由知其善惡而力行之故
不明乎善不誠乎身乃學者第一義天下未必皆
甘爲不肖之人緣無窮理之功則自以爲是而實
非謂人爲非而不知其是也

子曰天生德於予桓魋其如予何懟也徒反。德天
而天自弗達患難不能傷也不言德可言天全天理
生我以德謙辭相魋也出於桓公故又稱
桓氏魋欲害孔子事見史記

附解人之生者德也無德則雖生而猶死人皆有可
以達天之德而弗踐其功則沒沒而生悠悠而盡
矣夫子平日一言一動莫不以天爲依歸所謂事
天如事親者也天祇此理天不能外
理即何能不與子之德生德者天全德則夫子之
自言則以爲天實生我之德不敢言德合天也天
既生子魋安能害子此必門人恐懼以此安之故
不覺自露其眞也後世不得其解則以爲聖人之
德本天授非由學力而自棄其德即自違於天矣
可勝慨哉

四書恆解　上論　下冊　塞仙　西充鮮于特圓藏

子曰二三子以我爲隱乎吾無隱乎爾吾無行而不
與二三子者是丘也隱隱秘與猶示也門人疑子道
幽深而子言已無事不與二三

附解前人謂夫子作止語默無非教其理是而出自
夫子自言則非也聖人無自譽之詞周家禮明樂
備小學大學之法至春秋人已視爲虛文
甚或厭苦而不爲之夫子身體以教其徒四方學

以詳無恨之狀欲人常自省察免於此也
子釣而不綱弋不射宿朱子曰綱以大繩繫網絕流
宿鳥聖人不以口腹戕生命釣弋以生絲繫矢而射宿
以為養與祭祀忍盡取襲取之乎
附解天生百穀以養民而禽獸魚鼈食之有時取之
有節義祭尊賢之外不以己故輕屠物命也義當
釣弋而不綱宿甘旨以毒生靈君子傷之戒
用無節滋味日新窮甘旨以毒生靈君子傷之戒
殺放生所以養吾心之仁而推錫類之孝孔子達庖
伐一樹殺一獸不以其時非孝孟子曰君子遠庖
廚聖賢仁至義盡自有權衡也佛家茹素戒殺以

四書恆解 上論 下冊 契如西充鮮于圜藏

戒乎貪殘暴珍之徒於人心不為無補然必以旦
為例而至豺虎亦可優容祭養不須珍饌則倒置
冠裳因噎廢食實非中道梁武之流不知代天理
物之大經妄期不死之異術未立綱常徒廢牢享
何堪一噱若夫佛經謬妄認假為真貽誤後人蓋
非一類即如捨身飼虎乃喻言涵養心性以性為
乾金養於坤土謂之乳哺西金而竟作實事豈知
佛當日為西方主忍辱化民慈悲立教不過如聖
人仁廉恭儉之意亦以夷情好鬪好殺故以此教
之所謂因俗制宜者也其實西域衣皮食鮮乃其

土風至今達賴喇嘛門下餐氂牛飲酥酪而誦經
不輟曷嘗蔬果為生耶中國僧流乃國家藉以收
養窮民彼既不知心性功亦不識經文多贗偏
執一說㝠不足辨若夫負罪引慝悔過己之一徑
五府之心外絕屠狗之緣亦未始非修己之一徑
而王公士庶致齊散齊清其神明以誠祭祀自古
聖人已然豈可與異端同誚愚因張南軒之言恐
人弗察而一概相量故詳論之
子曰蓋有不知而作之者我無是也多聞擇其善者
而從之多見而識之知之次也而言此欲人務窮理

四書恆解 上論 下冊 毛忤西充鮮于圜藏

附解聖王在上禮樂法度修明小學大學人習之以
成德而賢才悉奮無家自為書者春秋
道衰學廢百家雜興大都未聞大學之道稍有一
得遂自以為奇而妄作以誤後夫子既不能有位
以其道正天下則取聖人之典籍而刪訂之以教
其徒非欲後世取法亦就己分內所當為者之當
刪訂之時議子者則以為僭聲子者則以為奇子
故言天下古今之義理有一定權衡吾人或有所
作必深知其理而後非妄世蓋有不知而遽作之

者我無是也惟是博探眾論或考之古或詢之今
多聞矣而自加詳擇必其善者而後從之凡古今
所遺多見而默識於心折衷成法精審無疑果其
瞭然於心而不謬乎天理人情之極則脗合乎前
聖後聖之心源然後敢語諸門人載諸簡策若有
一毫未精必不為也此乃某平生區區所得力豈
敢謂與聖作同符哉亦自心酌理稍求無愧知之
次也然而擇也非中有權衡安能知之無差故
在夫子為即本以達未在學者當即委而竊源未
可專憑聞見而不存義亦不可空言心性而弗博
哉

四書恆解

上論 下冊

牽州 西充鮮于
氏特園藏

涉尊德性道問學固不可偏廢也三代下書籍汗
牛充棟而存聖人之真者幾何夫子蓋有以預憂
之厭後言龐事雜卒召秦火豈非妄作者階之厲

互鄉難與言童子見門人惑見賢遍反○互鄉今徐
鄉之惡而子曰與其進也不與其退也唯何甚人潔
己以進與其潔也不保其往也
竝疑童子子曰進謂見來退謂入於
已甚上三句釋見童子之意下推言之意凡人
潔己皆當許其自新不僅一童子也往前日
附解此章本無錯簡與進三句貼童子言下人字推
開說聖人視天下無不可化之人第患其不知向

善耳既來見即有向道之心尚計較其習之惡
豈復曲成之仁哉後世儒者或高自位置而令少
年負氣之流激而入於不肖然後歎聖人之量遠
也互鄉一統志在商水縣春秋為陳地王伯厚援
王無咎以為亳州鹿邑縣今從寰宇記

子曰仁遠乎哉我欲仁斯仁至矣仁天理而具於心
諸也自心而不徇天
知循理是達於仁者由不欲仁也故示之

附解仁即性也以其為天地生生之理如果有仁故
曰仁人心未生以前粹然渾然性本善也心皆仁
也既生以後氣質拘七情擾心雜陰邪私欲以動
欲習於惡俗便其私情而不顧義理之安則以仁
為難能夫子即曰諄諄焉不能從也此章故翻切
曉之言仁即我身之理全其為仁實我自全我之
理耳特患縱其有覺之心昧其虛明之性則仁即
己有亦無由安於其宅苟能一念欲仁則一念之
轉機即天瓦之無失仁斯至矣甚言克復之非難
以詔及門但此欲仁之念必持之至堅守之至久

四書恆解

上論 下冊

堯州 西充鮮于
氏特園藏

心不皆仁矣聖人教人復性之學由下學而上達
其中功夫次第非一言可了然皆本人心天理之
自然而為之節文非有身外之事也奈人溺於嗜

即有溝洫經洫水而復堙禹既平水土矣及其在位又復詳加經畫使野無不耕之田民無不獲之利故曰盡力其制則九夫為井井間廣深各四尺曰溝十里為成成間廣深各八尺曰洫宮室第以安身溝洫所以便民示以法制責成有司非必日溝十里為成成間廣深各八尺曰洫宮室第以親愻宮室天子自有制度非是故為齊陋與齊民等服愻宮室天子自有制度非是故為齊陋與齊民等但粗足規模從其樸儉不於此用心耳觀禹不以載飲食衣服宮室之財用甚備蓋聖人不以累民未嘗不以天下自養特去取彼此適得乎中

四書恆解
上論 下冊
堃 西充鮮于特圓藏 氏

有斷不可與常例者耳非夫子表之禹之無間何以明於後世

子罕第九 凡三十章

子罕言利 句 與命 句 與仁 也與示之詳子曰吾無行也與
附解自漢人誤註此章歷代因之於是人以求仁為妄想志仁者無貪求記夫子敎人防弊固正其本如此
難知命為未務即欲人不求利亦不可得其貽誤非淺鮮也今正明之常人言命謂窮通得喪生而已然此大惑也夫子繫易曰窮理盡性以至於命

四書恆解
上論 下冊
堃 西充鮮于特圓藏 氏

五十而知天命祇此天理命於人曰性主於天曰命先儒分義理之命氣數之命說是矣然竟謂二者判然則又非蓋天以一元之理一元之氣而流行於品物萬古而不窮此天之命也人得天之真理真氣而生果能全其所賦則天之太極我之太極統於義理之命而非氣化衰之理悉悖乎天心而氣化衰正則失其所以為人之理不能相囿苟其心理固全備而命由我立氣化不能相囿苟其心理壞必不能支是氣化之命悖乎天心而氣化衰生而已分兩端也從古聖賢言命曰天命靡常峻命不易盖天雖高明莫測然祇一理而已此理命不易盖天雖高明莫測然祇一理而已此理
天為太極在人為性人者天地之主也盡人道而天道備焉天與我同此理安得不與我同此命故
順命立命至命皆以在我之理合乎天心孔孟之命不必富貴福澤也即貧賤而亦享天心而是也故曰久不在兹匪人其如予何信己之命必如聖人之至命立命然苟知天之命止此一理則天之命蓋純乎義理而氣數不足言矣其次未能順理而行正諒不謀利計功雖未必皆合天心亦必有善無惡而天固將維持安全之若以命為有定幸而聰明富貴則侈然自肆悖理蔑義

章首夫子發問之意又以曾點之問三子是證典己之故又不知三子者之言何如一節是夫子許三子亦何孟浪也張氏椿曰營有二沂水經注沂出蓋縣艾山東南逕東莞縣故城西與出黃狐山之小沂水合至下邳縣入泗此大沂水也又泗水注泗逕魯城西南合折水出魯城東南尼上山西北卽顏母致禱處平地發泉此小沂水也愚按周正建子而民事仍從夏時此言莫春仍夏時也詳見春秋註

顏淵第十二凡二十四章

四書恆解　下論　上冊　壬姓　西充鮮于圖藏

顏淵問仁子曰克己復禮為仁一日克己復禮天下歸仁焉為仁由己而由人乎哉請問其目子曰非禮勿視非禮勿聽非禮勿言非禮勿動顏淵曰雖不敏請事斯語矣

顏淵問仁子曰仁卽性也以其為天理故曰仁己私欲根於心陰陽非由外附者也兼內外而言謂天理自然之條理復其理萬事萬理莫不統於仁一以貫之義由己不由人欲顏子以實用其力殺其性分之私而成天理之全故顏子進道之始功以其寶美故夫子詳之特詳

附解仁者人之所以為人卽性也在天曰太極第此理在先天渾然粹然者無稍欠闕有生以後氣質

四書恆解　下論　上冊　癸㑰　西充鮮于圖藏

有諸己而充實而光輝而化神有許多功夫次第求放心而歸於中極至虛至靜以生浩然之氣由陰火之靈動不息故也為仁者以安止之法理存乎心而心體賜中含陰為善難為惡易皆此滓也人身秉天地之氣而生其異於禽獸者理之大為仁一句言其在我己者何氣質中之陰己復禮為仁語其本末之道也終功效總括言之及再問而後示以下學之功效非一端顏子問仁之寶夫子因其天資高明將始使之靜而存養動而省察內外交修本末交養功拘而七情擾天理不勝人欲矣夫子以求仁教人

心非可以強制也必虛靜以養之克己者天理充實之後渾然在抱陰私之氣全無有覺之人心悉聽命於純一之天性如克而勝之耳非天人交戰無不善因以攻之復禮者復性也人未生以前性本有衡為以氣質拘累物欲牽引遂失其本來之性克己至淨而天理返乎性始故曰復也然夫子不日理而日禮者理之本體渾然耳著於外而始有迹象禮者天理之節文其見於百為而莫不當理卽禮也仁者人之在心無可見必於禮見之仁禮之

本禮仁之用言復禮而後內外兼盡非空空守靜
如告子之不動心也一曰克復天下歸仁極言克
復之不易而性量之該括無窮此一日乃仁極熟義
精之候非忽然了悟而已其克復實功必親相授
受不能悉著於文夫子必為顏子示之而記者略
之非故為略之實不能以文字傳之也非禮四句
白交明言其目可知綱領有在而後人執以為克
復之全功抑思禮隨時而變通聖人因心而作則
即交武周公之禮在當時已多不可行夫子言禮
未嘗拘拘成法況後世禮制益疏未必矩步規行
便可以修齊治平故非禮四句只是當乎天理而
已而凡聖人之禮亦該其中為仁禮二字若德造
其極則合天地而通神明若得其一端亦有神於
人紀但此章以全體之仁言禮字亦該本末精粗
不可以他處言仁禮者相槪也夫天則陽性之純
於人而為仁具於心而心在後天則陽性之純
不敵陰私之雜故一心而必以禮宰之克
心者知覺運動之靈非可無也而必以禮宰之克
復之後無心非理即無一非性矣先儒言心而但
以持守克治為主持守克治不可少也而氣質之

四書恆解　下論　上册　西充鮮于嶽氏特園藏

私非可以力攻智取故孟子發明養氣不動心之
義孔子登不以此教人哉春秋雖衰禮法猶存故
孔子以禮為先而養氣之功不載於遺文至戰國
而禮教裘矣孟子乃明示之夫氣者質為心之郛
而心者氣之帥天理為心之本體氣質為心之鄰
郭浩然之氣天之所以為天故養之而德可合天
克己復禮能外此圖功哉人為萬物之靈受氣
於天成形於地先天得乾性坤命而生故性無不
善後天以坎離情為質故性不盡善而夫子亦
曰相近不明乎天地之奧與成形成性之原安能
知仁之實際與克復之功能哉程子四箴於義未
全愚嘗擬之附識於此其視箴曰五氣精華神聚
於目眈逐喪明迴光若谷誠以守中謹義志箴曰
色若儳惟恐汙顙志氣如神日月雙沐其聽箴曰
氣應坎精惟耳為靈神泉響答五音瓏玲心為之
宰應感靡甯嚴凝天德愼擇涇渭聞如未聞非禮
勿聽其言箴曰吾心籢動與神俱義謹出悖心
矢嘉謨必愼必戒若愚禍機德應善惡分途
神明內隱誠一不渝表裏中正闐此靈樞其動箴
曰四體百為應乎天則動惟厥時心理協極禮度

四書恆解　下論　上册　玉嶽氏特園藏

四書恆解 下論 上冊

為之性靜而虛定必使一念不起渾然在中所謂致中也動而省察必使念念合理力除邪妄所謂致和也孔子曰為仁以性存於氣質之中如果核之仁存於深密之際而實生機之本耳孟子曰養氣以理不外氣質而寓如金玉之生必藉沙石而成故返氣於虛靜耳至於動而為萬變以義禮智信行之皆純必不能外之良而發者當中也者天下之存於內者純必不能外之良而發者當中也者天下之大本也和也者天下之達道也致中和本於至中萬理歸於一理孔子以為仁詔門人原思其亦聞之

察克治之苦耳然所謂仁者必涵養功深先天一元之性由有諸己而充實而大而化此身之私累外誘之來堅持不動遂以為仁子以為難謂其省矣因心不易制於其動而嚴加克治治之至久覺

泛應各當故曰仁則吾不知也抑此理也其義本於羲文先天乾南坤北而後天離南坎北者何哉乾坤無功以日月為功六子皆乾坤所化而坎離獨得其真陰真陽人心先天為乾後天為離離中之陰即人心之靈也而天地則至陽之離以陰為

輔人心則不能渾然故心之陰常蔽其性之明而克己復禮者必克陰累以全陽性因後世邪之術託於是取坎填離人不知為克己復禮而以為爐火交媾種種怪誕則天地之性人為貴所以然者無從而知矣夫天地不過一陰一陽闔闢而生萬物人得陰陽之正者在先失陰陽之正者在後天此心所以分為人心道心性所以有善與相近也不明乎天地之原與人身受氣成形之本然安能知性與心之分合立命事天之實功哉第其功夫次第非文字所能傳必有明師授受恆久不息乃可知耳

四書恆解 下論 上冊

子曰士而懷居不足以為士矣 居非禮而苟便於己者懷思戀也此必有

附解居不是居室凡意所便安處皆是士之名至貴聖人屢言之後世將此一字看輕故自勉為聖賢者實矣

子曰邦有道危言危行邦無道危行言孫 危行皆去言行以道無可危也矯激者流危其言行以自禍故子言有道則可無道則否蓋為泄治之流而發

附解危字不是好字面君子秉德中和言行以道求自異於人而自無入不得何危之有昧者矯激之陰即人心之靈也而天地則至陽之離以陰為

四書恆解 下論 上冊

我哉蓋孔子告哀公時胷中已有成竹沐浴誠敬
冀其事之必行非徒嘗試一告及哀公畏齊之言
出則非其心不欲討第慮其力有不能子安得不
卽彼此情勢曉之且以營衆加齊牛可克正就義
理中曲直成敗而言非他計利害可比奈哀公卽
不畏齊又畏三子故夫子出面自歎深惜其言之
不行也如程子之言可杜後世計功謀利之徒亦
易啟迂執不情之諭蓋詞未達耳至胡氏先發之
聞謂身愛權爵便宜討賊毋貽君憂權而得中然
夫子實無其位亦不可行也獲麟事杜元凱謂所
感而起故以爲終較說得好後世附會朱子集註
成圖書現亦公羊之陋識

子路問事君子曰勿欺也而犯之 以道事君念無不
忠愛之至也不阿諛
曰犯非顯直之謂 誠而贊時納諫

附解子路之學升堂奉職盡公其素所能又性剛正
犯亦易事而子告之以此何也人臣念念勿欺其
君縈是難事已能然矣而又以犯之爲吾心已盡至於
君之從否不必深究則非愛君之至故曰勿欺也
自返無慊而又犯之惟恐君或踣於過失則其忠
愛乃至以是爲子路戒蓋勿欺者其平日忠信篤

敬必有許多翼翼君亦信之犯之則易入於不然徒犯
弗能強君之從也古今人臣緘默者固非顓直者
多取禍正爲此章之義不明

子曰君子上達小人下達 君子盡性希天日進面盆
上小人偷欲忘身日卑而
幾希而其後霄壤

附解天命之謂性性卽天理人之所以爲人聖人盡
性以立人極而天命通焉故詩曰帝謂文王予懷
明德夫子聖不自聖也而曰知我其天天生德於
予天未喪斯文匡人其如予何不嫌自夸何哉天
人一理理造其精卽可合天故曰天且不違而況
於人但天理止在吾身身心清明廣大純一不已
天卽在是動而爲言行事業無處非天理斯無事
不享天心悖理久久盈則名雖爲人實已非人夫
事任心悖理久久盈則名雖爲人實已非人夫
子此言蓋爲門人示也上達之功該窮理盡性本
末內外之學在中非篤實深造不能後世儒賞譽
言天命不知一念而天理去留係爲卽天命賞罰
從焉是以致飾於外無以清其本原面純一不已
之功克諧者少僧羽之徒妄想合天不知天理莫
大於倫常盡性者敦倫之本人倫不修天理已亡

四書恆解 下論 上冊

傳不知君子本末則以聖人為無所不能者幾疑其無書不讀無事不為抑思百工技藝天下古今傳記之繁風土人物之狀雖一覽無遺豈能周知而窮盡哉且有材技藝能玲瓏穎異而倫常心術大不堪問者故夫子曰不可小知而可大受也言君子於材技藝能未必能優於人而誠正修齊治平之學所以裕其大本大原者至周則內聖外王之業非君子莫能任也至於小人窮理正心之學無有斷不可受大任而一長一藝效能於奔走見試於事為輒有成效是可小知也有君子總其大而小人亦不廢所長天地尚安有棄材哉

四書恆解 下論 下冊 西充鮮于氏特園藏

子曰民之於仁也甚於水火水火吾見蹈而死者矣未見蹈仁而死者也仁即性也以其為天地生生之人無仁則物非水火之可養身尤急此也且水火不可蹈而蹈仁則物鬴非為天地之心而完人尤有益而無損死不可富死而死也勉人為仁因此言之若夫義當死而死則全仁者也雖死亦如乎生仁者死也

附解天命之謂性其在人如木果之有仁故曰仁也秉於生初本無虧缺奈有生以後氣拘物蔽則失其仁之本體聖人教人盡性修身全其仁乃成為人也無如糉情背理者多甘失其本心而不惜故子言此舊說言殺身以成仁與未見蹈仁而死

四書恆解 下論 下冊 西充鮮于氏特園藏

終有不合以為言各有當此章特為凡民發均非也蓋仁者壽大德必壽夫子言之後世因顏子三十二而卒遂謂仁者不必壽則夫子言為無憑不知顏子特天資純粹精進不已故夫子屢贊之於其卒也歎曰惜乎吾見其進未見其止原非謂顏子已造於神化之域其卒也因稟質羸弱秉受於先天者一氣不固觀其年二十八頭髮皆白可見夫子以其質美而勤學故嘗類之寶則未到聖人地位也宋周濂溪氣恬靜類於顏子故首推顏子以為發孔子之教萬世無窮者顏子夫顏子之足發孔子之道固不待言然曾子以忠恕明一貫子思以至誠闡中庸子貢以日月喻仲尼孟子以時中推孔子其發孔子而教萬世亦不後於顏子若以顏子為已到聖人粹處而不免夭亡致天下後世以聖學為不能立命此則大不可也此章未見蹈仁而死煞有至理今為詳言之庶千古聖學可以復明而顏子之不幸短命固亦無害於其大賢也蓋人之生也得天地之正理正氣而生故獨靈於萬物此人性之所以善也其稟山川父母之氣而生賦質不無昏雜此壽夭之所以不齊也夫其

四書恆解 下論 下冊 堯曰 西充鮮于氏特圖藏

八卦皆從此出實無分合之可名萬物皆秉之以生而得其渾然全體者則惟人而已得太極之理而後可以為人否則為物故曰五行之秀而天之心第太極之理氣在天地者未嘗有駁雜而一氣之屈伸變化感於隆汗清濁者則有異焉母有形之天地實無形之父母受氣於天地父母者同而不同非氣質之所由來歟故性在先天純粹無疵孟子道性善也性在後天性梏於形孔子故曰相近也太極之理既生以後其在人身中者如水在瓦缶金玉水晶琉璃盂之質異而水之明暗異性之拘於氣質者正猶此矣惟後天不及先天故聖人教人以學謂為復性之功但氣質亦有清濁之不同如金在沙上智八分金中人質亦有清濁之不同如金在沙上智八分金中人五分金下愚二三分去其氣質之薇但須披其沙耳若知覺運動固心之靈人所以貴但須披其沙得賢父師以教之而習於善久則性復其內有習之一字不可以一言盡也存其心養其性遠以葆其中和外有以熟其義理下學而上達則氣質皆為規矩不然安能復乎性之本然哉故此章乃言有生以後氣質之中求性無論智愚皆有之

四書恆解 下論 下冊 辛 西充鮮于氏特圖藏

是相近也孟子曰人之所以異於禽獸者幾希即指此相近者而言奈人不知此相近之性即先天太極之真縱情悖理習為不善遂至相遠二也字不同上決詞也慨從令於性無為心有覺使有覺之心悉從令於無為之性則心不離心而性無為心心不踰矩也誠知性則知心之本體乃知心性原無二而人自二之愚必深造自得其心者知其性也然此非空言可了必分言心性非於心外求性正欲人以正心復性毋偏任其心遂謂為性耳

子曰唯上知與下愚不移 知去聲○不移於惡即為上知不移於善即為下愚

附解此章向來誤解謂氣質之中又有美惡一定而非習所能移既非性善之旨謂天下可移者多惟上知與下愚不移亦非夫子勉人之意蓋天命之謂性率性之謂道天理有不善否必曰無之人性即天之性何以有不善則孟子性善一語無可移易矣後儒因不明先天後天之義以後天知覺之心為性而不明先天人合一之原遂令此等書義不明書義不明猶其小也令天下後世以聖人為不明

子游曰吾友張也爲難能也然而未仁

仁矣表章子張之賢而規其未仁愛之非刺之也爲語辭

曾子曰堂堂乎張也難與並爲仁矣

謂言志趣高明也難與並爲仁自謙其資之遜而不敢以堂堂求仁戒乎學堂堂者也

附解子張自是光明闊大人故夫子亦稱其光耀而列於四友子游意帶規勸曾子則直贊其堂堂而言己才遠遜難與之共爲仁蓋恐不如張者畫虎不成反類狗也記者連記之又以戒乎不如子張而妄爲堂堂者子張晚年進德篤實此二章所言蓋其少年時事然而未仁有深望其歛才就理深

四書惄解 下論 下冊 臺灣西充鮮于圓藏

造於仁意難與並爲仁言其高明之資己不敢學步以戒妄爲堂堂者如後世文字之學有等穎悟不煩力學者中下以之爲法必至自誤聖門造道亦是如此勿作輕刺語

曾子曰吾聞諸夫子人未有自致者也必也親喪乎

自致自獻其天良而不容已
逃子言以勉人識其本心

附解人心之良乃天理也因嗜慾錮蔽遂爾消亡然天理種子不能盡滅若滅盡則非人矣故聖人爲難

人力學以復其天良奈人多暴棄反以聖人爲難學己必不能希聖曾子特述夫子此言言人有能

自盡其誠者必也親喪乎爾時天良發現不能自掩人能長保其天理之良則無時不用其誠矣此

曾子立言徵意

曾子曰吾聞諸夫子孟莊子之孝也其他可能也其不改父之臣與父之政是難能也

莊子名遠魯大夫能因其臣遵其政故子特遜之以賜有位也非爲臣與政之不善者言其他此外孝行

附解張甄陶以爲愧季孫非也夫子言其他者愧也其父文子之賢不及獻子且夫子言此時季孫宿已卒何自愧之則爲當時父言賢而子不肖者愧也其父二字當認眞若獻

開論人物及之非必有他意而曾子述之則爲當

子不賢而莊子不改其臣與政反爲大夫不孝大禹之幹蠱宋哲宗之紹聖何是何非學者切當明辨

孟氏使陽膚爲士師問於曾子曾子曰上失其道民散久矣如得其情則哀矜而勿喜

陽膚曾子弟子孟氏士師魯司空兼官
曾子告以仁民之意道教養之王道朱子曰散情義

四書惄解 下論 下冊 冀縣西充鮮于圓藏

乖離不相維繫

附解天生民而不能使之自遂其生皆全其性也故立君上以教養之有教養之任而曰民難化者誣也雖麟之意官禮之法自誠意正心始以暨於平天下理萬民一以貫之各得其宜此非可責之庸

之六經外此並無置郵字太史公時孟子書尚未
大行而其言若此當從之為是

公孫丑問曰夫子加齊之卿相得行道焉雖由此霸
王不異矣如此則動心否乎孟子曰否我四十不動
心孟賁勇士告子名不害丑以為難告子先我不動
心相去聲。不異不足怪異勵而劇而暇逸如常度也孟子言
則夫子過孟賁遠矣曰是不難告子先我不動心音貢
告子未詳孟子言告子未得為心之害而不動心有道乎曰有北宮黝之養勇也不膚撓不目
逃思以一毫挫於人若撻之於市朝不受於褐寬博
亦不受於萬乘之君視刺萬乘之君若刺褐夫無嚴
諸侯惡聲至必反之黝伊糾反撓奴效反朝音潮刺七亦反去聲。心不動由於養勇以敵之盡黝以貢其被剌猶其貢挫刺皆毛布寬博寬緩也嚴畏憚刺毛
者也舍豈能為必勝哉能無懼而已矣。舍去聲下同孟施舍
名也專言舍者以嘔之黝以敵勝乎人為主舍以無懼為主而不動心孟施舍
似曾子北宮黝似子夏夫二子之勇未知其孰賢然
而孟施舍守約也 情堂養勇者可比持籍以引出守

四書恆解《孟子 公孫丑上 盩厔氏特園藏于西充鮮

夫志氣之帥也氣體之充也夫志至焉氣次焉故曰
持其志無暴其氣聞與告子曰不得於言勿求於心可不得於
氣不得於心勿求於氣可不得於言勿求於心不可
聞與告子曰敢問夫子之不動心與告子之不動心可得

四書恆解《孟子 公孫丑上 盩厔氏特園藏于西充鮮

反而縮雖千萬人吾往矣孟施舍之守氣又不如曾
子之守約也以守孤守氣之心惶惶然不足恃恐懼也引曾子之言大勇
夫子過孟施舍守約以明其養勇者之端反亦不異子曰子好勇乎吾嘗聞
大勇於夫子矣自反而不縮雖褐寬博吾不惴焉自
反而縮雖千萬人吾往矣孟施舍之守氣又不如曾
子之守約也
聞與告子曰敢問夫子之不動心與告子之不動心可得

持其志無暴其氣朱子曰此一節公孫丑問孟子誦
告子之言又聽以己意而告之也蓋其氣敢然而守既節但以志為至志動心也然兩相須必更持志而又無暴其氣然後內外交相須而心無不動志固從之
亦不動其心志動氣氣動志耶此皆即不
志也今夫蹶者趨者是氣也而反動其心夫蹶僵下句蹶腳蹶逆也趨走也孟子言
志壹則動氣氣壹則動

惡乎長曰我知言我善養吾浩然之氣問孟子之不

勤心異於告子者何所長而孟子自言其實知言知人之謙若得失見於其言窮理盡性全乎天地之氣究極乎事物之宜能善養其養浩然內有以絕于彊擾行貌其實無下文敢問何謂浩然之氣曰難言也身心所獨隱喻而不可以迹象言也其為氣也至大至剛以直養而無害則塞于天地之間大氣者本一而二不可離也此二節申言直養無害之氣過故至大乾坤一元所以能配如其本天地全此氣也稍于中卽不能害人之氣卽理所謂浩然也義靜者本一而不可離此二節中言直養無害道無是餒也餒如飢餓之餒配合一而不可離也此二節申言直養無害之義理之總名二者之相發言其為氣也配義與道其為氣也集義所者外著者易見卽可以知內勤致和故曰先言義與道而後者充實於中故必由內勤致也此氣所由生也義靜者外著者皆以知內故曰先言義與道而後

四書恆解 《孟子 公孫丑上》 奚以 氏 特圖藏子

生者非義襲而取之也行有不慊於心則餒矣故
曰告子未嘗知義以其外之也慊口箅口短二反。集義由少而多以至
備朱子曰今攻取如齊侯襲莒之襲可見而掩取非朱子曰拈取也如齊侯襲莒之襲可見而天理人欲之義內外一原道不可見而集義之時以事見外義之未能見告子不能集義不能直養浩然之氣
義必集故曰必有事焉而勿正心勿忘助長也
者以宋人然朱人有閔其苗之不長而揠之者芒芒
然歸其人曰今日病矣予助苗長矣其子趨而往視
之苗則槁矣天下之不助苗長者寡矣以為無益而
舍之者不耘苗者也助之長者揠苗者也非徒無益
而又害之氣長上聲揠烏八反舍上聲此乃正言義
之實事也

四書恆解 《孟子 公孫丑上》 奚以 氏 特圖藏子

然則夫子既聖矣乎此公孫丑又從行去聲辭命辭命達而辭言語誨諸侯德行孔子兼言語諸德行已造於聖人已矣朱子曰公孫丑四者雖有不同而其理則一政徒其偏陂不免於政事之偏陂也其事聖人復起必從吾言矣宰我子貢善為說辭冉牛閔
子顏淵善言德行孔子兼之曰我於辭命則不能也
子顏淵善言德行孔子兼之曰我於辭命則不能也
然則夫子既聖矣乎行去聲
曰惡是何言也昔者子貢問於孔
子曰夫子聖矣乎孔子曰聖則吾不能我學不厭而
教不倦也子貢曰學不厭智也教不倦仁也且智
夫子既聖矣夫聖孔子不居是何言也惡平聲夫音扶
而朱子曰惡歎辭也昔者以下孔子之言也學不厭者智之所以自明教不倦者仁之所以及物故丑再言之以曉孟子何言以
人矣故丑故孟子曰惡是何言也
昔者竊聞之子夏子游子張皆有聖人之一體冉
牛閔子顏淵則具體而微敢問所安此亦公孫丑問之

善也故聖人教人克己復禮化其氣質而歸於中和則去其蒙晦者而已孔子之時周室雖衰文武周公之禮樂猶存特人厭苦而不爲者或徒爲觀美孔子身體力敎特人厭苦而不爲者或徒爲觀美孔子身體猶存特人厭苦而不爲者或徒爲第使循循於規矩之中卽可以窺過其上智孔子第使循循於規矩之中卽可以窺過其上智人其一班也特其時禮樂蕩然學聖者莫由問津至孟子之時禮樂蕩然學聖者莫由問津孟子因公孫丑動心一問發出知言養氣之旨夫心本動

四書恆解 《孟子 公孫丑上 辛》 西充鮮于特圓藏子

也何以不動且心與氣何以相關此非實致其功者不能知也道心人心祇此一心人心從何而來道心從何而來氣之本平先天後天者有別而心之分乎理欲者異也先儒亦言復禮卽克去陰質之私而復乎乾元之性克治擴充先儒亦言復禮卽克去陰質之私其私擴充其善夫克治擴充存心之要也而知克治足盡復性之事孟子曰存其心養其性所以事天也於心言存而復於性言養其義始周而此章養氣則以清平心之源而復乎性之初告子之學卽之質世釋家所祖其不動心也靜存其空明妙有之質

四書恆解 《孟子 公孫丑上 辛》 西充鮮于特圓藏子

而於心之動也則强制其憧擾之端自宋以來儒者多是此學特儒者靜心而亦以物理爲要故重格物而補傳其實踐倫常不欺暗室亦有合乎聖人矣而理氣之原不明故其所謂不動心者亦非夫理不虛附氣載以行氣非空渺理爲之宰靜而養其未發之中得乾元之本體則太極渾然一氣也動而得平中節之和著時行之妙用則一氣散爲萬物也孟子之不動心內外交修動靜交養其功非可淺求其理難以形狀故先曰難言以爲像形容之切實指陳之集義者擴充其天理以爲養氣也氣之原必有事焉涵養其正氣以與理相比非但集義而別無養氣之功也三代下三敎分門僧流靜心有似告子羽流養氣則似勤舍其所守者後天虛靈之心非純一不已之性其所養者後天血氣之質非乾元太和之氣而儒者亦以心爲性其所謂不動心者亦强制頑空而已孟子若有見於後世之失而預爲之防先言勤舍之養勇是後世養後天之氣者類也然後言告子之不動心由於養氣而原其剛大之本體申以必配道義蓋內養

四書恆解孟子卷七 晚年定本

盡心上凡四十六章　　　雙江劉　沅輯註

孟子曰盡其心者知其性也知其性則知天矣心者氣之靈受中之始有善無惡後天理雖己後而理故知此乎先天本然之體則知性即天理故指明心性與天此承上而指其用功之實存養其性所以事天也則後天之神明皆先天之一貫存其心養其性所以事天也或殀或壽氣數之不可也殀壽不貳修身以俟之所以立命也心者氣為命而存養修身以事天則理純而氣亦固是神而壽之數不能拘此為自立其命貳謂惑於氣數亦固是

附解此章為當時言心性者直揭其表裹語簡而義該全部大學中庸歷代聖人心法皆具於此直是

四書恆解　《孟子　盡心上　一》 嵋西充鮮于圜蠡子

渾成雪亮而猶有謂孟子之文不簡密者何哉通章皆指點之詞人皆知心為一身之主而不知心有先天後天之分未生以前秉天地理氣之正而後為人物則偏駁矣故人心之量原是粹然在先天則渾然無名象如天地太極之渾含此時心即是性迨既生以後則氣質之心足以梏其浩然之氣而心之本體非舊矣故孟子言人知心為身主不知自來盡其心之量而無所不通者皆由知性也性即天理而人得之以為心心蔽於欲則先天渾然之性不全人遂日與天遠能知其性則天

四書恆解　《孟子　盡心上　二》 嵋西充鮮于圜蠡子

之理體備無遺而洞然於人之所以為人即天之所以為天則知天矣舍性言心而以為天命之本然可乎惟性為心之質而後天之心常足以擾其先天之性故聖人教人存其知覺之靈不使逐物而紛養其本然之性不使為心所役久久則後天有覺之心皆純乎義理而為先天渾然之性天之所以與我者始全所以事天也舍存心養性求事天可乎夫天者理氣之宰也人生受氣於天秉理為性天原以可大可久者付之於我而不能存養於是神為欲昏氣為欲耗見殀壽之不齊而疑天之不可恃矣念吾身之不久而或懈其修存矣我之得於天而主宰乎吾身者尚能立乎性心存養確然有見卓然有主知吾身有與天地並壽者而殀壽不齊不足惑之兢兢焉惟恐吾性有未純心有未安一息尚存不敢息其修身之學以俟乎天命而自樂其性分則心通乎造物生徒而識超乎天下之先不似他人囿於氣化虛生徒死此所以立命也自古聖人盡性之功可以參贊由此其選獨奈何舍心性而不務自外於天也哉語意如此心性命三字道得十分了然而人無實功徒

以臆測分首節為知次節為行至末節疑為另是一意煞是謬妄明者當必知之或曰先儒皆言心為身主性即心之理虞延亦但言心子何云先天之心為性也不足為性也曰虞延言心而之心為性即心之理虞延亦但言心子何云先天分人心道心是明明有二心也性本純一不雜安得有二人心之發氣質之累為之而非天之本然也五官百骸必待血氣而存而血氣之靈多於天命之性故非養浩然之氣至於不動心則先天之純一之性不敵情識之擾所以存養之功必造其極始為事天立命而為仁不熟亦不如荑稗也況縱其有覺之心有不喪其粹然之性者乎儒者知人心之危防閑之靜存之而不得養浩然之學則血氣之靈如樹心蟠蟓終無術以去之而文王之德之純孔子江漢秋陽之喻皆莫得其所以然故愚嘗反復而明辨之也究竟心性之實如何姑即易見者以譬之天與人以理氣之全此渾然粹之在吾身者如金在沙中心固未嘗無性而亦甚僅矣上智之聖心無私欲則猶是先天之本來然此曠世一逢矣其次則心皆涸於氣質之非性之本體故聖人教人復性之功而夫子則曰克己復禮

四書恆解 《孟子 盡心上 三》 西充鮮于特圓藏

為仁孟子則曰存心養性所以事天若心即性矣而又何復之有乎即心即性矣而又何存與養乎惟先天之心即性而後天之心多欲故命存於道心之乃以養其本然之性而人心悉聽命於道理則純一矣道言存神養氣即是存心養氣不曰心而曰神以心之靈妙言之也佛言元神元神即道心性之本體故曰元識神即人心知覺之神故曰識神而僧羽之徒言存神養氣者僅保其有覺之神呼吸之氣固宜儒言存神養氣以此為性猶是彼家說也至命之一字尤難辨程子之言命而不知天理之主宰為命愚嘗有說論之而論語命諸章亦詳茲不贅矣殊毒不貳修身以俟一句緊承說下其義始全程張朱三子言心性天命惟張子較純然言由太虛有天之名亦非也天即理也不虛而亦不實以形言之曰天以理言之曰性其靈變曰心分而觀之合而一之誠賦於人曰性其靈變曰心分而觀之合而一之非盡心知性立命事天者不能表裏洞然姑即二字形義言之性字從生從心蓋人所得於天之正理以為心者也心字從三點從斜鉤蓋人既生

四書恆解 《孟子 盡心上 四》 西充鮮于特圓藏

周易恆解序

一理也而天地人物莫不由之故曰道其散為萬殊者其歸於一本者也人為萬物之靈其氣得陰陽之正而其性即天地之理窮理盡性以至於命則人一天地而凡萬事萬物悉有以得其中和顧其功非易致徑尤多歧不有以標其極則天人合一之旨不明而民生日用之倫不著也庖犧以前非無神聖然朴榛初啟禮制未詳氣運所區勢難驟備天浪圖書以開聖人之智聖法天地而立卦爻之文於是萬象咸包萬理咸具而天下後世性命倫常之事幽明始終之情莫不畢範於斯矣六十四卦特陰陽動靜之所推然其窮幽達顯占變知來大之極乎天地之高明小之盡乎物情之纖細以一爻通於千萬爻以一卦通於無窮卦分之則事事各有其宜合之皆於一是辨其異同中之異異中之同四聖人各有其意四聖人實無二意拘而求之鑿而益之非能讀易者也夫禮樂教化唐虞三代之法已詳而伏羲以前尚無規範易之設卦觀象固為後世發蒙也詩書名象悉由繼起窮神知化必有心源易故為文字之祖王功聖德之全而歷代諸儒或僅貌玄

《卷首序》

一　西充鮮于氏特園藏

虛或徒求術數即言理之家亦每舍經而從傳顧此而失彼信聖人之教不其隱乎愚謝陋無文非敢以註易自明也顧嘗深求其旨極之於天地準之於人倫以孔子為宗而折衷前人之緒論不敢雷同不敢好異要以平心酌理無失乎天地之常經聖人之軌則雖詞多訓詁不免為有識所軒渠然鄙意竊欲人人皆曉而不使視為畏途也故顏曰恆解以俟將來云

嘉慶庚辰年九月初一日雙流劉沅敍

《卷首序》

二　西充鮮于氏特園藏

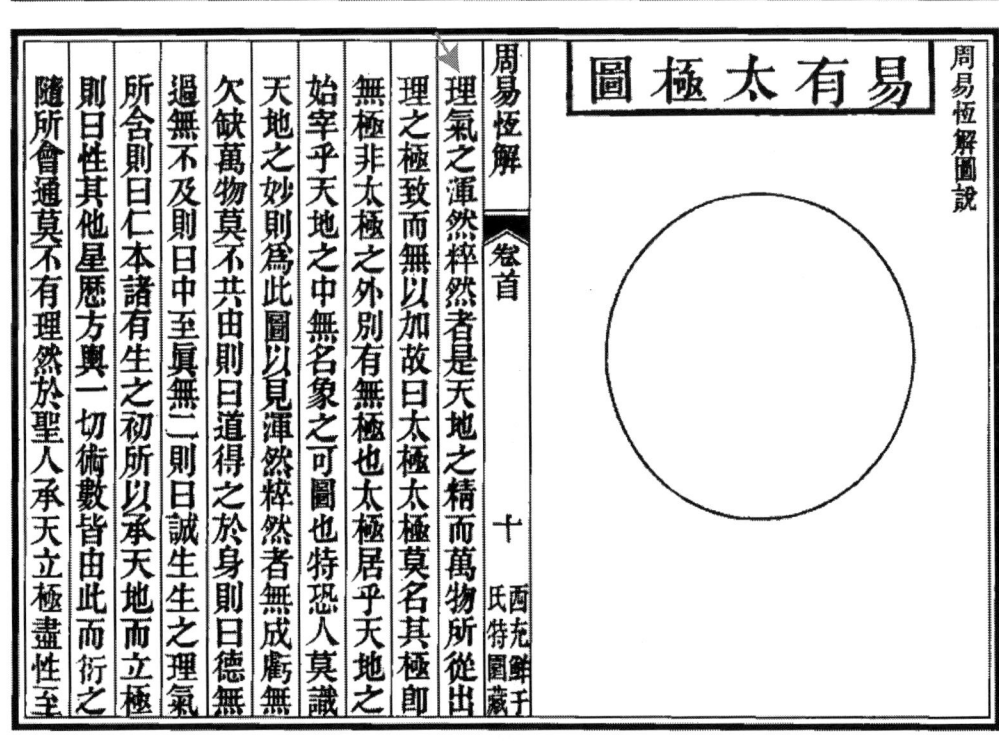

炎武言之甚詳其說以唐韻爲正義頗優於前賢然聖人本意恐人以爲純言義理不喜誦習故多用韻以諷之葢亦不得已之苦心而今世古音已晦學者勉強求叶必至遷就義理以就音韻其失轉甚故茲集於韻略之

　　　　　　　　雙流劉沅識

周易恆解 卷首　　　　　九　酉充鋒于氏特圖藏

周易恆解圖說

太極圖

周易恆解 卷首　　　　十　酉充鋒于氏特圖藏

理氣之渾然粹然者是天地之精而萬物所從出理之極致而無以加故曰太極太極莫名其極卽無極非太極之外別有無極也太極居乎天地之始宰乎天地之中無名象之可圖也特恐人莫識天地之妙則爲此圖以見渾然粹然者無成虧無欠缺萬物莫不共由則曰道得之於身則曰德無過無不及則曰中至眞無二則曰誠生生之理所含則曰仁本諸有生之初所以承天地而立極則曰性其他星應方輿一切術數皆由此而衍之隨所會通莫不有理然於聖人承天立極盡性至

兩儀圖

▬▬　▬ ▬

周易恆解　卷首　　十二　酉充鮮于氏特園藏

命之學為釁爪矣舊傳周濂溪太極圖內圖白黑二氣以象陰陽由中一點運化蓋取生陰生陽之意然太極者理氣之總滙陰陽合於其中本難名象故曰無極者無極者狀太極也非太極之外別有無極太極既無極矣而又可圖耶故茲但列一空圈以象渾然粹然之意

天地未兆太極在天地之前天地既分太極卽在天地之中謂天地之外復有太極者非也惟天地卽太極之體故天包乎地而以陽施陰孕於天而以陰承陽陰陽直而專則為一奇陰闢而翕則為偶此兩儀之象所由名也然奇者天一之數也偶者地二之數也陰儀陽儀祇是天地之體叚天一地二其數得三兩奇一偶則為四兩偶一奇則為五故數止於五以其為天地之交而陰陽奇偶所會也六七八九十卽倍一二三四五而成非有加於五之外也天地無一息不交陰陽無一息不和故成為太極渾然之體而陰靜陽動陽靜陰動互為其機互根其宅於是屈伸消長而生五行五行分布陰陽之功用以宏實則太極陰陽之理氣如環無端亘古不息故五行祇一陰一陽仍一太極耳河圖五行分列金木水火各居其方而中土為之運用卽是此理但聖人畫卦卽有形以象無形由兩儀而重覆錯綜之遂生八卦前人以陽動陰靜為生兩儀不知陰陽各有動靜夫子已明言之且於陰何以偶之義不明又似太極生天地者總緣不知天地之妙耳今特明著之

周易恆解　卷首　　十三　酉充鮮于氏特園藏

禮記恆解序

天以一元生化而品物流形各得其所自然之秩敘即禮之原也人秉五行之秀而其性則太極之在天地者播而為五行著而為萬物人性之秉太極者分而為五常著而為倫紀其理一則其所以順其自然盡其當然者無不一也第人汨於物欲喪其本來則以禮為苦人之具而不知吾性中之本然必如是而後安不如是則不安也目義皇以來代有制作至唐虞而成功文章乃煥然其可觀世變所趨人情所向既踵事而增華必多方而補救故三代聖王忠質交互用而其禮乃詳周之興也益出於播遷流離而數聖人以忠厚承之以至德永之觀於詩書所載孔孟所言文武周公實能以天地育物之心為心故其禮亦能以天地生成之道為道傳世久遠上既無聖天子持其綱下亦無賢公卿維其緒及春秋而事雜言龐有莫知禮之所以為禮者矣夫子聖德天縱尤嚴矩規凡禮之可以宜古而宜今者盡靡不身體之而其或有當變通者則有志而未見諸施行也當時諸賢習聞其說而不盡得其指歸一二好學深思之士貞輯羣言彙為此書雖其分編纂敘出

於戴鄭之徒未必遂得聖人精意而其文存卽其義存不得謂折衷時中不藉此而彰也先儒以周官儀禮為經此經為註又因其列學取士始於荊公爰多嘗議之者然究考其所言無非探賾聖賢書見聞意其精者出於七十子之徒而其淺者亦秦漢篤學之士非於道概未有聞而能剽襲為之者也書中如月令王制作者顯有姓名其他前人所疑多由未達文義敎而遽相詰詆我
朝禮敎昌明
欽定義疏廣大精微無美不備於前儒之是非判然瞭然益
聖人建中和而修百度不似書生空談曲學也沅謏陋於禮意毫末未窺而幸沐休明積久微覺有得篇慮承學者或苦於繁否則拘晦其旨爰於誦習之時隨文詁義以便參稽閱年忽已成帙以愚困之留未忍捐棄也敘而存之後有作者其或弗哂為妄誕也
夫

道光八年初夏日雙流劉沅識

鄭康成曰大听早昧爽擊鼓以召眾警眾也用樂大胥以敌學士興秩猶使有司擽其事不親徵也報禮畢非郊之尊卽於此而行一獻之禮亦釋菜禮輕也序所存於俊士者以其未命為士故曰俊序卽大學也天子曰辟雍諸侯曰頖宮此則諸侯之學也退脩之序卽東序也亦謂之東膠東序東膠皆文王世子之名故退脩之於此也

適東序釋奠於先老遂設三老五更羣老之席位焉適饌省醴養老之珍具遂發詠焉退脩之以孝養也反登歌清廟既歌而語以成之也言父子君臣長幼之道合德音之致禮之大者也下管象舞大武大合眾以事達有神與有德也正君臣之位貴賤之等焉而上下之義行矣有司告以樂闋王乃命公侯伯子男及羣吏曰反養老於東序終之以仁也

禮記恆解 卷八 文王世子 古氏特圓藏于西充鮮

老年數茂者為更又皆入侍天子親命迎勞三老五更之禮酒醴發詠奏樂歌眾工登堂清廟之詩所以脩身也
對老更而言既語即席
既歌而後乃語
反登歌入堂下管象吹武王所以伐紂之樂也
至進而省饌者親視饌之備否
老更乃迎老者三五約其尊者為之
敬道其德以告何以示孝
徒舞為文武有所勸
曲禮興乃以神興也
有德則為貴
公神興及諸侯
等反于其國皆當如此養老於東序遂推以及官司鄉皆若
是終于其仁心也以

禮記恆解 卷八 文王世子 古氏特圓藏于西充鮮

世子之記曰朝夕至於大寢之門外問於內豎曰今日安否何如內豎曰今日安節則內豎以告世子世子乃有喜色其有不安節則內豎以告世子世子色憂不滿容內豎言復初然後亦復初朝夕之食上世子必在視寒暖之節食下問所膳羞必知所進以命膳宰然後退若內豎言疾則世子親齊玄而養膳宰之饌必敬視之疾之藥必親嘗之嘗饌善則世子亦能食嘗饌寡世子亦不能飽以至于復初然後亦復初
陳氏澔曰世子之記古記篇名也鄭康成曰朝夕之禮親俯視之制親自所視齊和所食齊和所

附解天下古今事變無窮而聖人日脩已以敬脩其
欲或異也按此篇本記教世子之法故終之以此
養疾者齊玄冠玄端立于側
夕也中又朝文王為世子加謹敬視疾者之多於前
不能无其儀親視寒暖乃止之

身而天下平何也萬事萬理皆本於心而心有人
心道心之異克已復禮去其陰私化其氣質使人
悉聽命於道心而又實踐倫常旁通物理內外
交修本末交養久之而中和在抱天宇澄清不特
平日之習而安爲者胥協乎則耳目所不及心
思所不周者一經見聞是非立剖執兩用中化成
天下凡有德者無不庸凡利民者無不至一日而一道風
同悉由主德此論教之法不可一日而不講也此
篇所記蓋其遺法後世昧此故天置之才英明而
略功業炳如而禮樂不興到隆難致大學言明明
德而即曰親民以親於此篇之義不明矣
蓋太學之地天子元子諸侯世子卿大夫元士之
子及俊選皆與爲而其平日之敎之也六德六行
六藝莫非本諸心性實踐倫常以及材藝便民之
事升於太學者皆成德之材猶恐其心性不能中
和卽言行未必純粹也又以神瞽爲師有德行而
深於樂者察其中心之安仁否使之蕩滌邪僞益
葆天眞故夫子曰成於樂焉至元子適子等下與
庶人同學凡三物所有皆力行之與天下賢才朝
夕居遊養成德性且周悉於物理人情異日加民

禮記恆解 卷八 文王世子 十五 西充鮮于氏特園藏

即以成已者成人此爲親民之實即明德之所由
精純也是篇特錯舉其儀文而本原所在誠正修
齊何以漸次而幾實踐而詣固未道及是必七十
子之徒授受相承得其緒論而爲此編其事蓋皆
周制其言世子亦以文王爲宗夫文王之德之純
固非特爲世子一節也而爲世子如斯其後武王
周公致治亦由斯欲爲文武之治必爲文武之人
豈不在後人之自奮哉

禮記恆解卷八終

禮記恆解 卷八 文王世子 十六 西充鮮于氏特園藏

生致其敬盡其（養而使尸不以
代死者爲嫌謙而不醉飽也
肆腥爓腍祭豈知神之所饗也主人自盡其敬而已
矣審反
肆陳也腍熟食也言陳腥爓及熟食以祭何以生親
迎陳蓋神處於幽豈知神之所饗亦主人自盡其
敬而已矣而已矣非
輕詞乃鄭重之詞
舉斚角詔妥尸古者尸無事則立有事而后坐也尸
神象也祝將命也
斚角皆爵名灌以降神之後舉斚角祝詔主人奉
尸神象也飽以神之當安坐爲妥
尸神不言故用祝將命達幽明之意
縮酌用茅明酌也醆酒涗于清汁獻涗于酸酒涗猶明
清與酸酒于舊澤之酒也

禮記恆解 《卷十一 郊特牲》 三十   西充鮮于氏特圜藏

醆側產反汁音十亦獻
酌用茅以茅縮體齊
之使清而後酌也
醆酒盎酒差清酒也
以寶尊彝被曰泲酌
盎齊泲酌也
以齊灌獻曰盥而獻
也器言其所以盛鬱
鬯者齊曰酌以和鬱
獻之器盥所用不同
造之器曰盤而不曰
盥計其物獻曰獻日
也計其事故經所用
獻以言其物齊以言
九獻於首故獻通言
之酸酒獻之以盥酒酌
酸酒於同罍以盥尊
明故於此明之不明矣然
以酸酒涗於酸酒乎
釀酒於舊澤之酒也
酸酒涗清與清酒之
澤理也酸酒亦指是
世故於涗清齊三者
所用常祀不過此
祭有祈焉有報焉有由辟焉
祈求也恕而降禍於民若祈穀之
類報咎也以荅神麻若祈邊年侵邦之
辟解辟去也

禮記恆解 《卷十一 郊特牲》 三十   西充鮮于氏特圜藏

者

孔氏穎達曰解齊服所以用玄衣玄冠之義以陰
祈氏穎達曰用桃弧棘矢之類
於辟言由者以非祭之常禮有所用之也
齊之玄也以陰幽思也故君子三日齊必見其所祭
也以神處於陰必幽深思而後可冀來格
故孔子三日致齊其思必見其所祭
者孔子三日致齊如在以平日德行既純臨時誠敬又
至怳怳乎以齊爲虛文
怳慌將行之者繆矣

附解 一元之理氣無始無終無聲無臭闢闔之機斡
運化爲耳有理斯有氣斯有神鬼神者陰陽
之靈而已而何以情壯不同情氣爲物遊魂爲變
而後天地成形然天地雖分仍此一元之氣彌綸
物之秉其靈者異即所以呈其態者亦異本乎天
者親上神之所以正而清本乎地者親下鬼之所
以濁而雜祭享之禮聖人所以通幽明而達忠孝
也惟牲牢一事大小祀皆用之以爲人神一理事
亡如存則以飲食之道事之亦固其所而天地則
至尊無可褻矣何爲乎郊特牲而社稷太牢哉天
地之性人爲貴生民之利牛爲先王者父天而母
地享以太牢人子之義云爾然亦有其義之至精
者一陽生於子而老於乾歲氣周流後天八卦象
之由一陽而三而五而七而九陽終於戌乾位乎

禮記恆解 卷十九 樂記 五 西充鮮于氏特圖藏於去聲

人生而靜者渾然在中此卽所得於天中正之理而為性至感物而動則七情繁繞然後好惡形焉性卽為於伐性之斧故好惡無節於內知誘於外不能反躬天理滅矣夫物之感人無窮而人之好惡無節則是物至而人化物也人化物也者滅天理而窮人欲者也於是有悖逆詐偽之心有淫泆作亂之事是故強者脅弱眾暴寡知者詐愚勇者苦怯疾病不養老幼孤獨不得其所此大亂之道也

人生而靜天之性也感於物而動性之欲也物至知知然後好惡形焉好惡無節於內知誘於外不能反躬天理滅矣夫物之感人無窮而人之好惡無節則是物於是有悖逆詐偽之心有淫泆作亂之事是故強者脅弱眾暴寡知者詐愚勇者苦怯疾病不養老幼孤獨不得其所此大亂之道也

是故先王之制禮樂人為之節衰麻哭泣所以節喪紀也鐘鼓干戚所以和安樂也昏姻冠笄所以別男女也射鄉食饗所以正交接也禮節民心樂和民聲

以鹽菜遺猶餘也愚接申言禮樂所以被民平其好惡非欲人極口腹耳目之樂卽清廟大饗陶之禮莫不偏而是也好惡偏而人道必亂故以禮樂

備矣衰麻哭泣所以節喪紀也鐘鼓干戚所以和安樂也昏姻冠笄所以別男女也射鄉食饗所以正交接也禮節民心樂和民聲政以行之刑以防之禮樂刑政四達而不悖則王道

禮記恆解 卷十九 樂記 六 西充鮮于氏特圖藏於禁暴舉賢則政均矣仁以愛之義以正之如此則

治行矣

樂者為同禮者為異同則相親異則相敬樂勝則流禮勝則離合情飾貌者禮樂之事也禮義立則貴賤等矣樂文同則上下和矣好惡著則賢不肖別矣刑

同其等相親不乖戾相敬不流蕩禮樂過勝偏而不全檢其外為之合使其情皆得其正而交又推其效於天下貴賤之分可明好惡之正可反此禮樂之事本人情之正而又制為禮樂其令於民是其所以治民也先王愛民故制為禮樂其行在於禮樂之中是以為仁也仁者此道也正者義也仁義卽禮樂之正

大樂必易大禮必簡樂至則無怨禮至則不爭揖讓

禮記恆解 卷三十 坊記 十一 西充鮮氏特圓藏

子云禮非祭男女不交爵以此坊民陽侯猶殺繆侯而竊其夫人故大饗廢夫人之禮

繆與穆通故大饗祭禮男女同之所以備外內之官而孝覲也非是不交爵賜候其事未聞或因燕饗而美其貌後因兵爭殺之而取其妻如趙滅息以媯歸也古禮大饗同獻無他證候助祭者此證春秋以後之事記者言男女無別廳堂至廢饗禮甚言其失耳

子云寡婦之子不有見焉則弗友也君子以辟遠也

故朋友之交主人不在不有大故則不入其門以此坊民民猶以色厚於德

有見實賄其材藝也同志爲友辟嫌遠之大故喪病也朋友之交以下謂凡朋友皆然不止寡也

禮記恆解 卷三十 坊記 十一 西充鮮氏特圓藏

子云好德如好色諸侯不下漁色故君子遠色以爲民紀故男女授受不親御婦人則進左手姑姊妹女子子已嫁而反男子不與同席而坐寡婦不夜哭婦人疾問之不問其疾以此坊民民猶淫泆而亂於族

婦之子厚於好德也愚按寡婦之子非盡不可友而亦非盡爲辟遠也第防敬杜漸之意

好德如好色見常人多篤好於色故之音逸遠法聲引子言好德如好色之漁取如遇好於色賤也下申明之但謂取於國廣取於故云下漁非但謂取於國故於國諸事皆涉嫌媟故結之以亂於族

子云昏禮壻親迎見于舅姑舅姑承子以授壻恐事之違也以此坊民婦猶有不至者

迎去聲 鄭康成曰舅姑之父母也妻之父母外舅外姑愚按承妻以授壻卽其女之所歸必由父母授恐事父母或違乎男女之正也男女重則如此坊民婦歸以禮而無私褻之嫌婦豈猶有不至者

附解

禮法以範斯民其制於外而勤靜咸宜者悉其存於中而渾然至善者也然人心之變化不時禮樂之流傳易失故文武周公之法旣折衷而使之子力行以教門人日用言行之禮積久而陵夷孔

禮記恆解 卷三十 坊記 十二 西充鮮氏特圓藏

子遵循克復歸仁之功尤詳示而使之實踐所以成就者多坊之爲言蓄德於內而檢察於外也不使侵內不使溢動靜交養之學固存乎其閒記者習聞聖論而彙記以爲斯名其意頁厚然禮禁亂之所由生猶坊止水之所自來防其流亦安可不清其源哉萬事萬理莫不咸具於心而心有人心道心正其人心純乎道心其功豈一朝而至人人皆以爲當然則順帝之則道一風同不必言者民之父母也已身正而因以正天下六德六行坊實無處非坊讀者其推類而求返身而思庶有

禮記恆解 卷卅三 緇衣 八

西充鮮于氏特園藏

子曰私惠不歸德君子不自留焉詩云人之好我示
我周行

私惠以私情相惠而不合德禮之公也不自留御之也周行喻大道

子曰苟有車必見其軾苟有衣必見其敝人苟或言
之必聞其聲苟或行之必見其成葛覃曰服之無射
射音亦
詩作斁

亦喻人有行必審其終服之無射言服之久也而君子言行必觀其始要於終可以類推

子曰言從而行之則言不可飾也行從而言之則行
不可飾也故君子寡言而行以成其信則民不得大
其美而小其惡詩云白圭之玷尚可磨也斯言之玷
不可為也小雅曰允矣君子展也大成君與日在昔
上帝周田觀文王之德其集大命于厥躬

下二行如字

聲周田觀文書作寧
割申勸文書作寧
言必可行行必可言
則徵信乃成信則民皆化
何夸美而飾惡引實民
得夸美而飾惡引書以
雅以證成信引書以證民皆化於善其說甚見詩小

禮記恆解 卷卅三 緇衣 九

西充鮮于氏特園藏

子曰南人有言曰人而無恆不可以為卜筮古之遺
言與龜筮猶不能知也而況於人乎詩云我龜既厭
不我告猶兒命曰爵無及惡德民立而正事純而祭
祀是為不敬事煩則亂事神則難易曰不恆其德或
承之羞恆其德偵婦人吉夫子凶

南人南國之人卜筮於人不足信也於人也即事取事可正巫覡作者取正蓋人事神事相因已不敬神事煩而已不敬神事煩而事神日瀆取其義非拘守恆言不恆德者羞來於人

附錄此篇與坊記表記皆篇記者其始有深意乎蓋
名此獨舉緇衣二字記者其始有深意乎蓋
人之所以為人者天理而已天理無不善而七情
之發見於好惡者往往乖宜登性有不善歟氣質
偏而物擾甚耳孔門以為仁教人正欲其復禮功非一朝
理之正而清乎好惡之源第克己復禮功非一朝
而事由實踐非賢君相持其綱明師友廣其化人
亦安能樂而就之此篇首言為上易事為下易知
而即繼以緇衣巷伯易事者親民如子親愛之則

春秋恆解 卷一 桓公

堯西充鮮于氏特圖藏于

公與夫人姜氏遂如齊 公羊無與字

會不書夫人無外會之禮諱之也而書與書遂明夫人欲如齊而公不禁遂與之偕失夫綱自取禍也

夏四月丙子公薨于齊丁酉公之喪至自齊

左傳公將有行遂與姜氏如齊申繻曰女有家男有室無相凟也謂之有禮易此必敗公會齊侯于濼遂及文姜如齊齊侯通焉公讁之以告夏四月丙子享公使公子彭生乘公公薨於車魯人告於齊曰寡君畏君之威不敢寧居來修舊好禮成而不反無所歸咎惡於諸侯請以彭生除之齊人殺彭生齊侯與夫人姜氏如齊謀而實未沒其于齊昭公見弑之事夫人非于齊昭公見弑之事夫人雖逝而實未桓弑天理所不容其禍自取之然諸

之惡不可怨故臣子之辦書甍書喪以尊君雖被弑而書其地以惡齊書葬以斥魯臣不能討賊禮各得而義綦嚴矣

秋七月

冬十有二月己丑葬我君桓公

附解孟子曰人之所以異於禽獸者幾希幾希者何天理而已天之理人得之以為人俗曰天理良心聖人亦止全此四字常人雖不能全亦必猶有此幾希而後為人天理良心仁也道也德也誠也其由日道實有日誠得於身日德本此天理

春秋恆解 卷一 桓公

良心施之咸宜節其過文其不及曰禮知之眞曰智行之恆且久曰信念念事事能存天理良心則慈讓敬愼一切自然俱有故曰仁者人也君子亦仁而已若親親敬其親則必愛敬其兄弟而女兄弟微別則以男女必有別也俗云萬惡淫為首百行孝最先孝則是仁仁必循禮而何至竟為禽獸之行然其原則必由父母善教也齊僖首敗王綱人且以為小霸而其家法不修至於如此其無禮也由其先不仁也子之告顏子也曰非禮勿視聽言動說者以為仁不外是制外即以養中也不知記者明言其目四者戒其非禮動察耳其為仁存養靜功不能以文字傳故記者未記益心至浮動性本虛明性即仁也存養其心知止有定矣而後動靜安相次而及靜能致中然後動而能致和非但兢兢克制防閑遂可為仁原思之難夫子所以僅可之夫七情之欲如水潰隄如火赴薪至難過也而天理固安能強持之文武周公禮制嚴且密矣不數傳而畔亂淫惡叢生豈禮之難行歟不仁故也無為仁之功則良心天理日就梏亡雖使之循規矩謹言

附解　天人一理也理之所在而氣數因之故積善必有餘慶積惡必有餘殃積之云者非一朝一夕之故也古今術士言禍福多中而不知以理為憑故往往自矜殃孽理者又專言理而不言禍福不知氣數統於天理理在而感應因之數乃理之昭著者也夢卜徵驗其幾甚微其事在若有若無之間乎左傳記災祥事甚多辨之不輕信亦非不言故曰知幾其神祉人以為曹亡徵數也否則謂其妄也豈知即此

春秋悮解　卷八　哀公　莘氏特圓藏

可以知修德迴天栽培傾覆之義哉陰陽迭為消長故盛衰本天道人事之常豈有久而不消歇者第有盛必有衰者數也而衰極必盛者理也理在天為元氣在人為善德人性本善全其天性者善人天道生生而不窮者一元之氣不窮實由一元之理無終極也人能存天之正理即可存天之正氣故盛衰有盛德可迴之堯舜之子不肖而堯舜有盛德知天下不可以天下與子作賓王家歷三代而不窮此以理迴氣數之道也曹將亡而振鐸示夢於人使其子孫知之而即戒

其暴也鄭能救曹雖無成功春秋所許也故詳書之

公孫彊竟見用而曹亦亡則人事相左非氣數不知懼自強豈何必亡哉奈夢者不言於眾朝廷不知必不可迴也曰何以不夢於其君臣曰富貴中人勢利薰心自謂高明豈信夢卜且人必有清明之志氣而後鬼神假信夢以相通夢以傳說文王夢非能孚有由來矣常人素無德行神昏氣濁與天日違下達者斷無上達之階亡其幾希安於愚蒙又何況夢之恍惚而可憑以言理乎孔子曰知我其天天生德於子天未喪斯文何其信天之確如斯周公頌文王曰帝謂文王子懷明德不大

春秋悮解　卷八　哀公　至　莘氏特圓藏

聲以色若與天相告語者豈為誕哉夫德固存於聲色之外所謂毛猶有倫必極之無聲無臭而後是也然無聲無臭者實不必求諸渺冥而近在身心心至隱微心全乎德又何人知之惟天知之耳存其心養其性所以事天心性在我而其原在天天人一理又安能不一氣故夢原是幻亦未必皆幻以理裹之則幽明始終之義未嘗不在焉若示夢其子孫亦未必信耳

哀公三十八年甲寅

春王正月宋公入曹以曹伯陽歸

周官恆鮮

鮮于道元題

辛未年八月刊

周官恆解序

天道不言而萬物生生化化流衍於無窮者何也一元之氣無終無始其流行於品物而大著於人倫者各安其所各有其宜聖人本此而立為治道是以裁成輔相俾天地之功用不虛而民生之性命各正蓋自義皇以來聖神遞興法制漸備至周而乃集其大成矣秦皇肆虐古制蕩然漢購遺經周官最為晚出疑之者頗多然皆未得乎聖人之德而即文字以相衡者也夫人為萬物之靈天地之心聖人全人道而通天道故無一念不合乎天卽無一事不當乎理而由是推己及人盡性參贊自郊廟朝廷以暨於民生日用無不為之制節使歸中和唐虞三代之隆未有不由此者也特養立而後教行已而後物正故大學之道無上下尊卑同之聖學不明則所以正心修身者無其本而徒求之文法曷怪其紛紜而錯謬哉王莽篡亂安石虛誕乃欲假此以欺當時而宇文氏之徒亦欲彷彿是豈知萬理統於一誠綱常必先自立塘寨所懷慚其見乎朱子以此書為自立塘寨所懷慚卽海隅所見乎朱子以此書為運用天理爛熟程子亦言有睢麟之意然後可行周官蓋皆有以見於其難矣而自買賣民田貪當不均

1924

周官恆解 卷三 春官 奎一 西充鮮于圖藏於

而行不自專也飾以殷之白色周承殷而酌定禮樂之眾及其長爲士承六而鄭都謀大夫士承六而鄭都謀士文明建旐故州里建旟及鄕遂建物各以其事如軍吏同象其官書某官之旟里所載旃某事如家同建物某里所載皆取其名爲象路載旞道車載旌隼迅擊象其急也鵰虎象其威也旗以爲期衆之所聚百法以治民象旗物也御案旗之別所載熊虎爲旗鳥隼爲旟龜蛇爲旐全羽爲旞析羽爲旌雜帛爲物通帛爲旜孤卿位卑先令旌而五色皆備焉

大喪其銘旌建廞車之旌及葬亦如之凡軍事建旌旗及致民置旗獘之甸亦如之凡射其獲旌歲時其號如魯之旗孟孫氏之旟叔孫氏之旗季孫氏之旌必建其象如門以爲識營德

鄭康成曰銘旌王則大常也士喪禮爲銘各以其物置旐旝民至則什伍之誅後至者同其葬云建之則行時揭旒之大司馬致衆之時同也獲旌獲者得舊旝予新

周官恆解 卷三 春官 奎一 西充鮮于圖藏於

都宗人掌都祭祀之禮凡都祭祀致福于國正都禮與其服若有寇戎之事則保羣神之壝國有大故則令禱祠旣祭反命于國

於地也獲旌更旝易舊予新常置旝旐民至則什之誅後至者同其葬云建之則行時揭旝之大司馬致衆之時同也獲旌獲者得舊旝予新

都宗人掌都祭祀之禮凡都祭祀致福于國正都禮與其服若有寇戎之事則保羣神之壝國有大故則令禱祠旣祭反命于國

其地而無主後者都宗人掌其禮旣祭致福于國在其地而無主後者都宗人掌其禮旣祭致福于國都王子弟所居之邑其地或有山川及因國之在不敢自私也獲旌更以獲者得都禮與其服有違越者得督之保羣神則之遺恐有陵犯也國有大敀禱羣神則之保于神之遺反命于王焉

家宗人掌家祭祀之禮凡祭祀致福國有大故則令禱祠反命祭亦如之掌家禮與其衣服宮室車旗之禁令

凡以神仕者掌三辰之灋以猶鬼神示之居辨其名物以冬日至致天神人鬼以夏日至致地示物魅以禬國之凶荒民之札喪

仕者則未受官而學蓺以待職用者也御案卜史祝宗巫人諸職皆有事於神其三辰之灋以神仕者別人辰日三辰此以神仕者掌三辰之灋以猶鬼神示之居辨其名物言致天神地示物魅者亦爲神所示而可見也示神必得此時而益壯也全乎可謹矣而冬夏至陰陽之精所聚鬼神分散然神明也天地人鬼之象雖能神於此時必生陰氣雖隱能仲陽氣雖衰能伸也致神物能則之國語古者民神不雜民之精爽不攜貳者而又齊肅中正其智能上下比義其聖能光照之其明能光照之其聰能聽徹之如是則神明降之在男曰覡在女曰巫使制神之處位次主而爲之牲器時服如此又能居以天法聖人用之何明哉何以見是以法令此正道賴令此正道減痛矣

總論
御案職掌邦禮而以祭祀爲主盖所以治神人而和上下故凡有事於禮及司神之官皆屬焉愚接天人無二理也天蒼蒼不可知而其理全在於人人道所在皆有天理循天理而行審於幾微久之卽念念無非天理則天道狂我故孔子曰知我其天而天且不違也後世禮樂不興人飢無以檢束其而天且不違也後世禮樂不興人飢無以檢束其

身心而又以天道為高遠神明為恍惚於是縱情茂理無所不為豈知悖天理而干罪殃自天子至於庶人心不正身不修而能倖免者蓋亦寡矣大宗伯所掌雖多祭祀巫覡之屬而其平日禮樂明備所以導民於中正者已詳然後人知人道即天道而敬鬼神省罪咎所謂非禮祈禱之事亦又免矣世或不信鬼神而縱情妄為或不修實德而專事祈禱聰明者既失之狂肆愚昧者又誤入於邪僻雖師儒之教不明亦枉上者有以使之若秦皇漢武佞妄想於神仙梁武道宗專求福於齋醮彼能為功豈不惑歟

周官恆解　卷三春官

　　　　　西充鮮于
　　　　奎
　　　　　氏特園藏

既不知正心修身仁育義正為天人相孚之本而歷代愚民為聞香為白蓮種種邪教煽惑為奸上之人既知其為非矣而不知其原由於大學之道不明也孟子曰經正則庶民興庶民興斯無邪慝夫經者豈非三綱五常敦倫盡性之實乎五倫本於五性原止一性盡其性而盡人物之性體樂刑賞悉杠其中矣為民牧者何不深思之而力行之至近世官吏素不能體上意以安民及民怨畔滋事則加以邪教之名期於免罪當宁或不察之亦以為果邪教矣覺民性無常平日教化皆不

周官恆解卷三終

周官恆解　卷三春官

　　　　　西充鮮于
　　　　奎
　　　　　氏特園藏

有明明德亦人人所能而莫知禂方無以成已何以成人孔曾此書將如畫餅登讀書稽古不負

君親之道乎

在親民

古貴賤無異學故天子元子諸侯卿大夫之子皆同一大學之道其力行德行道藝亦由上庠下庠漸次而升大學記曰小學在公宮南之左大學在郊小學即上庠下庠等也大學所以在郊以便體天下招致四方賢士之意二者與民相親以一概然而五方風氣異齊民生其間異俗非可以一概而施必與民相親人情物理細心體察卽一隅以反三隅久之然後隨時隨地隨人隨事斟酌而合乎時中大舜好問好察邇而用中由斯道也故明德必須親民親非但親近親愛此中有許多功夫在愚夫愚婦一能勝子無眾寡無小大無敢慢察言觀色慮以下人一切取善之法皆在其中聖人

大學古本傍言 九 西充鮮于氏特圓藏

明德雖止在一心而其理散著於萬事萬物事物不可勝窮以五倫爲大民生日用之事爲切明明德者性已盡身可以措諸天下無不宜矣察人情物理爲出身加民之本蓋萬理統於明德

明於庶物察於人倫亦由乎此高宗舊勞於外文王卑服卽康功田功爰暨小人則知小人之依能保惠於庶民卽周公待以告成王惟恐其不知民依後世理學與事功殊途高言義理而鮮經綸卽有勤名未臻純粹至箸書立說尤多偏駁降而愈下詞章記問之學至老不能盡工人倫日用之理或反視爲尋常矣六合之遙民生之眾古今時勢不同弗觀其會通而衷於至是日未大行也無知己也然而聖人陶漁版築卽終身匹夫亦有可法可傳一官一邑亦能安人濟物又何以故夫人固未有子然一身與世相違者也一室之中父子兄弟夫婦一日之內凡言行交際往來其人其事固已不齊觀我觀人明辨義理求其無愧於心已非易易而況大學之地貴賤賢愚無限天下人材羣集相習相親增廣智識者何窮豈必盡天下之事而知盡天下之民而求之哉所以明明德之人卽誠身之人誠者非自成已而已也所以成物也成已仁也成物知也合外內之道也故時措之宜成已能明其德已可以俯齊治平而更親民以廣其識耳俯其身而天下平聖人無兩副本領盡其爲學時卽講

大學古本傍言 十 西充鮮于氏特圓藏

止至善似乎駭聽而實則周易已言之鼎之大象曰君子以正位凝命艮之大象曰兼山艮君子思不出其位即至位即至於至善也當時門人學於夫子無不知之曾子亦特逃其詞而記者載入論語誠以其為學之要耳不知而以為凡事止於至善然不知止至善則憧憧往來朋從爾思物欲交感何從而定靜安故夫子慨之而曰天下何思何慮有欲止其心而不知至善之所者艮其限厲薰心夫子以為至危凡此皆與此書之言互相發者惜罕從事其學故不能會通其義

大學古本質言　 西充鮮于圓藏

耳夫子言知止即孟子所云養浩然止安止此志氣之主氣志之用持其志無暴其氣久而定靜安下文必有事焉而勿正心勿忘勿助長言養氣之法即止至善之功集義生氣則以義理之心生浩然之氣非但空空靜坐即曰明德其功次第甚多示人以知止初效益必知之眞而後能然故知字十分吃緊愚亦另提明二字許之至止至善何以即為養氣亦久鮮人知矣許見下文而後有定定而后能靜靜而后能安

學所以明明德其功不外靜存動察知行並進凡身心內之存養人倫中之言行知其是非即力行其是屏除其非學問思辨以致知篤行所以力行義盡於斯矣而皆以止至善為基故必先知止知止者致知之原也天下古今事物不可盡知亦不必盡知盡行故予言有弗學問思辨行惟當行者則弗能弗措知行必本於心而人心多私妄能不欺不息不肆惟知止則能收已放之心入虛靈之舍持其志無暴其氣至虛至靜一念不生則為知止矣心本浮動強制之而愈紛亂知止非用力

大學古本質言　 西充鮮于圓藏

強持也存神養氣守中不動使心凝然渾然虛無清淨之至則爲有定不曰能定而曰有定者心善動如子午定盤鍼即至靜亦有動意惟聖人性定而心不動乃能常定譬如靜坐凝有一息之定神凝有兩息之定一時共八刻十二分有一二分定時即為妙境志氣之帥氣體之充神為氣主神凝即持志非用力持之志心而言神以其靈妙言耳神養氣便是存心養氣不言心而言神神也存神養氣即氣聚入於虛靜曰虛無清淨寂滅者則寂然心不動滅盡私欲

緣物感而起繼而外物與知覺相習則遇事物而妄動無事物而亦憧憧矣初學知止至善養心之久而有定靜安氣象則存有基矣能靜然後能知意之發動一念之動善則擴充惡則克治久久物欲漸少靜存者愈固然後志與氣一浩然之氣自生而有諸己充實漸次以至神化因平日先有格物致知一段功夫乃能知其意之是否而誠之非不知止至善專求誠意便可誠也此處功夫先儒未知故似是而非反疑曾子之言錯簡今若再不贅言後人何從致力也蓋人心浮動非有以養

大學古本質言　　西充鮮于氏特園藏

之不能沈靜心之靈靈以氣而氣囿於質心運於虛虛故靈妙質故滯濁志為氣之帥以此矣持其志無暴其氣非俗所謂凝神靜氣乎神於何凝則止於至善也宅心於密常凝常靜一念妄動隨即斬除前人云不怕念起只怕覺遲隨起隨即放心之法即所謂格物也心斬除之故知求清明一有物欲之萌即真心斬除之故知止之功其源誠意以謹其幾不可偏廢若無知止之養心浮動無已時欲屏去物欲而欲生愈其意而意不能定雖竭力瘁神一生亦何由盡性故誠

大學古本質言　　西充鮮于氏特園藏

意而意不誠者多也其致知格物功夫兼內外而言致知該博學審問慎思明辨等功格物該非禮勿視非禮勿聽等功非空空強持其心死而後已安能細細體貼層層實踐使意無稍雜哉意不誠則循生迭起憧擾不盡又何以漸求正心之後則大學之序所以先教人誠意若正心之後則念念天理無事有心操持而意自誠聖人之不思不勉而從容中道由此其選焉

欲誠其意者先致其知

大學之道知行不可偏廢人知之而其用功知行一時並到人或不知也先儒重在先知聖人則曰知之匪艱行之維艱盡天下事物不能盡知亦不必盡知蓋不必知夫子所以言有弗學問思辨行之惟其有弗知弗行者所以為擇善而可不慎乎知蓋知弗行也知之無益於行或反有害於德安乃以物物窮理為知哉道雖無窮五倫為大天下皆五倫中人聖人言行制作止是經緯五倫雖時勢異宜民生異俗而隨時處中其要不外乎此必知者知日用人倫言行動靜之理耳實踐人倫必

大學古本旁言

人又何以為天地鬼神者陰陽之靈卽天地之
天地無為而二氣流行生化消長卽鬼神為之易
曰知變化之道者其知神之所為乎聖人統一
天至誠如神夫子言誠字以鬼神明之鬼神理氣
之靈特誣多偽託之儒者遂竝天地之正義而
亦以為誣子曰知我其天詩曰帝謂文王豈怪妄
之詞乎聖人事親如事天事親如事幽獨渺而
必嚴指視如人子不敢一毫欺豫其親耳明明在上
赫赫在下日旦無敢戲豫馳驅自古聖賢皆
然登詔顯鬼神妄測天道廢民義而求諸幽渺哉
未解天人一氣之實欲防閑邪誕而不知為慎獨
本原則不但不知天命而不畏且物怪人妖乘人
心之邪妄而作小人傾家喪命又旣而信鬼反召巫蠱
漢武始而求仙繼而求神又旣而信鬼反召巫蠱
之禍白蓮聞香等教咸世無窮若知鬼神不外天
理則敬鬼神以糾心遠鬼神以杜妄念事事依
於天理又何至為邪妄所愚乎周易一書多言吉
凶悔吝吉凶非禍福乎餘慶餘殃積善成
名積惡滅身教人避禍求福實教人誠意正心而
善禍淫者天道司天地之功化者鬼神天地人神

大學古本旁言

一氣相通由其本一理相貫歧而視之誕而置之
更何能慎獨曾子先言誠意必慎獨而乃承明所
以當慎之由曰十目十手指視卽如在其上如在
其左右之義耳曾子曰三字承上交一正一反之
義而以己意斷之指出嚴字見天人一氣誠意者
不自欺卽所以不欺天常解謂意之所生己知人
卽知之故必慎獨然畏人知而不敢為惡猶是聞
居為不善之小人曾子之言不自相矛盾歟至曾
子誠意五章首句皆有所謂字割裂原文增出明
新止至善本末四章又補一五章移此章於第六
章突然而起俱無所謂字末章以此謂知本句作
結刪聖經此謂知本二句以為衍文凡若此類以
文理言亦屬不合愚何敢計而令此書舛錯後人
孔子耳得罪與否亦何足計而令此書舛錯後人
無從問津則大學之道不能盡人而為品學何以
精純修齊治平何由不負孔子之訓邪
富潤屋德潤身心廣體胖故孔子必誠其意
人心易放難收易動難靜故自欺者多收心而凜

畏神天則人苦其難矣曾子故特言其效以歆動
之提出身心二字見意即心之勤者心爲身之主
者果能誠意雖未必即可正心而自慊者心亦安
心安則形神自暢即有廣胖之美人無不愛其身
而每多疾厄困苦雖氣化不齊亦無由積咎之多明
明德者止至善而常覺安誠其意而無敢欺肆
則志氣清明愧怍漸少禮曰四體既正膚革充盈
小則卻病延年大則精明強固孔子言愚者明柔
者強孟子曰盎於背施於四體四體不言而喻
下文引詩言赫喧皆是此義夫人無論賢愚貴賤

大學古本傍言

未有不願身安境順者大學之道初知止誠意便
有此效以此開示後人煞是苦心亦是實理實事
先儒未賤聖人之學遂覺人生天折窮困無可如
何則道亦似乎無用心廣體胖之人皆誠意中人又大不
誤解而謂世閒癡肥之人皆誠意中人又大不
惟意爲心之發動誠爲正之要功故特言先言誠
之效以歆動人下乃詳言其功以潤屋喻身就
淺近指點人此富者無心潤屋而多財自不居於
茅茨有德豈必張皇而氣象自不覺其光昌德潤
身中便有養浩然之功在浩然之氣乾元之氣天

之所以爲天也由善而養而充實即可以立命明明
德者心與天通氣與天合浩然者塞乎兩大而何
慮短折飢塞乎誠意之心廣體胖非遂乎常不同耳
光輝乃神安氣靜欲寡心淸已覺與尋常不同耳
然有此效驗不懈其功則美在其中而暢於四支
發於事業亦不俟他求以上三節言誠意之故及
功夫初效義已無餘因恐人不知誠意足該明明
德之事故又將夫子所言歸併發明一一梳析之
而前人不得其義竊易添設於是曾子之意隱矣

詩云瞻彼淇澳菉竹猗猗有斐君子如切如磋如琢
如磨瑟兮僴兮赫兮喧兮有斐君子終不可喧兮
上文言自慊好處自欺不好處教人嚴指視而愼
獨並及其效大義畢矣但誠意必先致知致知必
內外交飭非專特守心日擴清明亦非泛驚見聞
求諸身外且致知格物誠意功夫雖有次第而莫
非所以修身卽明明德誠意爲首恐人疑其罣漏故
可太歧視曾子獨標誠意及明德親民等義一
引詩之美武公者將格致誠及明德親民等義一
一歸併在誠意中而分析之後儒不知妄爲竄改
實學何以明卽詩人摹擬武公之德表裏兼到曾

-3317-

子引來自爲之解所以發明夫子格致等義不可
以詩人之意爲即曾子意也
如切如磋者道學也
此句言致知之功也善惡是非百出其途淺深大
小經權常變尤非一致安能一一而知之惟日用
倫常言行動靜自一念以暨念念一事以暨事事
不得參雜此二字中便該得博學審問慎思明辨
必審察精細得其是非之正始爲美惡雜陳剖厥
是非如切骨角分爲兩下使再不能相混再加詳
審如切而又磋去其渣滓使是中之非非中之是
不得參雜此二字中便該得博學審問慎思明辨
此句言格物也是非之心人皆有之何以多昏昧
而少明明私欲爲之也耳目口鼻四支之欲由七
情而紛不審天理任意而行則氣質之累生物欲
物欲之心横平且致知者非內有義外有學不能
漸銷其私欲而漸擴其聰明惟止於至善常使靜
安則志氣日清又能愼動不敢一毫恣肆然後知
日以致如治玉石者琢石而得玉矣又加磨礪使
成美器動靜交養久久此心定靜不爲外物所誘

大學古本廣言　竇氏特圖藏
功夫在內故釋之曰此言學以致知也

雖未必純乎天理而言行動靜覺合理者多不合
理者少則德日崇惡日修故曰自修也修二字
古通修治也美也致知所以爲誠意之地而必去
物誘之私知始能致一念之非必格知日以致動
而行其所知即是誠意修除去物欲卽即格字意
蓋曾子已如此解格字
瑟兮僴兮者恂慄也
此句言誠意也瑟縝密意僴閑制意恂誠也慄敬
也誠意者必先知止有定靜安之象矣然後一念
之動即知之卽去其非者行其是者此爲誠意
之動而審幾不遺罅隙由靜而鎭定少有疏虞故誠
意之內外交修一時並到故嚴密之意瑟兮間兮
而曾子釋以誠敬之意恂慄信也卽誠也慄敬懼也
赫兮喧兮者威儀也
此句言德潤身也上文言誠意之效以心廣體胖
言謂神安形適非遂至於充實光輝也詩人美武
公威儀則以其盛德在躬誠中形外與曾子言廣
胖不同雖由誠意而正而身修廣胖者即威儀然此
章釋誠意則威儀止可跟德潤意說盡此書言大
學功夫句句皆有實義不可混也

大學古本廣言　竇氏特圖藏

無不格知誠爲修身之外更無功業乃爲知修身之本也故結之曰此謂知本此章開端大聲特呼言誠意者毋自欺曾子因人多自欺卻又想修身不知一自欺則入於小人大學格致誠正等功倘安能一一力行末節引子言聽訟仍發明毋自欺之義其意曰毋自欺則誠其身已修明矣誠而無情之人皆可感化而修齊治平於此矣誠字原於孔子而曾子得誠身之傳特標誠意一章爲首細細發明使千秋後世力行其學必以一誠爲主又釋正心下四章此大學一書爲

大學古本廣言   㙓
                氏㹅輯圖叢

曾子之書而孔子聖經乃益明也不料後人妄爲竄改今若不詳辨聖學功夫塵封何時開乎曾子言大學以誠爲本依然夫子修身爲本不知而刪去夫子此謂知本此謂知之至二句抑妄矣

右第一章曾子標誠意爲學之本而竝舉孔子所言錯雜釋之因意與心有別誠與正心功不同故下章又釋正心身修則可以齊治平矣而家國天下施爲不同故又釋齊治平三章通計五章蓋惟恐學者有誤而然雖先述聖經自爲曾子之書原文本無石傳等字今將

存孔曾之舊於每章後僭增右第某章等字明曾子補孔子之意本止五章竝非十章惟恆解則云又傳幾章以此書自程朱竄改後效尤者眾以傳字別之於聖經杜人又妄改者所謂修身在正其心者身有所忿懥則不得其正有所恐懼則不得其正有所好樂則不得其正有所憂患則不得其正
學者常云身心性命之理日用倫常之道二語足該大學中庸矣第日用倫常之事本於身心性若非靜存動察久而純化豈能實踐倫理時措咸宜正心也修身也盡性至命也其功非旦夕必

大學古本廣言   窗
               㨿氏㹅輯圖叢

明師指授久而不逾方可性命之理詩書及孔孟所言愚爲恆解已各就本文釋之茲不贅身心字此章至爲分明惜前人妄改身字爲心字遂使後學憫然欠不得不詳論也萬物皆天地所生而人爲最靈者以其獨得天理具於心而有先後天之分先天之心卽性後天之心爲情情有七而心始紛物交物而情滅性矣孟子言惻隱等四端之情可以爲善非謂凡情皆善情卽是性也先儒誤認於是卽心卽性而正心之功亦不

槐軒雜著 《卷一 時中論》

建而至今卒不可興棄禮義詩書而不久依然復故天理民彝之正固無終窮而因革損益之宜則非一轍亦可依類而推矣後世法制之密有聖賢不能加然而窮理盡性之學罕有真修則刑名法術之煩者一於穆之命既生以前渾然粹徒增奸蠹王莽以篡逆而行周官安石以乖僻而創新法本源既非妄作皆謬夫豈修古道之不足憲章歟晚近之學者泥古則失於拘墟守成則憚於變制蘧子不云乎瑟不調甚者必取而更張之變其所當變而弗變也四民之業有祖父所傳子孫明之非人所固不能政舉其所不當變化而裁之神而明之非人所之者況天下之事期於教養合宜豈必株守成法然或藉口於時中詭隨以徇物在上則輕違乎典則在下亦變亂乎舊章此叉害於人心風俗之甚者君子安可不明辨而慎擇之哉時不同而中同堯舜以下之聖人皆是自人避變法之非而拘守前人學術治術往往貽誤不少先生嘗舉似以示吾徒此論引而不發感嘅不少

業編芽志

虛無清淨說

天以一元化生萬物理宰乎氣氣寓乎理其流形於品物者有名象之可言而上天之載則固無聲臭者也人為萬物之靈其氣質之欲著於視聽食息者與物無殊惟天命之性本於維皇而未生以前渾然粹然者一於穆之命既生以後憧憧往來者乃雜形氣之私聖人教人復性以去其氣質之私而全其本然之性必由養氣存神神即心之靈也人心易放道心難純非至虛至靜莫能養其性也求放心而致中一念不生沉潛靜處無私不雜執中精一即此其是未發之中存神於虛一私不雜執中精一即此其是故存心養性非至虛至無則無以致其中非至清至淨猶不免雜於欲以此四字狀其至靜之意而豈廢人倫遺日用之謂哉聖人德造其極泛應曲當之妙本於至虛至明明故萬理皆徹虛故含己從人而其原則由涵養之熟天理渾然夫虛非於穆不已之天乎文王之穆一天之穆詩人歎想其純而曰不顯之德不顯者乃穆穆文王以此而名乃訓以為豈不顯是徒知顯者為德而不知不顯者乃德之源則其以虛無清淨為非曷足怪焉夫不顯之德所謂闇然者也然而篤恭天下乃平合乎上天之載是故理著於萬物固有形有象之可名理舍

槐軒雜著 卷一 存眞辨異說

西充鮮于氏特園藏

夫豈公論唐人佞佛太過闢之固宜憲宗有唐令主其迎佛骨不過惑於異說欲求長年文公當以寡欲修身仁民事天之學告之至於朽腐之骨雖聖人亦屬無用此理之易曉者乃不以為言而謂信佛必至短命豈不為抵觸君上乎孔子曰老耼博古知今則吾師稱為猶龍而昌黎以為坐井觀天何小視孔子如是因佛老之員失其傳而異端競起而知心性倫常之鮮能踐而憎道益張誠使反身而求之實外無聖賢佛老俱有妻子則凡託於佛老以為好貌子言其是者不可以為非則其非者乃不至以為中庸之道遂百出其途可慨也已襲聖賢以為學者可一掃而空之惜乎明者甚而佛老之眞者無異聖賢其偽者皆流傳之謬先生嘗言其是者不可以為非則其非者乃不至以為是此篇所以名存眞辨異也

感應論

楊芳

一元之理氣流行而不息生生而不窮者曷為之主宰哉上天之載無聲無臭而其仁覆萬物無終無始者昭著於耳目之前各得其所日禮各有其宜日義不爽日智不息日信五性皆本於天五倫亦由斯出

槐軒雜著 卷一 感應論

西充鮮于氏特園藏

人為天地之心無一非天所賦而況有善無惡者本天之理而人之性乎善與善相感而善事應之惡與惡相感而惡事應之天亦何心惟其人之自為哉吉培之傾者覆之感應捷於影響大易全書所以藉身凶誘人於善也後儒不知天人一氣之原誨人修身不言禍福孔以以禍福為天理之自然而純避禍為人情所同然欲使一念之動必歸天理純知善福本富然而有希福之心未知惡不可為而有畏禍之念則因勢而利導迄乎行之久而志之所而天人自知感召正不必盡為上智即中下之材未為而為者亦可以無所為而亦為夫子所謂勉強之久歸於自然也善不積不足以成名惡不積不足以滅身餘慶餘殃諄諄致戒而何乃以感應為異端之學乎聖人不敢謂天下皆小人而亦不敢謂天下皆君子明天理以正人心示災祥以嚴修省固覺世牖民之要義豈可以為妄談若夫忠臣孝子遭遇艱難致命遂志正氣與天地相參馨香合萬姓同享正其善之至而天命申之人極賴之不得以為意外之禍也惠迪吉從逆凶虞廷已早言之但畏禍求福必當以改過遷善為心不可存希翼之想耳

使來獎借多端且以前賢講學相例聞之不勝愕然夫道者天理而已人人皆有天理則人人可以為聖人聖人亦祇全乎天授之正耳達而為君相以禮樂陶成天下窮而為師儒以中庸裁成後學皆本成己者以成人及其功用既溥敷化大行後人尊而信之寶而傳之其人則本無壽世留名之想也史臣陋劣則為道學文苑等名岐交行而二之一二有志之士以聖賢之事淑身遂高自位置生徒復相標榜於是門戶之見以興學聖人之途以雜益嘗私心慨之而顧蹈其覆轍乎古禮古樂不可行於今矣而斤斤欲踐之不知周公之禮孔子已多所折衷使生於斯時亦惟遵一王之制酌時俗之宜不外乎中正而已世事日增情形日異法制之密民生日用所循蓋有古人所不能及者而其不逮古人則五倫之不修耳道以五倫為大五倫由心而起心之不正心性不除由天命之全體未復復性者有動靜交養之功始終本末之序以昭昭靈靈識神為先天乾元之善性此儒學亦類於禪宗而告子之不動心非是原黑之克伐怨欲不行亦非仁也愚分卑學淺安敢妄言聖人之道第研窮六經有年覺天人本無二理困勉亦

槐軒雜著 《卷三 復王雪嶠書》 巴 西充鮮于氏特圓藏

可成功居常以言動規矩語人必先令其靜坐收心心本浮也而沈之本顯也而潛之中者天下之本也致中而後可致和一念之善而擴充一念之惡而克治此動察之功耳喜怒哀樂之未發止於其所委志虛無久而渾渾淪淪者一先天純一之性則動而言行踐閱者亦少矣故曰苟志於仁矣無惡而大學之明明德孔門之為仁中庸之盡性孟子之養氣不動心皆自此而臻前人以禮法教人未嘗非是而不即現今行習之事示以是非使其易循必違稽古制迂視聖人施之既不順而為之亦苦難小則誤身大則誤世安可不辨耶自來以虛無清淨罪佛老而不知心至難持凡存養之時非虛靜不能疑道虛無者一念不生渾然在中清靜者私欲淨盡天理純全耳心在後天氣質之欲恆多義理之性恆少存有覺之心養無為之性必有事焉而勿正心勿忘勿助長也惟至虛至靜而後浩然之元氣乃生日月合璧保合太和由有諸己而至化神其功效次第一一可據特非師不傳非人不授故孟子以為難言也不然念念而防之如治棼絲終身豈有復性之日哉今儒修偏於外鶩僧道習為頑空而本原之學罕有識者愚為此

槐軒雜著 《卷三 復王雪嶠書》 巴 西充鮮于氏特圓藏

為聖人理義之邦由義皇以來神靈疊出禮樂制度昭明矣外裔則不能然置無知赤子於物類而不立之君師天心豈安故毓秀鍾奇鴯民覺世四裔之有賢能亦猶乎中國也佛不待言若觀音大士為佛門之領袖其靈異尤彰南史載朝士癇疾觀音示現療之而瘳則其由來已逺考諸載籍大士氏妙水罷夷人少而穎異長厭塵勞靜參性命遂達心源由瀾滄江入南海棲於落伽山民間有求無不響應我朝百靈效順觀音常為福護廟祀已遍海隅頌之者曰救苦救難觀世音而已不知其德之純亦如吾儒

槐軒雜箸 卷三 培修白衣菴碑記

莘 氏特圖藏

仁者慈悲救苦即悲憫之意耳而豈有異術哉乾坤覆載萬物各著其功男女同此秉彝各成其德閩閫原多聖流邑羡所以崇於十亂也又於容誕而置之省垣白衣菴舊祀觀音乾隆甲辰寺燬於火而觀音之像巍然道光癸卯復遘回祿像亦無損是非其神有不朽者歟孟子曰仁也者人之所以合而言之道也全乎仁即道光乎仁也者人純乎天理而已理即天理即無愧乎聖賢耳聖賢而民尸祝之於瑘豈之佛菩薩中土日日聖賢耳聖賢而民尸祝之於瑘豈有戾乎諸善士捐募重新此寺其樂善良不可沒愚

故為表而出之並述大士崖略以免淺議者之瑕疵

觀音廟祀遍天下靈蹟亦多第人罕知其出處及其實德先生以仁字詁之以南史事證之理確而事非無稽可使俗流織口亦可使事觀音者返而求諸此心之仁矣 受業姪孫鴻典志

青羊宮善工碑記

天者理而已人為萬物之靈秉天秀氣以生即得天正理為性故盡天者必盡性盡而念念事事合乎理即時時在在通於天此聖人之所以為至人而凡餘則惟時稟相在不忘敬懼而已人倫日用之事無一而無天理故凡人皆當 畏乎天命之三畏豈冀天佑而然乎天不知以詔來茲而解者誤以中庸一書言盡人合天之學以詔來茲而解者誤以大德受命為作天子不知受命即栽者培之之意耳近入尊上帝為玉皇而復有經說其言河漢其事類於矯誣而其競業業不敢褻天之意則固君子所不廢青羊宮道人日日課經亦拾殘字以免穢污兩端皆為善行薛鳳池等又為捐金若干以助可不為

莘 氏特圖藏

正䚦 卷一 六 西充鮮于圖藏

已治人之道不絕如綫太宗命世之才而無師作則人倫不端啓後世妖淫之禍豈非天惡其無以作率而反導民䙝倫乎人君統三綱之責如此開創何以明大學而作育人才昌黎天姿高曠有志聖學而亦未遇明師因闢佛之故後世翕然宗之以原道爲不刊之論學者知道在倫常而不知常必本於心正身乃能脩若不正心而徒言日用倫常則一切皆浮而眞心天理不純盡天理性也盡性知天而人倫日用巨細精粗乃協其宜夫豈但如原道所云已哉至闢佛而不知佛之實又橫詆老子竝孔子亦不足信實爲武斷愚常力辨僧道可闢佛老不可闢矣今將破千載之疑不得不又贅言以列於後

一正䚦兼及佛老者不知佛老之眞則其合聖人者亦非之而學聖無從始基也

盈天地皆人則皆天之赤子天豈不安養之佛者天生異人以綏靖外地者也去中華萬餘里曷嘗欲惑中華因中華聖教漸微儒修多驚名利甚而蕩棄禮法民之秉彝覺其不安聞清淨慈悲等說乃欣慕之然固未從其教也太宗遣元奘求經元

正䚦 卷一 七 西充鮮于圖藏

奘人品頗高太宗又重其人經至又加珍重民乃靡然從風然佛之行誼中華不能知也佛如聖人豈尚喜人媚禮降福愚民不知士大夫亦以傳譌於是不脩德而徒求福利佛豈同於羲舜堯舜之昌黎進諫憲宗言佛卽聖人不過同於羲舜堯舜朽骨卽不足貴陛下以羲舜之道脩身卽以治世䣺年自古聖人皆如此佛必不能有加也如此享遐年清心仁覆天下天心必眷之民安而己亦立說憲宗當亦豁然而乃君欲求壽以信佛短命觸之豈臣子之道乎故佞佛當禁而僧流非佛之眞妄爲附會尤必當辨佛有妻有子不廢人倫明心見性卽盡心知性之義慈悲廣大方便清淨亦聖人仁義廉讓之言耳眞空不空妙有不有理至虛而至實費而隱微之顯其意亦同所謂不垢不淨不廢宮室衣食男女不爲所累也不生不滅因物付物不生事亦不廢事也不增不減恰得乎中無過無不及也流俗誤解別爲之說亦如解釋孔孟之書者大失其義豈足爲佛咎平四夷多無人倫非佛倡之中華寺宇收養窮民不能更蓄妻子則事理之不得不然凡誕妄之說考諸佛籍亦無其

正譌 〈卷二〉 五

乃有善不善學道者欲求復受中之始必存心養性如何存養人身有竅為有妙為天地生化萬物非物物而生化之也有竅為陰陽五行全滙聚於此無聲無臭無始無終而陰陽生焉五行布焉生而不窮變化而不息是為天地之中無可名也以其為萬物之原理之至極而名曰太極天地之太極至虛而至實一元之理氣渾於一竅人則之生以前受中者亦如天地既生以後神氣散布於欲動時收放心入竅而使之定安是為有觀竅百骸此竅空無有矣黃帝內觀此義皆此義竅妙雖有二名止於至善也

存其心之功也若無嗜欲時則默守中宮一念不生至虛至靜氣寂而理趣自生是為無欲觀妙其竅之功也亦易闢闔通平造化當觀竅觀妙時果能觀妙至和亦易闢闔通乎造化當觀竅觀妙時果能實止一處故曰同出而異名元者幽深之意觀竅著之和亦易闢闔通乎造化當觀竅觀妙時果能一念不生太虛同體則妙趣有難言者所謂元也再內外交脩仁義同熟中庸云天下之大本故曰元穆穆之德元之又元通乎帝謂皆由是基故曰元王

正譌 〈卷二〉 六

之又元眾妙之門而夫子謂成性存存道義之門亦斯義也成性者盡其性也允執厥中守其精一是為存存萬事萬理所會歸曰道義之門自聖學卒傳解者妄為之說遂以老子為異端不思孔子所敬禮豈稍有不合而稱以猶龍乎昌黎第沿俗說儒者宗之錯解老子何足為老子病而不知竅妙之說致中正而明明德養浩然平昌黎第沿俗說儒者宗之錯解老子何足為老等語全不得其端倪其實聖人之學隱矣人何從盡性至命全入道以合天道乎

周道衰孔子沒火於秦黃老於漢佛於晉魏梁隋之間其言道德仁義者不入於楊則入於墨不入於老則入於佛入於彼必出於此入者主之出者奴之入者附之出者汙之噫後之人其欲聞仁義道德之說就從而聽之

自羲農以來聖人遞興成已成人之道至周大備後雖衰微而文武之道在人議大議小孔子且因而成聖則天下未嘗無人持功利富強日競至戰國而放恣益甚上無君相持綱下而儒衡分裂處士橫議至來焚書坑儒之禍然而孔孟之言因爐餘而大顯則毀糟粕而存菁華冥冥中亦有深意

後世孔子大顯於世孟子之言遂確而儒者亦云云然夫子所以為萬世師者何止春秋不實踐孔子言行則雖尊孔子而不得其真亦無益有損況徒工文字誦詩書而不敢實行者乎
道德高厚教化無窮實與天地參而四時同其惟孔子乎
凡聖人皆萬世師不獨孔子也孟子生民未有等語皆因當時無人知孔子而云然不然孔子祖述堯舜憲章文武而謂賢於堯舜百王皆莫之及祖述憲章何以通即後人欲學聖等夫子於天原不

正鵠 《卷三》 壽 西充鮮于氏特園藏

為過但夫子亦不過盡其人道不期而合天耳人之所以為人即天之所以為天聖人人中之至人非有奇異自漢至今須孔子者難以枚舉惟先孔子而聖者非孔子無以明後孔子而聖者非孔子自言非生知十五志學三十而後立豈果絕人以學步哉尊聖太過使人不敢學聖大非天生人之意聖人望人之戒之
童蒙求我我正果行如筮為筮叩神也再三則瀆瀆則不告也山下出泉靜而深也汨則亂亂不決也

慎哉其惟時中乎艮其背背非見也靜則止止非為也為不止矣其道也深乎
水性流行而山阻之如人性本善而欲蔽之昏蒙之象故卦名蒙然水出於山初出之時必清也又有泉象故卦聖人恐人自安於蒙則以童蒙喻之言水本流行雖暫為山阻而終必達如童蒙不久於蒙且卦體二剛中與五相應五為君位是蒙之主阻水而使之蒙者五也然能阻之即能通之水善流行不安於蒙必求出蒙於何而求之五而已故以童蒙求我為象教人自求出蒙但求教於人必

正鵠 《卷三》 壽 西充鮮于氏特園藏

以誠聞教即力行不可徒口耳而多瀆如求神然以筮求神信之者真則初筮所告即誠信遵行不再疑惑若再三瀆則疑貳不誠神必不告也故蒙有可亨之理以其有剛中之誠與五剛柔相應必不終於蒙而能求五以出蒙夫子言初筮皆以剛中也謂初筮之時心必至誠使以疑貳之心而屢筮不誠則不告者亦蒙告之時故曰瀆瀆蒙也屢告是求者蒙告者亦蒙蒙將無已時故亦疑告以亨求時中者發蒙之人告不告隨時蒙者既而多疑則不誠再三瀆合宜乃得善教之法故可以養童蒙之正而為聖

日月寒暑萬古不移所謂天有常道也至常而
神知日月之妙乃知天地聖人亦未嘗言張子豈
能知之陰陽不測之謂神夫子所指非日月寒暑
也範圍天地曲成萬物通乎晝夜故之曰神無方而易無體以神無贊易而乃引來
之曰神無方而易無體合神與易為一已謬言寒暑晝
云神易無方體合神與易為一已謬言寒暑晝
又云陰陽不測結曰所謂通乎晝夜之道寒暑
夜陰陽之顯著者而其原皆在日月引用聖人語
雜湊不分明由其苦心思索而言非有實得也
晝夜者天之一息乎寒暑者天之晝夜乎天道春秋

正蒙　卷四　芸　西充鮮于圓藏

分而氣易猶人一瘧疾而魂交為成夢百感紛紜
對瘧而言一身之晝夜也氣交為春萬物糅錯對秋
而言天之晝夜也氣本之虛則湛本無形感而生
聚而有象有對對必反其為有對必反斯有仇
必和而解故愛惡之情同出於太虛而卒歸於物欲
候而生忽而成不容有毫髮之間其神矣夫
晝夜天之一息寒暑天之晝夜也其有一定乎晝
分如人一瘧疾大誤人之常不有晝而亦寐者即寐則有夢
作夜息固人之常不有晝而亦寐者即寐則有夢
出於七情七情本於氣質紛紜變態神識所為心

正蒙　卷四　堯　西充鮮于圓藏

虛即太極太極本無極而有七情之根乎且以卒
歸物欲倏生倏成而為神鳥知天地之神純乎理
物無無陰陽者以是知天地變化二端而已萬物形
色神之糟粕性與天道云者以是知天地變化二端而已心所以萬物殊
者感外物為不一也天大無外其為感者絪縕二端
而已

一陰一陽之謂道謂無一物無陰陽是也形色皆
天性非神之糟粕性即天理性與天道非二易該

天地人止一神氣凡氣之所在皆神神之所已得而知之矣此君子所以慎獨也
氣天之神不盡於日人之神不盡於目瘤則神著
寐則神隱讀謂棲心棲腎亦非
圖雖無文吾終日言而未嘗離乎是蓋天地萬物之
理盡在其中矣
終日言未嘗離是殊爲妄語
圖益言河圖然邵子未能知易何能知圖書哉謂
先天之學心也後天之學迹也
先天後天四字始於孔子止言未有天地之前既
有天地之後耳義文八卦方位名曰先天後天未
正譌　《卷五》　堯
　　　　　　　西充鮮于
　　　　　　　氏特圖藏
知爲聖人語乎爲後人語乎其名與義合固可不
朽若康節以數爲先天則妄矣先天之義不
一以天地言則未有天地之謂既有天
地矣則天地是先天人生物爲後天之言人
生以前爲先天既生以後爲天以生我者言天
地是先天之父母父母是後天之天地數雖起於
一以天地而天地不可以數盡也窮理盡性以至於
與天地合德乃爲先天之學何乃妄言之且以心跡
分屬即
凡人之善惡形於言發於行人始得而知之但萌諸

心發於慮鬼神已得而知之矣此君子所以慎獨也
人之神則欺天地之神人之自欺所以欺天地可不慎
哉
人之神即天地之神自欺則欺天所以當慎此條
義極精當
人必有德器然後喜怒皆不妄爲卿相爲四夫以至
學問高天下亦若無有也
人必內重內重則外輕荷內輕必外重好利好名無
所不至
天下言讀書者不少能讀書者少若得天理眞樂何
書不可讀耶何堅然不可破何理不可精
正譌　《卷五》　甼
　　　　　　　西充鮮于
　　　　　　　氏特圖藏
此三節皆粹然有德之言
漢儒以反經合道爲權得一端者也權所以平物之
輕重聖人行權酌其輕重而行之合其宜而已故執
中無權者猶爲偏也王通言春秋王道之權非王通
莫能及此故權在一身則有一身之權在一鄉則有
一鄉之權以至於有天下則有天下之權用雖不同
其權一也
惟聖人能權此條近是
先天學心法也故圖皆自中起萬化萬事生乎心也

心法二字始於邵子後儒相沿言之然學以明理
全天理而爲人即爲聖人何得云法云心法哉此
淺學者之妄言河圖五土生數居中以象太極人
心在後天已非先天純一之性不得同於河圖之

中

知易者不必引用講解是爲知易及孟子之言未嘗及
易其間易道存焉但人見之者鮮耳人能用易是爲
知易如孟子可謂善用易者也
易該天地萬物之理人能內外交養至天理極熟
無處不協於中則無事非易之理凡聖人皆然豈

正譌 卷五 塱 西充鮮于氏特圓藏

獨孟子哉孟子學已至於聖人避孔子而名曰大
賢人多不知然不明孟子之言則必不知孔子矣
謂孟子非聖大誤

總論

堯夫天資明敏志量和平不汲汲於仕進猷猷終
身有郭林宗氣象故當時人多愛敬之且同鄉賢
公卿如文富司馬諸公皆相與交遊程張諸子亦
共推重考其平生瑕疵甚少當爲一代高人然未
遇明師實踐大學之道但工於數學談言偶中人
遂以爲奇而朱子且爲詩美其爲神仙皇極經世

等書或本有此意而伯溫與門人附會成書然聖
道本中庸除卻心性倫常外無他事術數之學聖
人不廢但必以理爲主善用之則有功於世誤用
之則有害於人聖人修身砥行全得天之
理盡倫物之宜以此成己即以此成人即以窮神達
化察來彰往洞達幽明亦不以之立教以其非急
務也天有常道無論君子有常行窮理盡性以至於命
則人道即天道無論窮達皆爲完人若匪匪言數
則罔念作狂克念作聖妄之徒效尤乎故今摘其甚者
況創爲新異令庸妄之徒效尤乎故今摘其甚者

正譌 卷五 塱 西充鮮于氏特圓藏

言之非必毀議康節爲學術人心計耳觀者諒之

正譌卷五終

不及特其目耳先儒不識中字源流又不知執中
本義將中字止說在事處而明德之實功止日因其所發
說成事物恰好處而明德之實功止日因其所發
而遂明之不止毫釐千里之謬矣然夫子何不日
執中而日止於至善蓋就人易曉耳天地之元氣化
特為此名特標止字使人易曉耳天地之元氣渾淪
流行無一毫絕續人所知也而天地之法言之
淪無動無靜止於其所則人不知也伏羲作易洩
天地之藏而其源實由圖書靜而無靜動而無動
圖書明著其機而知者甚寡姑以易象言之大禹

正誤 卷八 芮氏特圖藏于西充

何以首連山益乾靜專坤靜翕而後有動直動闢
靜者動之源止者天地之奧也禹以首艮止言其義
湯首歸藏言其所文王易為乾坤以兩儀既定萬
物生成皆本乾坤於法象為易言而象艮卦則盛
言艮止之義位坤曰安貞之吉未嘗敢外禹湯而立
說也夫子彖傳曰艮止也止其所也時止則止時
行則行動靜不失其時其道光明於大象又曰君
子以思不出其位其敎人靜止中之意何窮大
學者夫子綜自古聖人盡人合天之功以示旨子
明明德至在執中子名之曰止至善止字前已言

正誤 卷八 芮氏特圖藏于西充

亦為異端矣
者言禪言元皆不外止至善而亦闢之遂並靜養
一錯講養氣之功由不知不動心之故而凡聖人明
德俯身之學俱惝恍無實際也
大哉乾元乃統天至哉坤元乃順承天二元止是
一元二元者氣也即理也理宰乎氣氣載乎理理
氣安可強分哉原氣之本始聲臭俱無尚何有跡
觀氣之散著萬象森列不為虛無然而有理始有
氣有氣始有質凡成形成象者質也氣之為也
在即理在無在非理即無在非氣而況人為天地

家言 二 西充鮮于氏特囧藏

凡人立志勝人易生傲慢惟立志學聖人則無害者何也學聖從小心敬慎入手已之惡惟恐不知人之惡渾然忘之質直而好義慮以下人無小大無眾寡無敢慢何有驕心也

度量要大心要小凡事要敬氣要利嗜欲要少理要明待人要慈禮要肅一切要誠守要久

人生福澤由天志於聖人念念不欺事事天理而塞患難者未之有也故程子曰仁義未嘗不利今人祇見得聖人難學一切快心逆理之事目前有利益則毅然為之不知天理無不善善人天心所繫行險

志於名利為身家妻子而已名本虛聲無德之名即時已不齒於君子何待身後利不過求安飽從古聖賢何嘗飢塞而死德儉而福自來天之定理彼蒼豈靳於君子也

百工技藝各修其職不欺其心決無凍餒之憂今人止是畏貧賤所以立志不堅反貽伊戚

困知勉行及其知之一成功一人皆可以為堯舜孔孟俱言聖人可學也顏子曰舜何人子何人有為者亦若是張子曰三代下學者求為賢人而不求為聖人是一大病此立志之法也

徼倖何如居易俟命也

學聖人而至於飢寒枕楛無此天理若忠孝節義則雖死而生配天不朽非凶禍也

職業

孔子曰執御乎執射乎吾執御矣謂人生不可無職業也孟子曰矢人惟恐不傷人函人惟恐不可不慎恐人職業之誤也自古聖賢耕稼陶漁釣築醫卜皆可托業無害於義理而可以贍衣食即為正業

第一好事是讀書但須讀有用之書四子五經天理家言 三 西充鮮于氏特囧藏

人情物理無不全備一一講明體諸身心無不可成之功業若貧性魯鈍止熟讀四子字字力行不可作紙上陳言觀已可卓然立於聖賢之林矣

近日書籍太繁然必以聖為歸心性倫常能實踐為要若第務淹博施之修齊治平不可者最當擇別乃為善讀書人

學字最能收心故程子曰非欲字工即此是學書家議論以柳公正則筆正之言為要人品事業無可觀工藝奚益此傳青主所以不屑子昂也

詩以道性情人心自然之音不可過抑非特流連光

槐軒約言

河圖洛書天啟緘機以明道伏羲仰觀俯察神明之德類萬物之情於是三才間奧悉具於斯自秦焚六籍道學罕傳周易僅為卜筮之用史傳別創儒林之名於是黃老六經判然兩途神仙為猶龍豈素隱之名於是黃老六經判然兩途神仙聖賢幾如秦越則以本原未徹而技藝多淆也夫黃帝垂衣裳而天下治子極稱之老子與夫子問答歎為猶龍豈素隱行怪之流蔑棄人倫之教而世儒不察徒見方士流假名竊似貽誤於時遂並其最初而詬之亦見其惑矣曰黃帝倚矣老子道德經語多不倫先儒疵之不一子曷以明其非偽歟曰然誠有之蓋未通其詞義而沿俗說以相訾嗷也老子曰道可道非常道名可名非常名言道之不可以常言盡也說者則謂其外別有道老子曰大道廢有仁義言大道將廢顯有仁義正之而說者則以為廢去仁義若此之類不可勝書子試觀純陽呂子之註釋可以悚然矣曰黃老皆聖人而古今學黃老者晉之清談唐之金丹朱之齋醮以及秦皇漢武方技術數百家之流歷歷為蠱其說安歸曰然人倫日用人有之人無二道身心性命之理日用人倫之道人人有之人可以行之外此無有天理外此有何聖人黃老而

槐軒約言

非人乎則或外別有教若猶是人也又惻於羑舜孔子之列而曰其道獨殊平心而論其可通乎其言必清必淨毋勞爾神毋搖爾精毋使爾思慮營營以保爾長生乃寡欲清心卻病延年之意豈言誠身必身曾子戰戰兢兢皆是此義豈希聖不必保養神氣乎虛無清淨乃靜存之時一念不生渾然在抱非廢去倫常一切皆同空幻漢承秦弊不得其真淮南王安之流惑於方士悖禮傷倫至武帝益務為荒怪民窮財盡繼以嚴罰史遷生逢其時難於顯刺以申韓黃老同傳謂形名之家原於道德遂為後世所藉口自是而方外而清談齋醮蕪雜多學者莫辨真偽至以幻術雜技遂為神仙誦經禮佛遂為好善然僧道之正者如達公如希夷輩固昭昭耳目之前並無奇詭之術況之黃帝老子恭已垂裳猶龍歎慕奈何以歧出之非為聖賢咎乎自漢至今誣謬相沿不特情事紛紜亦且書籍淆亂吾以天理二字定人性以中庸二字概聖賢實踐心性倫常之人謂之聖賢可謂為仙佛無不可否則異端聊以匡末俗而明大道耳曰先儒言道至難能聖由天授故民可使由不可使知而佛老以其教惑人故當先闢佛老後學禮

日月合明鬼神合吉凶聖人知我其天配天皆是此理自孔孟而後無眞師指授卽有眞師文人多自恃已見所以其心三月不違仁存心養性事天無人知之此當實踐其功非可以口舌文字傳也

問儒言心性子獨言神氣何也曰神氣者心性之實心在先天純乎天理宋儒祗知人心道心而不知人慾則心不盡性知人心道心而不知人愚四子五經反覆詳明皆是發明此理毋忽道心一心何以有二且不識仁字不知仁卽天理

問性無爲心有覺人生百爲全憑有覺之心至無爲之性聲臭俱無矣又如何養法曰心性言理之虛明神氣之靈其純一者性浮妄者心養浩然之氣以虛無之神養虛無之氣求放心而入於中田寂然不動百日先天神氣凝結有諸己更加養之功多行陰功德行使浩然之氣日日充滿謂之充實內而常靜養一切妄念消除外而檢點言行一毫非禮不作則神氣穩於丹田貫乎周身粹面盎背不言而喩謂之充實而有光輝始焉養其丹田兼修德行內外兼修本末交養迄乎德修而足先天神氣積中而發外凡氣之所在皆理之所

又問

禮意附

何難不幸短命可歎耳

在清明在躬志氣如神與天地合德日月合明由此其選也自孔孟而後竟無人知所以敎人學聖人人以爲學聖如顏子不免於窮與短命不知顏子未到仁人聖人地位也使天假之年仁聖抑又

心是也人人有此天理見於言行一切太過節之牛之死乍見孺子而悲卽是仁世俗所謂天理良道也德也誠也包萬善而爲名以一端言不忍仁義禮知信爲五性仁字以全體言卽天命之性

又問

不及文之卽禮合宜曰義知之眞曰知行之久且誠曰信自義皇至於春秋聖神迭起禮之明備莫過於周而其本則在於仁大司徒以三物賓興六德曰智仁聖義中和至春秋而專尙繁文禮遂流於浮華故孔子曰人而不仁如禮何禮云禮云玉帛云乎哉而林放問禮之本卽深喜之聖人之意可見矣後儒不知夫子曰以爲仁聖人之言夫子以禮敎人罕言仁道不思論語言仁四十八章苟志於仁矣有能用其力於仁矣乎譚譚以仁聖人而聖門諸賢問仁者不一其徒且禮因時而制

居脈理證之。即脈名。亦甚多。不外浮沉遲數
四者。初學人手。記名人之方。及藥性。又分
陰陽。審虛實。為要
人身內養不足。元氣虛而癘氣乘之。發於四時
者不同。寒熱偏勝之端不同也。春時有痛首
疾。夏時有痒疥疾。秋時有瘧寒疾。冬時有嗽
上氣疾。問而知其氣。望而知其色。聞而知其
聲。診視非一處。病情非一端。望聞問切。交
盡其術。而察其生死。分而治之。蓋古之醫
者。皆明於陰陽造化之理。達于人情物理之
全。而後神明其術。今但以四脈言之。水火之
所以濟。與溺竅精竅食喉氣喉。前賢俱不敢明
言。以其為人之妙。即天地之機也。何必拘拘
以求。亦知其理通臟腑而已。

醫理大概約說 望聞問切捷法 八

醫論

醫道雖多。不外乎氣血。氣。血之主。而神。
又氣之主也。故補血必補氣。氣行則血行。無
補血法也。至神。則心之靈。尤非可以藥補。
但審其病從何起。如用心太過而神耗。則宜靜
養。用寧神之藥。色欲太過。而水不濟火。則
宜用滋水之藥。然皆必自加靜攝。非可專恃藥
餌。故愚嘗謂心為身主。人必養心。以為生神
之本。病不可治。皆心未養而神離身也。疾之
不可以藥治者甚多。惟風寒暑熱。藥可以療。
七情內傷。則必調平性情。冤孽魔祟。則必修
德祈禳。陰陽二宅冲犯。則必改造培修。醫書
專言方藥。實多不效。要在神而明之。變而通
之。不可拘一以求也。且精氣神三者。有先天
後天之別。先天之強弱不同。後天之戰養各
別。三者還相為宮。不可以強弱分。一強則俱
強。一弱則俱弱。古人所以重攝生。不其此以
歟。

醫理大概約說 醫論 一

至于傷寒。古有成書。然冬三月。方為正傷
寒。窮苦人。無衣。無火。少食。少酒。又多

醫理大概約說 醫論 二十

希敬之。

醫道分內外科。此大謬也。人之所以生者。血氣調和。百病不生。凡瘡瘍。多由不知保身。虧了血氣。一遇飲食不慎。受寒受火。道不時。便發為瘡瘍。治此症者。必須勤其人。寡慾清心。保養身體。然後審其病根由來。或是酒色。或是飲食。知道其病根由。將血氣培補。久久。乃用藥治病。或散寒。或散火。風火便是瘡毒。散風火。便是解瘡毒。世人不知此理。一遇瘡毒。祇是用藥解毒敷貼。誤了多人。更有不肖之徒。見人瘡毒。用藥使之破爛。伊得逞其私見。萬一治好。便是功勞。若治不好。說是病本難治。人為所惑。說是瘡本難治。可惜可嘆。凡有患瘡。毋論大小瘡毒。起初有痕跡。便服補氣解毒藥。如人參敗毒散。荊防敗毒散之類。將其寒火去了。外面。用生甘草銀花黃連為末。調敷。便可解散。切不可用艾火燒。用針打。往往誤事。傷人性命。戒之戒之。至於女流。血氣行動之時。食生冷之物。或心性少平和。動輒生氣著

醫理大概約說 醫論 二十一

惱。氣憤。憂愁悲哭。以致血氣凝滯。結成包塊。久必難治。其本原壞也。不可誤用治瘡法。所以凡保養人。必須自家貴重身體。十分信神。不作惡。一遇此等病。即改悔心腸。再請明醫去治。而凡事寬仁厚德。忍讓耐煩和平。要想人命在天。天所佑仁者。修德善人。凡事守理。天自默佑。使其全愈。醫治時。一切保重謹慎。自不待言。此話。須醫者細細開導勸化。即是善事大功德也。病何窮。祇有隨宜用藥。譬如用兵。奇正相生。而其身前後左右。又有多少之不同。如遇瘡症。即以人之受病在何經。細為用藥。即如脾經。須有生白朮懷藥。而所蓄帶有火症。則必施以生大黃黃連等。即其所受病之時。亦須參得幾分。必有卓見。莫妙於多看書。細思其理。而書中所言經絡。亦不盡合。經者。大大一條。而最是緊要。絡者。即經之所分。隨經去做事。不須太分。如肝經肝之絡在肺始。絡又在脾始。凡看瘡。先以顏色為要。再審其夜間如何。須看其所得之病。夜來是如何象。

學聖人局量

大慈悲心 慈悲仁也。仁人心也。天理良心也。凡人必有仁。然後念念事事。惟恐得罪於人。至於忠孝友悌。大倫所在。其不忍一念相欺。不敢一念恣肆。更無待言矣。仁也。而曰大慈悲者。由一念以及於念念。由一事以及於事事。俱是此不忍人之心。所謂昆蟲草木不可傷。盡其性以盡人性物性。參贊化育。皆以此為根本。

大廣大心 廣大謂度量也。古人云。有大量者。始有大福。量小者。居心狹隘。見理不明。氣質剛躁。止知有己。不知有人。己。不顧損人。自恃而不服善。自私而不諒人。自小而不容人。能有度量。必自平日反躬自責之人。一言一行。惟恐不合乎理。損傷於人。刻刻檢點自己不是。雖外人怒我罵我。分毫我。多不理他。止是自家反躬自問。無愧了。任他無理加。都全然不理。至於君父大倫所在。以及弟兄朋友。犯而不校。更不待言矣。

醫理大概約說 〈學聖人局量 一〉

大方便心 方便者何。敏於事也。勇於義也。人世相與同居同游。同往來晉接。無非五倫中人。五倫中人。有尊卑大小。貴賤親疏。竭誠竭力。敬慎服事。君親而賢。能象其賢。君親而不賢。匡救諭諫。能幹其蠱。做到十分周到。遠近之不同。如君父母。至尊至親。竭誠竭至使其君親為聖人。忠孝事業。做得無古無今。此臣子分內之事。不足為功。此外。凡事君親。十分周到。不得言方便也。弟兄朋友。其中親疏厚薄。賢愚是非。斷不能一同而視。事兄愛弟信友。先自家各盡其道。愛之敬之。不欺不苟。久久不變。不管他說我是非。我止盡其心。盡其道。求無愧於我心。若他有事。止要不悖義理。則真心代勞。盡心盡力。委曲成全好事。此便是方便之道也。易。境有豐嗇。時勢有常變。雖當方便。也要對的義理情事。必不可一概冒昧而行。至於從井救人。危身辱親尤非。所以古人云力量做得來的。盡其力量。力量做不來的。亦必用心周到。此所言者。謂事情大理所關

醫理大概約說 〈學聖人局量 二〉

也。若夫平日檢身修德。一言一行。一步一
趨。隨身方便。其事難以枚舉。其功亦簡而易
行。止要肯留心。不怠不肆。便可處處方便。
如行路。見一木一石礙腳。恐妨人行。去之。
饑寒困苦。一切不佳之事。惟恐人有。飽煖安
全得意之事。無處不可方便。此兩字實心奉行。
之間。無處不可方便。此兩字實心奉行。
二字。都在其中矣。一日之內。斗室。仁義
大清淨心。如何清淨。見財不貪。見色不愛。
一念一事。不縱情悖理皆是。止知安分守己。
心。事事體貼而行。無論德行道藝。擇一合義
之愛人者。止此天理良心。我念念不失天理良
勤職業。修心術。念人生萬事。總由天命。天
理者為之。如耕讀商賈。專心學習此藝。勤而
不懈。儉而不奢。廉而不貪。如此。無論何
念檢點。不肯一毫虧損天良。又念
事。俱可以謀生度日。此即俗所謂靠天而行
也。人心妄想無窮。不可任心行事。止要一生
不受饑寒。仰事俯蓄。可以粗足。便是第一美
境了。至於富貴榮華之人。彼有積累善德。上

醫理大概約說　學聖人局量　三

天方纔賜之福祿。我無他積累。如何妄想與他
一般。果然存心恬退。時時芟除妄想。則久久
習為固然。無論貧賤困苦。都安心住下去了。
此乃尋常人刻持私心。勉強學為清淨之法。若
夫讀書明理之人。能存心養性。履仁蹈義。內
而涵養有功。久久。鄙俗之見自消。外而動循
禮義。久久。美惡之情渾忘。則必有靜存動
察。始終本末之功。聖人非道非義。一介不取
予。萬鍾千駟弗視。由斯道也。此清淨二字
上之。則希聖希賢。敝屣天下。中之。則有守
有為。行藏不苟。下之。亦雲水心情。無處不
可自適。是在人自為之。而自勉之耳。
大柔和心　和者。喜怒哀樂皆中節。是天下之達
道也。措諸世者。恩誼浹洽之謂也。以其上而
言。修於身者。天下中國如一人。是天下之達
宏深也。此和之至者。非聖人不能。以其次而
言。五倫之內。各盡其道。各得其所。恩明誼
美。情義不相乖離。此和之切要。不可無。亦
人之所當盡者。再次。則不忍為不仁。不敢為
不義。小心敬慎。平心靜氣。惟恐傷人。惟恐

醫理大概約說　學聖人局量　四

債事。惟恐取禍。謙虛忍讓。縱有大不平。大不堪之事。大可恨。大可誅之人。也置之不問。將自家好勝好強。剛躁之氣。極力柔服下來。故曰柔和也。寬柔以教。不報無道。君子居之。此之謂也。不然。柔之一字。乃不好字面。善柔也。柔奸也。柔弱也。柔佞也。柔靡也。安得而為之。凡人不能忍辱謙讓。俱是血氣剛強。心情躁暴所致。故柔其氣以從理。和其情以同物。然後倫誼可以浹洽。動履可以無災。

右五言。本佛道書中語。而其義理。實與聖人之道無殊。聖人言行。不外乎此。即四子六經。名賢議論。亦不外乎此。但世人忽而置之。迂而笑之。甚且以為異端而闢之。是以學聖學賢。無從入手。愚嘗舉以訓門人。謂此五言。乃學聖之局量。必先有此五言心思。實行五言義理。然後可以希賢希聖而希天。惜乎遵行者罕。今老矣。不得已。書示兒曹以為一家之授受云爾。

先君子平生教人。言語甚富。無非性情心

醫理大概約說　　學聖人局量　五

術。施於日用倫常。右五言。看是二氏之言。實吾儒真實學問。茲因刊布醫說。特附於後。昔人云。治病當治未形。此五言之理。果能實體。又有何病。習醫高明。受病苦人。請以此治未病焉。
　　　　　　　　　男棖文謹志

醫理大概約說　　學聖人局量　六

Index

A

abuse 118, 120, 131, 187-8, 222
acupuncture 7, 120-1, 152, 155-6, 158-9, 162, 167, 204
ages 12-13, 65, 145, 175, 177, 185, 199, 239
agitation 98, 145, 147
allotted years 185
Analects 3, 52-3, 103, 114, 118
ancestors 48, 144, 200
ancestry 22, 219
ancient China 3, 57
anger 25, 28, 47, 61, 67, 69, 77, 81, 95, 97-9, 102, 112, 149, 151, 160-1
  excessive 98
anxiety 69, 127, 156, 163, 167, 227, 235
  overt 156
aperture 203-4, 219
Apex 85, 165, 167-70, 172-7, 180, 184, 196, 200, 202, 228
  creating 175
Apex of Unification 93
apple 95, 119, 125-6, 128, 152, 222
apple tree 155, 176

B

baby 35, 56, 74, 159, 162, 174, 188, 203, 239
bāguà 37, 62, 108, 182
Bāi Yù Kāi 36-7, 39, 44
balance 6, 29, 55, 78, 94, 176, 180, 229
  correct 50
  restore 78
Barefoot doctors 125
beggar 19-23, 48
Bèiwén 231, 237
belief 53, 75, 132, 149, 151-6, 158, 162-3, 167, 191, 198, 226-7
believing 66, 140

benevolence 24, 39, 67, 73, 105-7, 149-54, 156, 162-4, 173-4, 177-8, 186-7, 196, 231, 233-5, 239
  pure 198
  sage's 118
benevolent 88, 106, 152, 155, 180, 231
birth 44, 56-7, 59, 61, 65, 67, 71-2, 78, 83, 99-100, 104, 106, 111, 168-70, 174-5
black beans 21, 29-30, 42, 50-1, 56, 71, 184, 229
Bladder 95
Bladder and Small Intestine 8
blame Heaven 21, 41
blood 3, 9, 44, 70, 80-1, 84, 89, 98, 123, 133, 197-8, 216-17, 236
blood stagnation 217-18
blood thinner 197
Book of Change 62
Book of Gàozǐ 158
Book of Mencius 53, 148-9, 161, 163-4
Book of Rites 171, 173-4
Botulinum toxin 122
breathe 6, 57, 92-3, 133, 180, 196, 201, 204, 223
  lungs 6, 93
breathes life 11
Buddhism 3, 13, 32, 49, 65, 236
Buddhism, Zen 58, 65
Buddhist and Dàoist scholars 65
Buddhist cannon 38, 135
Buddhist monk 26, 30
Buddhist path 35
Buddhist story 91
Buddhists 16, 33

C

calm 21-2, 36, 77, 89, 127-8, 156, 190, 235
calm Heart 32, 133, 210, 234-5
canopy 14, 240
Cáocāo 48, 200

capacity 32, 72, 89, 102, 119, 126, 132, 145, 152, 175, 231, 236
  body's self-healing 198
  boundless 44
  fertile 97
  generation's 125
  perpetual 132
  recharging 6
  scholarly 13
  vessel's 177
Cardinal Relationships 189, 223
cell 64, 151, 153, 155, 175, 177, 180, 226
  single living 63
cell division 177
cellular body 152, 178
Centered 2, 10, 25, 28, 32, 44, 47, 49, 70, 132, 143-4, 158, 200, 223-4, 228-9
Centered physician 155, 188
character qi 69
cheat 25, 34, 141
cheating 23, 25, 48, 83
Chén Zhōnghuá 85, 186, 238
child 3, 35, 44, 46, 49, 56, 125, 158, 177, 180, 184, 194, 222-3, 226-7, 229-31
Chinese herbs 125
Chinese Medicine 1-4, 11, 68, 79, 95-6, 159, 218, 224-5
  dialectic 93
  modern 93, 110, 170
circle-ation 7, 97, 102, 111
circles 8, 60, 77, 92, 96-8, 124, 158-9, 161, 166, 168-9, 172, 175, 201
circulation 57, 97, 161, 170
  internal 99
  liquid 89
Classics 15-17, 54, 60, 75, 81, 88, 135, 224, 236
Clearing Heat 110, 170
compassion 11, 54, 65, 70, 73, 100, 103, 106, 112, 132-3, 143, 166, 175, 180, 230-1
  father's 32
Compassionate Heart 36, 231
compendium, ten-volume 52
Concealed Circle 85, 90, 129, 173-5, 177

Concealed Separation Outward 7
Concealed Words 93, 215, 219, 221-2, 237
concealment 120
Confucian 16, 40, 57, 65, 67, 73, 183
Confucian Analects 156, 158
Confucian Classics 12
Confucian philosopher 160
Confucian rules of benevolence 67
Confucian sages 236
Confucian scholar Zhū Xī 52
Confucian teachings 16, 52
Confucian texts 54
Confucian values, defined 88
Confucianism 13, 16, 31, 52, 62, 65, 73, 223, 236
Confucius 3, 30-1, 42, 52, 56, 58, 61-2, 65, 70, 72, 87, 102-3, 106, 108, 112
connectedness 59, 80
connection, original 145
connection Heaven 218
consciousness 4, 11
Consciousness of Heart 149, 153
constancy 76, 111-12, 119, 164-5, 172, 224
constant connection 93, 149, 201
constant rotation 196
constant thread 239
constant transformation 6
constant Unification 5
constipation 125
contemplation 9, 11, 45, 68, 170, 196
contemporary Chinese Medicine 1, 9
continuous life 177
continuum 199-200
contradiction 4
convenience 232-3
Convenient Heart 232
Correcting Errors 16, 183, 194, 201-4
couple 24, 125, 154-5, 158-9, 161-3, 226
creation 62, 73, 75, 83, 104-5, 108, 119, 167, 169-70, 177, 195, 204, 231
Croizier 225
cultivation 11, 16-17, 23, 28, 35, 44, 47, 65, 74, 82, 84, 88, 143-4, 217-18, 234-5

accumulating 40
benevolence–the 13
inner 50-1
true 40
cultivation activities 60
cultivation process 17, 85
cultivation techniques 219
cúnxīn yǎngxìng 203
curved line 175, 180
cycles 6-7, 89, 112, 114, 170, 177, 180
  balanced 185
cyclical motion 5
cyclical movement 5

D

Dà Xué 52
dāntián 203, 220
Dào 31, 33-5, 37-42, 72, 76, 83-4, 88-9, 104-5, 108, 145, 166-8, 170, 201, 213-14, 235-6
  great 31, 42
  human 179
  nation 17
  natural 197
  sage's 29
  true 80
Dào Dé Jîng 19, 21, 33, 36-7, 39, 55, 70, 72-3, 81, 168, 170
Dào Guāng Emperor 18
Dao heart 172
Dào Heart 8, 58, 63, 65, 71, 83, 85, 90, 97, 104, 149-50, 171, 173-5, 225-7, 237-9
Dào of Confucius and Mencius 112
Dào of convenience 233
Dào of human relationships 221-2
Dàoism 13, 37, 135, 236
Dàoist 13, 16, 33-8, 63
Dàoist master 35
Dàoist monk, elderly 13
Dàoist poem 132
Dàoist priest 22-3, 67
Dàoist recluse 35
death 5, 19-20, 24, 30, 41, 45-7, 55, 85, 99, 111, 119, 186, 202, 224, 227
debt, repaying 208

deeds 28, 49, 198, 208, 210-11, 217
defensiveness 131, 155, 186, 197
deficiencies 142, 168-9
dehydration 187
delicacies, new 118
Delusion 31
demons 17, 24-5, 44, 50
desiring 61, 69, 160, 211
destiny 36, 41, 61, 113, 146, 150, 178, 213, 218, 221, 234
  human 41
  life's 43
Dialectical Materialism 225
diarrhea 100, 125, 130, 152
dichotomy 68, 93, 129, 145, 152, 170, 175, 177, 221
  emotional 229
  life's 239
diet 100, 115, 128, 213
dietary choices, poor 128
digestive tract 115
dis-ease 154, 188
disaster 22, 25, 36, 48, 136, 143, 210, 235-6
discharging emotions 196
discharging movements 82, 98
disease 9, 11, 31, 39, 48, 50, 64, 114-16, 128, 130-1, 135-45, 155, 167, 213-17, 236-7
  chronic 214
  cure 146
  external 90, 130
  hundred 69, 135-6, 143-5, 160, 214
  inner 130, 213
  physical 126
  true root of 144, 170
disease-free life 94
disease processes 131
disharmony 128, 161, 175, 216
disillusionment 227
dislikes 10, 59, 149, 160-1, 164, 166-7, 172-7, 187, 217, 219, 221, 226-7, 229, 239
disorder 131, 162, 193, 195, 216-17, 230
  internal 190
  medical 79
  menstrual 98
  observable Outer Water Circle 131

psychological 155
disposition 191, 202, 232
distastes 166-7, 173, 175, 180
distract Xing 110
distractions 103, 170
distress 111, 121, 218
  psychological 102
disturbances 62, 81-2, 202, 222
divine 36, 39, 71, 75, 78, 81, 83, 106, 114, 118, 179, 189, 201, 224
divisions 1, 63, 78-9, 102, 160, 174-5, 177
doctors 25-6, 44-5, 50, 103, 116, 123, 125, 146, 158, 178, 218
  biomedical 197
  good 116
  local 122
  passionate 115
  traditional 225
  well-intentioned 158
Dǒng Zhòngshū 66
dream 22, 24, 99, 174, 177, 214
  emotional 174
  patient's 178
  women experience 174
drink water 223
drinking 6, 33
drugs 103, 113, 125, 155, 167, 216, 218-19
  lifeless 125
  poisonous 140
dynasty 12, 48-9, 67, 112, 143, 200

E

ears, deaf 23, 87, 226
Earth 20-1, 41, 43-4, 56-7, 61-3, 66-8, 70-2, 76-7, 83-4, 86-7, 89, 104-10, 163-5, 168-9, 202-4
  kūn 62
  physical 89
  true 37
Earth and Natural Character 56
Earth form 171
eczema 170
eggs, old 158
Elixirs 9, 33-5, 37, 77, 86, 102-3, 110, 172-3, 175, 204
emotion springing 196

emotional comforting 100
Emotional Intelligence 122
emotional reactions mask 78
emotional systems 115
emotional underpinning 166
emotional well-being 109
emotionless 116
emotions 60-2, 69, 77-81, 97-100, 102, 109-11, 115-16, 123-4, 126-9, 144-6, 149-56, 162-3, 202, 216-17, 226-8
  discharge 60, 78
  excessive 111, 115, 128
  human 13, 58, 61, 75, 100, 111
  human Heart discharges 123, 185
  invoking strong positive 155
  movement of 81, 114
  observable 97
  purest form 98
  selfish 94
  stretching 155
emotions harmonious 236
emotions move outward 126
Emperor Fire 96
energy 6, 8, 56, 67, 69, 79, 83-4, 89, 95, 97, 107, 110, 115, 126-7, 167
  moving 89
energy source 86
enlightenment 33, 41, 78, 191, 207, 229
environment 6, 95, 120, 130, 221
  external 98
error 3, 13, 16, 18, 21, 34, 47, 170, 179, 224
essence 4, 13, 30, 32, 58, 72, 83-4, 87, 89, 104-5, 113, 168, 213-14, 216, 220-1
evil 11, 17-18, 21, 24-5, 28-30, 36, 42, 44, 46-9, 51, 60, 138-9, 142-3, 197-8, 200
  eradicating 65
  small 29, 136
evil affairs 197
evil deeds 42
evil doings 43
evil emotions 234
evil mistakes 213
evil thoughts 29
evil trickery 27

excretion 95, 99
exhaust 20, 35, 133, 168, 173, 233
exhaustion 84, 167, 203
  reaching 197
existence 9-10, 19, 70, 72-3, 75, 83-5, 109, 111, 171, 182, 191
experience 9, 14, 35, 61, 99-100, 111, 123, 153-4, 170, 180, 190, 192, 201, 205, 222
experience emotion 180
experience life 146
experience longevity 13
experience objects 223
exterior 8, 59, 90, 110, 149, 155, 166-7, 170
exterior attachments 81
exterior distracts 81
exterior material world 172
exterior observations 9
exterior substances 124
exterior world 114, 145, 175
extremes 113-14
extremities, cold 197
eyes 6-7, 27, 30-1, 33, 59, 68, 75, 84, 99-100, 106, 121, 123, 125-6, 132, 193

F

fame 17, 40, 49-50, 211
family 2, 4, 14-15, 22-3, 25, 32, 35-6, 42-4, 47, 49, 73-5, 157-8, 219, 223-4, 227-8
father 12, 31, 34, 43-4, 49, 56, 61, 70-3, 88, 125, 144, 219, 221-2, 226-8, 231
  bad 222, 227
father-in-law 23-5, 27, 29
female 66, 78-9
Féng Zhìqiáng 184, 186
fertility 97, 125, 154-5, 174, 226
fertility specialists 100, 154, 157
filial piety 34-5, 38, 41-2, 49, 70, 118, 201, 231
Fire 24, 37, 57, 64, 90, 96, 99, 102-3, 105, 108, 110, 112, 125, 142, 170
  internal 219
  leakage of 99, 115
  leaks 103

Fire trigram 37, 107, 110-11
firewood 19-20
Five Cardinal Relationships 16, 31, 73-4, 88, 112, 171, 232, 235
Five Cardinal Relationships in Confucian teachings 90
Five Elements 9, 66, 72
Five Hearts 231, 236-7
Five Kinships 37
folly 224, 227, 239
  youthful 13, 194, 222
food 19, 33, 36, 41, 45, 49, 64, 93, 95, 97, 109, 115, 118-19, 128-30, 177
  denatured 93
  good 223
  industrialized 95
  tainted 130
forebears 10, 48, 143, 200, 219
forefathers 18, 47
formless 89, 236
fortune 27-8, 48-50, 195, 197
  bad 87, 197
  good 23, 197-8, 232, 234
friend 18, 45, 108, 128, 177, 180, 221, 230, 233
friendship 231, 235-6

G

gain
  eternal 49
  personal 137
  self 139
  short-term 49
gain perspective 129
gain profit 184
Gallbladder 95
gametes 177, 206
Gān Liǎo 147, 214
Gàozǐ 156, 158, 163
garden, walled 108, 113, 116
Gazing 79, 196, 203-4, 219
generations 3, 10, 13, 20, 36, 47-9, 56, 58, 87, 106, 118, 143, 155-6, 200, 203
Gentle Harmonious Heart 235
géwù 70, 74-5, 186, 188, 192-3, 199
ghosts 17, 24-5, 43, 120

gōngfu 3, 8, 28-9, 37-8, 50, 106, 143,
     177, 189, 192, 196, 202-3, 229
good deeds 26, 28, 38, 42, 48, 209,
     212
grandfather 36, 48, 228
Great Learning 16, 52-3, 56-9, 61, 65-
     6, 71, 75-6, 80, 82-3, 86-7, 189,
     192-3, 202
  ancient 189-90, 192-5
Great Purified Heart 234
guarding 65, 128, 188, 190, 203, 235
guards 43, 46, 66, 75, 78, 125, 169,
     187-8, 190, 196, 204, 213, 218
Guǐ Gǔzǐ 40
Guōdiàn Chǔjiǎn 150
Guōdiàn yǔcóngèr 160

H

habits 17, 56, 111-12, 114-15, 131-2,
     215, 226, 234
  bad 56, 61
  changing 133
  internal 123
hàorán zhīqì 67, 149-50, 163
happiness 23, 32, 63, 67, 69, 77, 99,
     119, 126, 151, 172, 180, 198, 212,
     235
hardship 19, 138, 210, 212, 215, 233,
     237
harming 24, 84, 109, 137, 139, 218,
     232
harmonious 10, 47, 67, 71, 80, 86,
     114, 144, 155, 164, 203, 229, 235
Harmonious Center 203
harmonious mind 210
harmonious state 123
harmony 52, 71, 86, 89, 116, 147,
     164, 170-1, 177, 198-9, 202, 204,
     220, 235
  gentle 235
  grand 104, 107
  restore 230
harmony rippling 237
hate 137, 139, 202
heal 10, 100, 116, 132, 135, 142, 164,
     187, 190, 192, 195
healing 3, 100, 115, 120, 146, 152,
     155, 159, 218

true 1, 133, 155
healing process 123, 131
health 1-2, 5-6, 13-14, 74, 97, 100,
     102, 109, 128, 143, 152, 164,
     186-7, 199, 210
ill 64, 175
improved 198
mental 155
patient's 159
physical 185
reproductive 125
healthy human Heart 144
heart 1, 24, 52, 61, 65, 80, 133
  baby's 228
  benevolent 72
  broken 112, 180
  complete 59, 164
  conscious 149, 151, 153-4, 156,
     198, 213
  corrupt 21
  defensive 203
  discharged 192, 196, 202-3
  disturbed 214
  emotional human 111
  enlightened 76
  eternal 37
  fake 173
  female 79, 81
  good 23, 29, 35, 178, 231, 233
  greedy 142
  hardened 35
  harmonious 144-5
  honest 42
  inharmonious 217
  kind 178, 188, 201, 211-12, 226,
     234, 240
  living 62
  lonely 159
  loving 207
  malnourished 216
  peaceful 204, 228
  person's 146, 156
  pure 83, 235, 239
  pure Dào 85, 174
  shame-free 233
  sincere 36, 48, 209
  tolerant 231
  true 94, 148, 192
  virtuous 24

wicked 36
Heart and Natural Character 59, 214
Heart diseases 130-1, 156, 162, 213
Heart medicine 213
Heart Method 3, 74, 90, 120, 131, 183, 187
Heart movement 55
Heart of Liú Yuán 5
Heart of Medicine 123
Heart of pure oneness 83
Heart of reproducing 20
Heart problem 115
Heart upright 60, 81, 202
Heart Yáng 83
hearts beat 6
Heart's emotions 235
Heart's movement 81
Hearts of humankind 78
Hearts of Xīnfǎ 237
heat 110, 170, 213, 216
  clear 110
heaven 54, 71, 75, 230
Heaven 44, 48-9, 55-9, 61-4, 66-8, 70-8, 80-9, 104-10, 149-50, 163-9, 171, 178-80, 197-8, 201-4, 234-6
Heaven loves mankind 234
Heaven movement 126, 130
Heaven principle 8-9, 63-4, 68, 79, 81, 112, 119, 121-2, 124-5, 144, 178-9, 184-6, 199-201, 220-1, 226-7
Heaven principle replenishes 114
Heaven trigram 37
Heaven's command 84-5, 104-5, 213
Heaven's Dào 179
Heaven's decree 58, 76-7, 87, 108, 150, 168
Heaven's Heart 78, 107, 234
Heaven's principle 35, 49, 60-1, 72-4, 78, 88, 90, 106, 113-14, 131, 178, 194, 224, 231, 234
  complete 82
Heaven's principle merge 112
Heaven's principle vanishes 173
Heaven's Yáng 83
hell 23-4, 30, 35, 45-6, 54, 230
Helping 139, 207, 209, 212

herbs 50, 103, 112, 115, 120-1, 146, 152, 155-6, 158-9, 162, 167, 187, 204, 216, 219
  bland 115
  expensive 116
  strong 162
Hétú 108, 182-3
hexagram, méng 194
Hóng Jūnshēng 186
house 20, 22, 24, 27, 34-5, 45
Huái Xuân 11-12, 14, 53, 70
Huái Xuān Academy 13-15
Huái Xuān Cultural Association 15
Huái Xuān Pledge 16, 221
Huái Xuān School 15
human beings 72, 105, 121, 124, 178, 239
human body 62, 67, 70, 72, 78-9, 81, 108, 177, 203-4, 216
human ethics 179
human Heart 8, 58, 65, 83, 85, 94, 96-7, 104, 106-7, 114, 129, 171, 174-5, 177, 202
human Heart discharges 193
human life 84, 234
human mind 110
Human Natural Character 73, 76
human relations 232, 236
human relationships 171, 201, 221-2, 231
human spirit 101
Human Xìng 185, 194, 197
humane 105
humanity 31, 52
  knowing 88
humankind 59, 78, 105, 124
humble 18, 22, 24, 35, 190, 207
humility 38, 41, 86, 208
Hùnyuán 11, 69, 112, 145
Hùnyuán circle 77, 84, 161
Hunyuan Fertility 159
Hùnyuán medicine 1, 7, 16, 57, 59, 63-4, 66, 80, 92, 102, 110, 158-9, 173, 177
Hùnyuán Research Institute 13, 15, 108
Hùnyuán Xīnfǎ 8

husband   19, 21-2, 31, 45, 47, 72-3, 76, 88, 157-9, 198, 219, 221-3, 226, 228-9
husband-wife   227

I

ignorance   13, 194-6
immortals   36-7, 39, 213, 224
impenetrable Yīnshān   213
in-vitro fertilization   125
in-vitro fertilization procedures   167
infertility   78, 154, 159, 177
  unexplained   158
innate ability   76, 187
innate wisdom   76
Inner and Outer Circles   99
Inner Elixir   33-4, 37
Inner Fire   112
Inner Fire and Outer Water Circles   90, 119, 126, 133, 162
Inner Fire Circle   8, 60, 63, 69, 79, 96-9, 102, 110-12, 120, 123-6, 128, 130-3, 151-2, 156, 159-60
intentions   9, 44, 60, 69, 81-2, 90, 121, 129, 135, 141, 145, 190, 192-3, 217-18, 234
  good   3, 9, 28-9, 50, 102, 137, 185, 187
  lofty   214
  patient's   199
  skewed   149
intentions sincere   192, 202
internal cultivation   82

J

joy   8, 22, 30, 55, 67, 69, 77, 115, 131, 144, 149, 160-2, 177, 190, 212
Juéyīn   7
jūnchén   31, 73

K

kǎn   62, 64, 105
Kèjǐ fùlǐ   171
Kidneys   8-9, 95, 97, 167
killing   20, 74, 118, 142

kindness   23, 36, 44, 65, 70, 73, 100, 103, 106, 112-13, 119-21, 132, 155, 166, 175
  random acts of   26, 164
kinship relationships, proper   179
kinships   31-2, 37, 112, 226-7, 232, 236
  close   158
Kinships of Confucianism   31, 73
Knowing   70, 81, 179-80
knowing Heaven   88, 161, 164
knowledge   6, 13, 16, 67, 70, 74, 79-80, 84, 88, 107, 109, 146, 149, 173, 192

L

language
  abusive   141
  harsh   119
Lao Tzu   165
Lǎo Yìyún   13
Lǎozǐ   72-3, 81, 83, 135, 165, 170, 178, 221
Large Intestine   96
laziness   166, 189, 231
leak   111, 115
leaping fish   76
learning   14-15, 53-4, 56, 87-8, 160, 176, 230-1, 234
Lǐ Bái   99, 133
lí Fire trigram   62
lí palace   37
licentiousness   173
life-definition   124
life leaks   185
lifeless body   126-8, 131
lifestyle choices   64, 109
lifetime   109, 119, 159, 175, 179, 191, 215, 227-8
Líng Chè   135
Liú   11-14, 16-17, 26, 50-2, 54, 56, 58, 61-5, 68, 71, 76, 170, 172-3, 182-3, 203
Liú Bǎigǔ   15, 53, 65, 74, 112, 116, 121, 126, 184
Liú Bèiwén   13, 123, 145, 215, 231

Liú Yuán   7, 11-12, 15-18, 26, 32, 52-4, 57, 59, 69, 73-4, 102-3, 148, 166-7, 169, 217-18
Liver   31, 95, 97-8
Lost Heart   8, 11, 82, 92, 186, 219, 224, 227, 239-40
Lost Heart of Medicine   2, 11, 90, 184, 216, 224
love   14, 18, 21, 35, 38, 41, 49, 67, 69, 73, 92, 120, 202, 222-3, 227
loving life   35, 49, 211-12, 231
Lǚ Dòngbīn   40
lust   112, 171, 173, 189, 207, 213, 234

M

mankind   42, 73, 76, 78-9, 85, 88-9, 104, 106, 113-14, 168, 171, 178-9, 188, 194, 197
master   3-4, 11, 17, 35, 45-7, 57, 75, 88-9, 108, 146, 148, 163, 216, 228, 236
material   27, 59, 95, 97, 99, 108, 110-11, 119, 124, 126, 128, 131, 171, 173-4, 192-5
material accumulations   61
material engagements   222
material interactions   120
material manifestations   123
material possessions   94
material substances   56, 62, 196
material vessel life   149
material world   69, 89-90, 111-12, 126, 175, 192, 216
  changeable   226
  external   112, 126
materialistic   202
Me-dictate-ions   156
medications   125, 131, 155-6, 167
medicinals   4, 64, 146, 196, 217
medicine   1-5, 9, 11, 96-7, 121-3, 125-6, 144-6, 158-9, 169-70, 184, 187-9, 206-12, 214, 216, 218-19
  accomplished student of   215, 237
  benevolent   240
  defective   1, 122
  effective   1, 122
  entry level of   120, 125
  external   216
  hundred   135, 144-5, 213-14
  modern   71, 131, 159
  modern fertility   158
  physical   131, 188
  reproductive   125
Medicine's role   198
meditation   33, 45, 50, 65, 129, 189, 191, 220
melancholia   220, 226
memory   78, 111, 131-2, 152, 155, 161
  distant   177
  traumatic   132
memory reemerges   131
Mencius   15, 26, 30, 52-3, 57-9, 61-2, 66, 84, 87, 92, 102, 106, 148-50, 161, 163-4
menstruation   98
merit   23, 27-9, 31, 33, 39, 41-2, 187, 223
middle   13, 19-21, 24, 32, 35, 37-9, 42-4, 50, 62-3, 77, 107, 110, 124, 174, 186
Minister Fire   96
miscarriage   161-2
misfortune   136, 138, 143, 197
misguided beliefs   152
mistress   26-7
Mohist doctrine   223
momentum   50, 97, 124, 177, 219, 226
money   15, 19, 22, 25-8, 30, 32-4, 39, 43, 45, 48-9, 208, 234
monk   19-20, 26, 30-6, 39, 49, 54, 66, 83, 103, 129, 134-5, 230
Moon   17, 57, 62-3, 83-4, 87, 89-90, 211
morality   82, 137, 207
morals   60, 81, 87, 109, 234
mother   4, 31, 34, 38, 43-4, 49, 56, 61, 70-2, 125, 144, 203, 221-3, 226-7
  good   222
  loving   239
  proper   222
mother-daughter   229
mother nature   72
mountains   13, 31, 38, 41, 43, 194, 213, 217, 240
movement   7-10, 21, 63-4, 66-7, 78, 82-3, 85, 89-90, 107-8, 125-6, 161, 164, 190, 192-3, 217

constant 85, 149, 205
continual 90
excessive 85, 98
extreme 123
forwards 175
habitual 226
internal 98, 123
inward 60, 97
large 44
provoke 90
strong 101
movement outward 125
myriad 8, 10, 19-20, 66-7, 69, 71-2,
    84-8, 90, 108-9, 163-4, 168, 171,
    179, 182, 194
myriad affairs 84, 86, 108, 171, 174
myriad applications 184
myriad attachments 152
myriad cells 174
myriad divisions 147
myriad emotions 160
myriad interactions 57
myriad juxtapositions 164
myriad layers 192
myriad materials 110, 179
myriad miracle 177
myriad relationships 239
myriad symptoms 110
myriad thoughts 63
myriad variations 167
mysterious 5, 17

N

Natural Character 29, 36, 41, 54-9,
    61-2, 65-8, 70-3, 75-9, 90, 152,
    213
  nurturing 58-9, 70
nature 8, 24, 35, 63, 74, 76, 81, 83-4,
    92-3, 95, 97, 123-4, 128-9, 171,
    198
  human 17, 234
  pure 61
  true 63, 76, 79, 121, 124, 149
Negative Concealed Words 229
negative connotations 236
negative narratives 53
negative thoughts 150
negativity 102, 121, 154-5, 217

nèibìng 130-1
Neo-Confucianism 52, 65
Niàn Hé 26-7
nose 7, 84, 99-100, 193, 203
nurture 14, 61, 64-5, 70, 81, 86-7,
    107-8, 114, 118, 149, 163-4, 187,
    196, 202-3, 220
nurture Xìng 203
nurturing 66-7, 84-5, 163, 171, 190,
    193, 218, 220
nurturing dāntián 220
nurturing life 84
nurturing Xìng 204, 220
nutrients 95, 119, 191
nuts 7, 156, 166

O

offenses 29, 43, 46, 179
oneness 71, 79, 83, 104-5, 168, 171,
    179
organs 6, 8, 80, 94-6, 120
  physical 126
  reproductive 79
orifices 44, 71
origin 11, 32, 37, 40, 62, 66-7, 72-3,
    84-5, 99-100, 107-8, 110-14, 171,
    173-5, 179, 203-4
ourselves unite 71, 159
Outer Circles 8, 95, 161
Outer Elixir 33, 115
Outer Water and Inner Fire Circles 7,
    64, 124, 172
Outer Water Circle 8, 63, 94, 96-9,
    104, 115, 120-2, 124-5, 128, 130,
    144, 151-2, 162, 167, 178
outward movement 8, 60, 69, 98, 123,
    128
ovulation 159, 174

P

palpitations 112
parents 3, 31-2, 35, 37-9, 42, 44, 49-
    50, 56, 70-3, 88, 124-5, 158, 200-
    1, 223, 228-33
  good 224
  proper 221, 240
partners 158-9, 174, 223, 227-9

path 1, 18-19, 23-4, 29, 31-2, 35-6, 41, 50, 145-6, 149, 154-5, 169-70, 174-5, 193, 199
  correct 1-2, 119
  proper 2, 4
patient 1-3, 99-103, 109-10, 114-16, 120-3, 144-6, 154-8, 161-2, 167, 178-80, 186-8, 198-201, 217-19, 229, 239-40
patient's body 180, 187
patient's Heart 101, 103, 111, 121, 146, 216, 218
patient's life 110, 240
Perfect circle image 240
Pericardium 96-8
perishing 78, 96
person
  bad 184, 187
  good 21, 74, 144, 147, 184
  kind 35
  noble 90, 235
  talented 140
perspective 3, 8, 25, 106, 115, 125, 189
  geocentric 175
  medical 2
  new 170
  regain 131
perspicacity, great 231
persuasion, theoretical 145
phases, five 108, 171
phenomena 70, 108, 192, 233
  external 78
  natural 70
  observing inner 74
philosophies 11-12, 16, 42, 52, 120
physical ability 126
physical action 151
physical appearance 83
physical body 1, 5, 34, 58, 60, 67, 78, 80-2, 84, 106, 110, 113, 125, 159, 174
  living 63
physical form 56, 59, 61, 78, 83, 163
physical malfunction 131
physical material 61, 79, 94, 106, 119, 126, 128, 158
  earthly 64
physical matter 106

physical origin 131
physical structure 127
Physical sustenance 239
physical vessel 6, 64, 77, 80, 83, 94, 124, 128, 130, 177
physical world 124, 153
physician 1-2, 100-3, 119-23, 143-6, 154-7, 177-80, 186-91, 194-6, 198-201, 203-4, 214-16, 218-19, 221-7, 229, 239-40
  benevolent 219
  good 116
  inferior 146
  modern 225
physician's ability 122
physiology 119, 124, 130, 152, 174
polarity, establishing 169
political correctness 224
Post-Heaven 56-7, 59, 61-2, 78, 81, 83, 86-7, 89-90, 99, 104, 106-9, 114, 119, 183, 202
Post-Heaven dichotomy of Yīn and Yáng 224
Post-Heaven Heart 58, 60, 65-6, 106, 185, 194, 217
Post-Heaven movements 82
Post-Heaven Qì 67
Post-Heaven Yīn 62, 64, 213
power 37, 48-9, 57, 137-8, 200, 208, 212
practices Heart medicine 146
Pre-Heaven 56-9, 61-2, 66, 79, 81, 83, 86-7, 89-90, 99, 104, 106-9, 182-3, 194, 202, 214
Pre-Heaven Dào Heart 65
Pre-Heaven Heart 57, 194
Pre-Heaven Natural Character 62
Pre-Heaven state 56, 59, 99
Pre-Heaven Water 84, 89
Pre-Heaven Xìng 81, 83
Pre-Heaven Yáng 64
precious 11, 111, 217, 239
precious truth 127
principle 4-5, 58-9, 61-3, 66-8, 70-2, 74-80, 83, 85-90, 104-9, 113-14, 150, 163-75, 178-80, 221, 236
  guiding 190, 215
progression 60, 150-2, 155

propriety 10, 38, 40-1, 67, 76, 79, 88, 107, 112, 114, 129, 141, 171, 179, 222-3
  refining 230
prosperity 22, 36, 136, 228, 239
prosperous, live 133
Protecting Xīng 186
pureness 71, 104, 107, 114, 174
purity 62, 86, 106, 149, 196, 213, 239

Q

Qì 9, 26, 67-9, 78, 80-2, 88-90, 95, 106-7, 163-4, 168-9, 190, 202-4, 216-18, 220, 235-6
qián 22, 62, 72, 83-5, 105, 163
Qīng Dynasty 13-14
quality 6, 68-9, 88, 100, 112

R

reactions 8, 69, 100, 123, 126, 132, 151, 162, 188, 220, 226-7
  emotional 10, 103, 112, 130, 172, 191
  external 112
  good 132
  overt 103
recharge 6, 85, 92, 99, 119, 128, 162
recharging 6, 50, 128, 131
Recharging Instruments 6, 8, 69, 84, 93, 100, 115, 119
recognition 11, 78, 109, 152, 155, 192, 220
relationships 6, 8-9, 72-5, 88, 90, 97, 107-8, 112, 119, 158-9, 187-9, 201, 221-33, 235, 239-40
  horizontal 228-9
  improved 198
  intimate 158
  proper 118
  vertical 229
  weak 128
relatives 36, 44-5, 49, 125
relaxed breathing 156
religions 2, 17, 35, 99
resent Heaven 41
resentment 32, 97, 107, 240
responsibility 2, 70, 99, 120, 139, 144, 188, 199
return 21, 24-5, 28, 37-8, 46, 49-51, 61, 71, 78, 106, 119, 124, 177-8, 202-3, 222
rice 19, 30, 33
righteousness 26, 35, 45, 67, 70, 79, 88, 107, 118, 164, 201, 204, 233-5
Rites 16, 171, 173-4
river 17, 21, 27, 30, 41, 52, 124, 134, 165, 167, 172, 185, 195, 205, 240
road 13, 16, 19-21, 23-4, 28, 30, 32, 35, 37-9, 42-4, 50, 89, 146, 174
root 2, 8-9, 66-7, 76-7, 81-2, 84-6, 104-6, 131, 162, 164, 167-9, 171, 178, 197-8, 201-2

S

sages 4, 16-17, 36, 41, 48-9, 58-9, 74-6, 84-5, 106, 109-10, 171, 190-2, 213-14, 221, 235-6
samurai 54, 230
scales 23, 25, 41, 44, 54-5, 78, 86, 169, 184
scholar tree, ancient 14
scholars 14, 17, 42, 63, 86, 91, 93, 113, 231
sea 114, 161, 190, 195, 213
self-cultivation 70, 73, 83, 87, 119, 193
self-deceit 193
self-esteem 69, 219
self-examination 186, 202
Self-forgiveness 120
self-investigation 192
Self-Knowledge 6
self-manipulation 153
self-protection 102
self-reflection 189
self-selected actions 197
self-smallness 232
selfish 56, 189, 193
selfishness 39, 50, 56, 64, 70-1, 73-4, 76, 80-2, 86, 107, 112, 116, 118, 159, 193
  pure 74
  trace of 39, 123
selfishness diminishes 60

Separation 5-10, 60, 62-3, 83, 93-4, 98, 105, 107, 110, 112, 126, 161-2, 171, 195, 216-17
Separations of Tàijí 171
Shào Yōng 182
Shàoyáng 7
Shàoyīn 7-9, 77, 90, 97, 115
Shí Xīn Dé 9, 18, 21, 38-9, 47
Shí Yīn 21-3, 25
Shí Yīn Fū 11, 16-18, 21-3, 28, 34, 39, 48-9, 51, 57, 59, 61, 64-5, 68, 143, 199-200
Shuāngliú 15, 18
Sī Mǎyì 48, 200
sincere 39, 70, 81, 192, 203, 208
sincere intentions 58, 60-1, 81-3, 193
sincerity 4, 13, 24, 44, 60, 74, 82, 84, 88, 106, 169, 178, 180, 196
  absolute 87, 105, 133
skill of nurturing Xìng 204, 220
skin 8, 66, 84, 92-3, 99-100, 144, 146, 180, 205
sleep 5-6, 45, 60, 90, 92, 97, 99-100, 111, 115, 128, 131, 161, 177, 188, 240
Small Intestine 96
smells 54, 93, 95, 100, 126, 132, 171, 220
smoke cigarettes 226
soil 20, 32, 41, 57, 89
son 13, 31, 44, 47, 73, 76, 88, 221-2, 227-8, 231, 237
  bad 227
  good 227
  proper 237
son-in-law 23-5, 48
Sòng dynasty 16-17, 52, 93, 224
sorrow 8, 55, 61, 69, 99, 112, 119, 125, 131, 150, 154, 160, 172, 176, 180
soul 155, 224
  transformed 237
sounds 21, 40, 78, 84, 92, 97, 100, 126, 132, 154, 171, 180, 220
source 52, 59, 62-3, 89, 92, 106, 121, 127, 182, 222
spending 26, 93, 96-7
sperm 71, 100, 102, 158, 174
  deficient 158

Spicy food 115
spirit 3, 22-3, 33, 36-7, 45-6, 62, 66, 78, 84, 87, 106-7, 111, 177, 202-3, 216
  generating 216
Spiritual Path 3
spiritual training 32
spirituality 107
Spleen 31, 95
spouse 44, 180
stillness 6, 10, 36, 63, 67, 83, 85-6, 90, 93, 107-8, 164, 178, 190, 196, 204
  creating 132
  quiet 127, 129
  reaching 196
stillness exchange 164
stimuli 69, 100, 111, 114, 126, 166, 220, 226
  external 123
Stomach 95, 100
stomach pains 97
stools 125, 167
stop 2, 25, 63, 70-1, 80-1, 83, 85, 87, 136, 189, 204, 224, 232-3, 240
stopping 80-1, 190, 192-3, 223, 232
streets, two-way 119, 222, 227, 229, 232
strength 6, 84, 90, 109, 154, 158, 188
  genetic 124
  inner 223
  physical 208
stresses 10, 94, 133
struggle 4, 9-10, 75, 85, 127, 197, 202, 207
substances 34, 95, 115, 191, 216, 236
sun 41, 44, 57, 83-4, 89, 111, 117, 128, 131, 133, 144, 162, 175, 180-2, 211
Sun and Moon 17, 57, 62-3, 83-4, 87, 89-90
Sūn Bìn and Guǐ Gǔzǐ 40
sword 54, 185, 230
symptoms 110, 112, 121-2, 125, 146, 156, 161-2, 218, 239

T

table 33, 186, 205

Tàijí 8, 59, 62, 66-7, 70-1, 83, 85, 104-5, 108-10, 164-6, 168-70, 172-5, 179-80, 182-3, 202-3
  complete 113
  explained 182
  principle of 64, 85, 164, 171, 183
Tàijí picture 169
Tàiyáng 7-8
Tàiyīn 7
teacher 2-4, 11, 34, 37-8, 40, 47, 50, 56, 116, 122, 127, 140, 145, 229-30, 240
technique 183, 187, 199
  modern fertility 125
technology 3, 127
temper 229
  bad 142
temperament 79, 111, 202, 232, 234
temple 26-8, 30-2, 35-6, 50, 65, 189, 191
texts 16-18, 33, 52, 54, 58, 65, 87-8, 135, 143, 147-8, 182, 213-14
therapies 4, 13, 43, 74, 80, 112, 132, 149, 152, 170, 214, 216, 224-5, 239
  complementary 1
  drug 158
  herbal 7
  manual 120, 216
tiān lǐ liáng xīn 天理良 226
time 4-6, 10-11, 13-14, 19-20, 26-9, 32-5, 38-9, 41-5, 56-8, 87-8, 111, 120-2, 154-6, 161-2, 219-22
timeless principle 11
touch 84, 92, 100, 132, 134, 205
traditional medicine 3, 225
transcend time 58-9
transformation 39, 62-3, 83-4, 99, 104, 106, 108, 113, 169, 185, 203
trauma 131-2, 154-5, 162
  emotional 162
treatment 7, 115, 121-2, 131, 152, 155, 158-9, 167, 198, 204, 217-18, 229, 240
  applying 170
  preventive 122
  water circle 159
trigrams 37, 60, 62-4, 72, 107, 111, 163

gèn 194
kǎn 8, 63-4, 94, 194
kūn Earth 72
Tripitaka 135
True Fire 96-100, 119, 125, 161
  accumulated 97
  loosing 100
True health 177
true Heaven principle 68
True medicine 123
True Words 16
trustworthiness 38, 41, 67, 79, 107, 141
truth 1-3, 5, 16-18, 22, 40, 48, 53-4, 58-9, 74, 79, 81, 87-8, 93, 169, 214-15

U

understanding cultivation 64
understanding Heaven's principle 73
understanding propriety 231
Unification 5-10, 92-3, 97-8, 110-12, 161-2, 188, 198, 217
  daily 92
Unification and Separation 90, 92, 94, 160, 177, 180, 185, 240
Unification capacity 161
Unification Instrument 7
unite 61, 97, 104, 177
unity 75, 99, 147, 204, 225, 227
universe 8, 11, 31, 63, 67, 76, 83-4, 87, 107, 143, 149-50, 165, 170, 220
upright 81-2, 110, 118, 129, 164, 174, 201-2, 207, 211
upright Heart 25, 58-9, 74, 82-3, 85, 113, 201, 219
upright principle 71, 201
uprightness 26, 60, 67, 81, 84, 86, 88, 104, 163-4, 168, 180
utter compassion 185
utter despair 190
utter disdain 54
utter peace 191

V

Vast Heart 232

vessel   1, 8, 54, 64, 84, 98-9, 111, 121,
    124, 151, 170, 174, 177-8, 186,
    239-40
  cellular   159, 199
  human   62, 224
  living   64, 89, 97, 125
vessel awakes   97
Vibrating   85
vibrating line   54, 80
virtue   11, 20-4, 27-9, 38-9, 42, 47-9,
    80-1, 85, 87-8, 145-7, 189, 200-1,
    211-14, 216-18, 220-1
  accumulating   28
  cultivating   220
  human   79
  inner   214
  misunderstand   75
  path of   25, 32
  ultimate   107
virtuous   42, 47, 49, 58, 72, 88, 138-9,
    208, 232, 236
virtuous actions   27
virtuous intention   167
virtuous momentum   221
virtuous slaughter animals   118
virtuous son-in-law   25
vision   71, 199
vital energy   95
  expansive   67, 149
vitamins   95, 125
voice   20, 23, 40, 54, 154

W

wāi mén xié dào   1-2, 170
wàibìng   130-1
wanting   24, 27, 39, 46, 137, 157, 161-
    2, 223, 231
warmth   6, 27, 30, 84, 96-9, 119, 128,
    156, 165, 170, 177, 191, 196,
    201, 231
  body diverts   198
  extra   159
Warring States Period   35, 58, 163,
    168
warrior   181, 185
  inner Wounded   184

Water   13, 57, 63-4, 89-90, 105, 108,
    110, 112, 142-3, 165, 167, 194,
    205, 235
  kǎn   62, 64, 72
water, nature of   13, 194
Water, obstruct   13
water, stagnant   194
Water, transporting   37
water circle   94
water flows   89
water trigram   64, 107
wealth   25, 27, 48-9, 209, 212, 234
weights   23, 25, 44
Western Medicine   1, 4, 218, 225
wife   22, 24-5, 31, 45, 72-3, 76, 88,
    158-9, 218, 221-4, 226, 229
winter   6, 239
wisdom   16, 110
Wǒ Zhī Yán   148
woman
  poor   46
  young   134
woman's decision   167
womb   44, 56, 65, 72, 99, 111, 145,
    152, 203, 228
  mother's   74
women   21, 43, 79, 224
  favored   224
  good   32
wood   43, 108, 199
words   20-1, 53-5, 57-9, 68-70, 108-9,
    131-3, 144-6, 148-9, 156-9, 162-
    4, 183-4, 215-16, 218-22, 231-3,
    235-7
  bad   184, 216
  empty   93, 110
  fancy   106, 201
  few   122, 146
  final   99, 231
  following   90
  gentle   162
  good   215-16
  harsh   100
  immoral   142
  irresponsible   137
  knowing   156, 164, 180
  obscure   141
  patient's   103, 123, 155, 159
  restrained   220

right 95
unfriendly 138
wounded 149
words of Liú Yuán 148, 200
worry 69, 80, 127, 163, 211, 235
Wounded Warrior 13, 25, 93, 128-9, 144, 174, 182, 185, 187-9, 195-9, 201, 219-22, 224, 227, 229
Wújí 90, 168-9, 202

X

Xīn Dé 21-36, 39, 44-8, 184
Xīn Dé and Yīn Fū 39-40
Xīnfǎ 3, 11, 50, 80, 82, 85, 102, 119-21, 148-52, 155-6, 182-3, 215, 221, 224, 226
  applying 56
  cultivating 111
  path of 11, 191, 229
  strong 115
  term 183
Xīnfǎ case 115, 122
Xīnfǎ cultivation 133, 199, 226
Xīnfǎ disorder 152
Xīnfǎ flows 219
Xīnfǎ patient 162
Xīnfǎ physician 159
Xīnfǎ problem 152
Xīnfǎ scenario 162
Xìng 79-84, 87, 94, 102-13, 122-8, 148-56, 158-60, 163-4, 173, 177-80, 188-90, 192-205, 213-17, 219-21, 225-7
  acquired 214
  completed 163
  doctor's 121
  domain of 149, 153
  form 149
  leaks 197
  mankind's 169
  parent's linking 229
  preserving 190
  recover 106
  scattering 218
  true 202
Xìng falters 102
Xìng of Water 194
Xìng outward 150
Xìng permeates 106
Xìng transmission 144
xiōngdì 31, 73
xiūshçn 60, 74
Xiùzhī 43-4

Y

Yáng 10, 62, 64, 72, 83-4, 89, 93, 95, 104, 108, 110, 169-70, 215, 217
  absorbing 109
  extra 97
  internalized 96
  midst of 60
  moving 170
  pure 62-3, 111
  pure True 124
Yáng, Heaven 57, 62, 64, 84-5, 95-7, 99, 110, 119, 123, 128, 130
Yáng line 62
Yáng movement 105
Yáng principle of pure Xìng 114
Yángmíng 7
yellow beans 21, 23, 29-30, 42, 61, 174-5, 180, 184, 197, 239
  very few 203
Yìjīng 8, 37, 62, 72, 108, 165, 168-9, 182, 194
Yīn 10, 58, 60, 62, 64, 72, 83-4, 89, 93-4, 104, 107-8, 110, 169-70, 215, 217
  midst of 104, 110
  pure 62, 112
  true 83
  ultimate 104
Yīn, Heaven 57
Yīn and Yáng 6, 68, 72, 83, 90, 93, 104, 108, 119, 145, 152, 164-5, 168-70, 172-3, 239
  interplay of 107, 110
Yīn and Yáng manifests 104
Yīn and Yáng merge 63
Yīn and Yáng offend 216
Yīn and Yáng transform 104
Yīn evil 213
Yīn Fū 21, 23-5, 27, 29-30, 47, 50, 184

  story of Shí 16, 34, 51, 57, 61, 65,

143
Yīn Fû and Shí Yīn 24-5
Yīn lines 64, 111, 120
Yīn material 105, 111, 124-6, 130
Yīn selfishness 114
  expel 171
Yīn to Yáng and Yáng to Yīn 62
Yīn Yáng 169
Yīnshān mountains 213-14
yǒudìng 190
youth 12, 35, 37-9, 45, 239
Yù Kâi 37-42, 44-5, 50, 154
Yuán Liàng 40-4

Z

zàngfǔ 8, 90, 95
Zen story 54, 120, 134, 205, 230
Zhōng Yōng 30-1, 52
Zhōu family 48, 200

Commentary on The Lost Heart of Medicine.

"I am sure it was no accident that this pair of scholars were led to the sacred and little-known works of the Heart Medicine master, Liú Yuán. Like the great master's works, Yaron Seidman and Teja A. Jaensch have created a mastery of cultivation. Far from a typical text of Chinese medicine, this work has a life and spirit of its own, the words penetrating deep into the Heart of the reader. Caught up in the journey, one finally looks up and sees their whole perspective and reality slowly changing, realizing they have been treating themselves with the medicine that comes from simply reading *The Lost Heart of Medicine*.

At one point in the text, the humble scholars recommend that upon completing the book, the reader review the story of *Shí Yīn Fū and the Ledger of Good and Evil*, which is provided an entire chapter unto itself, to find previously hidden meanings. I would add that the same is true of the entire text, each read providing deeper meaning and further insight for the dedicated scholar. Like all living things, the more we invest into it, the more we receive from it. Modern medicine, Western, Eastern, or otherwise, needs healing. That job begins within the Heart of every medical practitioner and the way can be found between the covers of this text. May your journey inward be met with understanding, kindness and gratitude."

Tristin McLaren LAc, CCE,
Bird & Bee Acupuncture, Bellevue, Washington, USA

"All ancient traditions regard the human Heart as the core of our existence, our mandate and purpose. In the classical teachings of Chinese medicine, the Heart is not only referred to as the *Emperor* of the organ networks, connecting the Earthly vehicle of our bodies to the Heavenly realm of spirit, but as the sacred domain where human destiny manifests itself in the process of cultivation. This development of the Heart-mind has not only been a concern of Dàoism and Buddhism, but constitutes the essence of the Confucian inquiry into the nature of humanity. Yaron Seidman and Teja A. Jaensch have made the outstanding choice of exploring the Heart teachings of the Confucian Classics by meticulously translating and elucidating the work of Liú Yuán—great forgotten scholar of the Qīng dynasty, lover of medicine and mentor of Zhèng Qīnān, founder of the eminent Fire Spirit School of Sìchuān herbalism. Seidman and Jaensch have made a magnificent resource for all physicians of medicine!"

Heiner Fruehauf PhD, LAc,
Founding Professor, School of Classical Chinese Medicine

"Every so often a book comes my way that causes me to reflect on my own healing practice and question my worldview. The authors, Yaron Seidman and Teja A. Jaensch, have indeed produced a scholarly book that does so. Surreptitiously titled *The Lost Heart of Medicine*, it is part historical discourse, part philosophical treatise and part clinical manual. The text reviews many aspects of Chinese medicine and culture that, if they are not already lost, may well become so. Exploring the stream of Chinese philosophy known as *Huái Xuān* and the philosophical writings of its founder, scholar Liú Yuán, the authors weave a narrative that includes the Dào, the Yìjīng, the human spirit and body, and their relationship to medicine. While the technician may search the text for prescriptions and acupoints, the healer will truly understand. Sprinkled with quotes, poems and stories, the text cultivates the development of a moral and ethical Chinese medicine perspective that tries to re-establish the Heart of Chinese medicine back to its rightful position. We can all benefit from reading and reflecting on such a book."

Associate Professor Chris Zaslawski
Director of the College of TCM at the University of Technology, Sydney

"In our tradition, the truest approach to classical Chinese wisdom always includes two aspects: Yáng 陽, which includes the physical, tangible, visible, somewhat obvious and that which is easier to understand and Yīn 陰, the invisible, elusive and mysterious, which more often than not slips by most, totally unnoticed. Xīnfǎ 心法 the *Heart Method*, holds true when we work with the art of traditional Chinese medicine. If we focus on the overt, emphasizing only our mechanical skills or intellectual prowess and allow the way of the Heart to elude us, it is (as we say in China) *yī tiáo tuǐ zǒu lù* 一條腿走路, as though we are using only one of our legs to walk. For those of us walking the way of the Heart in our healing practice or spiritual journey, I recommend reading Seidman and Jaensch's Hùnyuán Xīnfǎ to help illuminate the path."

Master Wú Zhōngxian (吳忠賢), a lifelong Dàoist practitioner, Master Wú is the recognized lineage bearer of many schools of Qìgōng, Tàijí and internal martial arts. He is the author of 11 books (five in Chinese) on ancient Chinese wisdom traditions and co-founded Blue Willow World Healing Center and Qín Jiàn Akademin (琴劍研究院).

"This text facilitates the physician through a journey of discovery that draws from traditional teachings and philosophy. It challenges mainstream application and rhetoric to questioning or looking deeper to find relevance to today's clinical practice; moving beyond eastern or western medicine to the provision of good medicine. Physicians are encouraged to develop effective communication skills to explore the issues that underlay the clinical presentation. This text promotes the premise that not all maladies are immediately apparent. Often there can be a deeper issue, requiring the practitioner to draw on their traditional knowledge, training and skills to be able to identify and know how to treat the patient as a whole. This is Xīnfǎ."

Robyn Bowcock, RN MN,
Associate Lecturer at the University of Western Sydney, Australia

"The message moving throughout this book is revealed in the bags of yellow and black beans. Without this knowledge of good and evil within oneself, there is no possibility of transformation. The physician must meet and be involved with humanity and only when they have succeeded to transform and develop themselves, can they properly judge the difficulties within another person. These *words* will be received gratefully by both physician and patient alike, awakening our Hearts."

Annika Andersdotter, philosopher and educator

"By recapitulating and expressing idiomatic ideas that form the backbone of ancient Chinese philosophy, this book both reaffirms and settles us back into Center, where medicine and life are rooted in spirit. This Center, manifesting as perfect action, is the pinnacle of art: of our art in medicine and that of life. There is no difference. This book is a lighthouse in a sometimes turbulent and bewildering sea of signs and symptoms that characterize most modern texts and a reminder of that single unifying principle prior to Separation in these ten thousand things."

Anthony Captain, Mountain Medicine, Blue Mountains, Sydney

"Dear Yaron and Teja, I cannot find a way to describe how your book awakens one's inner self."

Master Robert F. Feng, Shaolin Ssu Kung Fu, North Fuquay, Varina USA

Scholar's Notes.

Scholar's Notes.